Sports Vision

Vision Care for the Enhancement
of Sports Performance

Sports Vision

Vision Care for the Enhancement of Sports Performance

SECOND EDITION

GRAHAM B. ERICKSON
Professor of Optometry
Pacific University College of Optometry
Forest Grove, OR, USA

ELSEVIER

Publisher: Cathleen Sether
Acquisitions Editor: Kayla Wolfe
Editorial Project Manager: Susan Ikeda
Production Project Manager: Sreejith Viswanathan
Cover Designer: Alan Studholme

3251 Riverport Lane
St. Louis, Missouri 63043

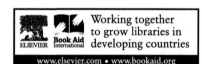

Working together
to grow libraries in
developing countries

www.elsevier.com • www.bookaid.org

*This book is dedicated to my wife, Dina, and children, Alexander and Maya,
for their enduring love and support, and to students and practitioners
of sports vision for their inspiration.*

Preface

The role of visual performance in sports has received considerable attention over the years. With the increasing participation rates in sports and recreational activities, interest in vision care services for athletes has intensified among eye care practitioners and sports personnel. Sports vision can be defined as vision care and consultation designed to protect, correct, and enhance vision in order to make sports and athletic competition safe, enjoyable, and more successful. It encompasses a broad scope of professional skills, including the prevention and management of sport-related eye injuries, identification and management of sport-related concussion, determination and delivery of appropriate refractive correction, determination of appropriate protective eyewear, understanding of filters and their potential application in sports, assessment and remediation of functional vision inefficiencies, assessment of sport-specific vision skills, vision training to enhance visual performance, and consultation with athletes and other sports personnel. Vision is the guiding sense for most sports performance, and sports vision is one of many disciplines that can contribute to the achievement of peak performance.

Personally, I have been involved in both the provision of sports vision services in a variety of clinical settings and the teaching of sports vision to optometry students and practitioners. This combination of experiences obligated me to develop not only the requisite clinical skills but also an understanding of the relevant professional and research literature. This book reviews the main elements of the vision care services provided to athletes by eye care practitioners, all of which begin with an analysis of the visual demands that are critical to success in sports. I have attempted to build a foundation from vision science research to guide the application of clinical care, an evidence-based approach. I am indebted to the many practitioners and researchers who have shared their ideas and insights on the burgeoning area of sports vision, for the concepts and procedures discussed in this book are the culmination of those collective contributions. While there are many areas where numerous questions remain unanswered, the combination of careful task analysis, review of related research findings, and logical deduction can guide the practitioner in determining appropriate vision care. I've included items in the Appendix that can help the practitioner to incorporate sports vision services in a variety of clinical settings. While this book is primarily addressed to eye care practitioners, other sports personnel may find useful information for assisting athletes with visual performance needs.

I gratefully acknowledge the following individuals for their contributions to the development of this publication: Drs. Bradley Coffey, Alan Reichow, Karl Citek, Fraser Horn, Lorne Yudcovich, Fred Edmunds, Keith Smithson, Amanda Nanasy, and Dina Erickson. I thank Pacific University for its encouragement and support on this project, and the students and research assistants have my enduring appreciation for the role each of them plays in my professional growth. I thank Kayla Wolfe, Susan Ikeda, and Sreejith Viswanathan of Elsevier for their assistance in development and production.

Graham B. Erickson

Contents

Contents

CHAPTER 1

Introduction to Sports Vision

Have you ever wished you could improve your batting average, lower your golf score, or just play your favorite sport better? Most people who participate in sporting activities love to win or at least improve their performance. Athletes at all levels of competition spend a substantial amount of money on sports, including equipment and clothing. Yet many performances that fail are not caused by poor equipment or clothing, or even by the wrong physical movement, but by the movement being performed at the incorrect time or in the incorrect place.

A significant percentage of the general population in developed nations participate at some level in sporting activities. The National Sporting Goods Association produces yearly estimates of participation by sport and gender for the United States (available at www.nsga.org). The eye care practitioner must recognize that sports participation crosses all lines of age, gender, race, and socioeconomic status; every patient is potentially a sports vision patient. In addition, a significant percentage of the population may not actively participate in sports but are avid spectators.

Considerable debate has taken place concerning the role of vision in sports. Vision is the signal that directs the muscles of the body to respond. The legendary football coach Blanton Collier is credited for developing the concept that "the eyes lead the body."[1] Vision provides the athlete with information regarding *where* and *when* to perform. Superior size, strength, speed, and agility cannot completely make up for inefficient processing of visual information. For example, if the eyes do not tell a batter where the ball is heading and when it will arrive, he or she is not going to hit it no matter how perfect the swing is. Even for the discriminating spectator, excellent visual function allows improved opportunity to enjoy watching sports. Little debate exists that vision is a critical factor in sports performance; however, even when conflicting evidence is taken into consideration, research clearly shows that successful athletes typically possess superior visual function that allows them to see and perform better than novices in sports.

The athletic community should be educated about the aspects of vision that potentially affect sports performance. To clearly communicate these aspects, the following visual elements should be discussed:
- Sight: The clarity of the image on the retina and ocular health.
- Motor/sensory: Fixation stability and eye movements, accommodation, vergence, and fusion; visually guided motor performance.
- Information processing: Quick and accurate visual processing, interpretation, and decision-making.

Understanding the relevance of these aspects to performance provides an avenue for effective communication of specific vision care recommendations. A better-informed sports community benefits by improved access to services that potentially make sports and athletic competition safe, enjoyable, and more successful.

OVERVIEW OF TERMINOLOGY

The term *sports vision* has been used to describe many vision care services provided to athletes. Practitioners working in this area are usually involved with one or more of the following professional activities[2]:
- prevention and management of sports eye injuries;
- assessment and remediation of functional vision inefficiencies that may negatively impact competitive consistency;
- specialized contact lens services with emphasis on environmental factors in sports, position of gaze factors, emergency care, and attainment of optimal visual acuity;
- performance-based ophthalmic eyewear services that address visual and environmental demands;
- assessment of specific sports-related visual abilities;
- enhancement training of specific visual abilities considered to be essential for competitive consistency for a specific sport activity;
- consultation with athletes, coaches, trainers, and teams regarding visual factors and strategies related to consistent peak athletic performance.

Many in the global community are dedicated to the pursuit of athletic excellence. A critical but often neglected aspect of peak human performance is vision. The information presented in this book should help

Sports Vision. https://doi.org/10.1016/B978-0-323-75543-6.00001-2

stimulate the inclusion of these specialized services in the care of athletes, no matter the level of sports participation.

In North America, the term sports vision has been associated with vision therapy designed for the enhancement of sports performance. The areas of sports vision defined earlier clearly demonstrate that many of these services are basic primary vision care services that are modified to address specific task demands. All eye care practitioners should consider visual performance factors when providing vision care services to athletic patients.

HISTORICAL PERSPECTIVE

The use of special eyewear for sports is perhaps the oldest application of vision factors to performance. Daland described the early use of stenopeic slit masks by Eskimos for hunting,[3] and many other special-purpose optical appliances have been described in the literature.[4] Optical protection from solar radiation and glare has been used to some degree for centuries. The use of optical refractive compensation for sports has not been as frequently used, most likely for a combination of practical and aesthetic reasons. The available eyewear was not typically appropriate for use in sports. Contact lens technology did not emerge as a reasonable option for most athletes until the latter half of the 20th century, and refractive surgery options did not become advantageous until the late 1990s. Today, the benefits of significant advances in technology and designs for the correction and protection of vision are enjoyed by athletes (see Chapter 6).

The evaluation of vision skills in athletes has also been an area of intense interest. The earliest literature citation found is an account of the sensory and motor abilities of the legendary baseball player Babe Ruth in 1921.[5] This report was followed later by an article discussing the role of vision in baseball.[6] These early articles produced suggestions for procedures to assess performance potential in baseball on the basis of vision skill analysis. Interestingly, debate in the literature exists concerning the actual vision profile of the great Babe Ruth. Despite the early report that Ruth had eyesight that was 12% faster than the average person,[5] a 1991 article reported that an ophthalmologic examination revealed amblyopia ex anopsia in his left eye.[7] The potential role of depth perception in batting is challenged by these discrepancies in Ruth's visual status; either he performed so well because he had superior vision skills or he was successful despite having degraded stereopsis as a result of amblyopia. Although no definitive

resolution can be made from these contradictory reports, some have speculated that the unilateral vision loss was likely the result of a complication of his nasopharyngeal carcinoma rather than an undetected congenital condition.[8] The exact role of vision in sports performance is still hotly debated, and many vision evaluation procedures have been suggested over the years in an attempt to discover the nature of this aspect of sports performance.

Because vision skills are generally recognized as a critical element to most sport performances, significant interest has been expressed in improving sports performance by using training procedures to enhance vision. Many of the visual attributes that have been identified as important in sport are amenable to training. The relevant questions are whether sport-specific visual abilities can indeed be trained and whether any improvements in visual skills transfer to improved sports performance by the athlete. Although the literature has few reports supporting sports vision training, and these reports often have significant flaws, enhancement of visual skill performance can be logically predicted to provide the athlete with a potential advantage when preparing for a competition.

The increasing interest in sports and the role of vision in sports has produced the impetus for the formation of organizations to facilitate professional communications. The United States was the first to form an entity through the establishment of the Sports Vision Section of the American Optometric Association (AOA) in 1978. Like many similar organizations, the AOA Sports Vision Section afforded practitioners a venue for continuing education, for obtaining updates through an e-newsletter, for a referral network through a member directory, and for gaining access to professional materials such as the *Sports Vision Guidebooks* and the *Sports Vision Bibliography*. The Section was also active in interprofessional relations with other organizations, such as the U.S. Olympic Committee, Special Olympics, Amateur Athletic Union (AAU) Junior Olympics, American College of Sports Medicine, National Athletic Trainers' Association, and National Collegiate Athletic Association. The Section provided practitioners and students opportunities to participate in sports vision activities, such as the sports vision screening program at the annual AAU Junior Olympic Games. In 2016, the Sports Vision Section was converted to the Sports and Performance Vision committee (www.aoa. org/optometrists/tools-and-resources/sports-and-performance-vision) and continues with many of the same goals and initiatives. There have been other similarly focused groups formed recently, such as Sports

Vision Pros (www.sportsvisionpros.com) and the International Sports Vision Association (www.sportsvision.pro). Ultimately, groups such as the AOA Sports and Performance Vision committee offer practitioners an opportunity to collaborate and advance the profession.

Organizations dedicated to sports vision have also been created outside the United States. The Canadian Association of Optometrists formed a Sports Vision Section in 1987, the European Academy of Sports Vision was formed in Italy in 1989, the Optometrists Association Australia established its Sports Vision Section in 1992, and the Sports Vision Association was formed in the United Kingdom in 1993.[4] These organizations perform similar functions to the AOA Sports Vision Section in their respective regions and have helped facilitate the growth of sports vision globally.

In 1979, Pacific University College of Optometry began providing an elective course on sports and recreational vision in the optometry curriculum. All schools and colleges of optometry in North America now offer some degree of education in sports vision as part of the curriculum.

OVERVIEW OF A CLINICAL MODEL OF SPORTS VISION

Vision care for athletes should begin with the identification of visual factors that potentially contribute to peak human performance so that these specific functions can be isolated and measured, if possible. The visual demands critical to success in sports can vary tremendously. Chapter 2 details an approach to the task analysis process, a process essential to provide appropriate vision care for athletes in any sport or position. Because sports performance generally requires the athlete to process visual information and execute an appropriate motor response, the practitioner should also understand how visual information is processed to understand the exact nature of the processes occurring in skilled motor performance. A model of information processing in skilled motor performance is presented in Chapter 3 to provide a useful approach for understanding the relevant aspects of sports performance.

Once the practitioner has identified the vision factors essential to the performance of the visual tasks critical for success in a sport, an evaluation should be made to measure the quality of those skills in the most appropriate, accurate, and repeatable manner. The visual skills that correlate with successful sports performance have not been definitively identified yet, so the practitioner must rely on the available literature and professional judgment to determine the most appropriate

evaluation for each athlete. Chapter 4 provides an evidence-based description of each potential vision assessment area and the relative value of each assessment area in an evaluation. Chapter 5 presents recommendations for performing team vision screenings and the unique challenges associated with providing vision care to a team. The results of a screening or evaluation should be summarized for the patient, and a performance profile is recommended in Chapter 5 to highlight areas of strength or limitation and communicate vision recommendations.

A fundamental role of the vision care practitioner is to provide expert consultation services to athletes regarding vision correction and the potential uses and benefits of ophthalmic products. Each athlete has specific variables that will affect ophthalmic recommendations. The gender, age, level of participation, combination of sports activities, and history of product use influence the choice of available options. Some athletes seek a single product to meet all visual performance needs, whereas others seek optimal products for a variety of highly specific uses. The eye care practitioner should advise athletic patients about the advantages and disadvantages of spectacles, protective eyewear, sun eyewear, contact lenses, and refractive surgery. Chapter 6 discusses the issues involved in the available modalities for vision correction, eye protection, and vision enhancement. The practitioner should help the athlete make informed decisions about the best options for his or her individual needs.

Participation in sports carries a risk of sustaining an eye injury. The vision care practitioner can perform a crucial role in the prevention of sports-related eye injuries, immediate first aid management if an eye injury occurs, referral of the athlete to an appropriate specialist if necessary, and follow-up care for the athlete who has sustained an eye injury. Chapter 7 provides an overview of assessment and management of sports-related ocular trauma from the perspective of both the athletic trainer and the eye care professional. The chapter provides recommendations for effective co-management of ocular injuries in athletes.

Sports also carry a risk for sustaining a traumatic brain injury or concussion. There is ample evidence that in addition to reduced visual processing speeds,[9] concussions lead to binocular vision deficits, oculomotor dysfunctions and visual field deficits.[10] Chapter 8 addresses sports vision procedures used to evaluate and rehabilitate sports-related concussions as part of a comprehensive multidisciplinary approach.

As previously mentioned, significant interest exists in determining whether sports performance can be improved by using training procedures to enhance vision. The athlete with identified visual deficiencies is logically expected to achieve improvement in affected aspects of sports performance if those deficient skills are improved to average performance levels. The athlete who possesses average, or even above-average, vision skills presents a more compelling and controversial challenge. Can the vision skills of this athlete be enhanced above the current level, and would this skill enhancement result in demonstrable improvements in sports task performance? A review of the literature concluded that most normal visual functions can be improved by specific training paradigms, although thousands of trials may be required to demonstrate enhancement.[11] There is limited and mixed support demonstrating that traditional sports vision training can improve sports-relevant vision or manifests into better on-field performance.[12] However, isolating one area of intervention as solely responsible for any changes in performance is quite difficult. Each sports vision practitioner develops an approach to visual performance enhancement that best suits his or her mode of practice; however, useful guidelines should be observed. Chapter 8 provides a sample of visual performance training procedures that have been used by sports vision practitioners, with a rationale and framework for developing effective training programs. Recent digital sports vision training instruments that have shown promising evidence for improving vision and sporting performance are included.

Athletes explore many options to improve performance; however, dietary intake modifications have seen recommendations vary widely over the years. Most of the focus has been on diets designed to enhance muscle performance, particularly strength, endurance, replacement and recovery. Recent research has demonstrated that certain nutrients, specifically lutein (L) and zeaxanthin (Z), can improve visual performance factors. Chapter 8 also includes an overview of modifications to diet to increase intake of carotenoids or to supplement with purified forms of L and Z. Placebo-controlled studies have found that for those athletes who experience difficulties with glare, photostress, and contrast judgment, increasing macular pigment density offers a potential method to improve these functions by enriching the natural physiology.[13-15] Macular pigment density is also linked to L and Z levels in the brain,[16] and the level present is related to functions such as cognition, reaction time, and temporal visual processing.[17-19]

The final chapter deals with the unique issues pertaining to the development of sports vision services in professional practice. Challenges of internal and external marketing are discussed, and specific methods for growing this area of practice are highlighted. Chapter 9 also provides many important suggestions for establishing consistent messaging throughout the delivery of sports vision services.

THE FUTURE OF SPORTS VISION

During the past 40 years a general increase in the use and provision of sports vision services by optometrists has been observed.[20] Eye care practitioners are a common component in the health care service team in professional sports and many collegiate athletic departments in North America. The range of vision care services includes vision screening programs, vision correction with contact lenses, eye protection consultation, eye injury management, and visual performance enhancement training programs. These services are provided either on-site at the athletic facility or in the practitioner's practice. Great interest in sports vision services exists within the sporting community, and the consensus is that this need is not being adequately met by eye care practitioners.[20]

The eye care professions have considerable room for growth in the delivery of sports vision services. Many high-level athletes have never received a comprehensive vision examination and are largely unaware of the potential impact of sports vision services on athletic performance. A review of screening data collected over 10 years from Amateur Athletic Union Junior Olympic Games in the United States found that more than 29% of participants had not received eye care for more than 3 years, with more than 20% never having an examination by an eye care professional.[21] Indeed, the rate of use of protective eyewear in sports demonstrates the limited impact that public education programs have had in the sports community. Significant growth potential clearly exists in all the areas of sports vision care listed at the beginning of this chapter.

Continued professional growth requires that the profession address some of the concerns and issues that may prevent fulfillment of the potential inherent in this area. Specifically, clinical evaluation procedures need to be ecologically appropriate, produce repeatable and reliable results, discriminate performance levels, be readily available and not cost prohibitive, and be practical for implementation in most clinical practice facilities. If such evaluation procedures are produced, these procedures must have sound scientific validity demonstrated by controlled studies. If this can be achieved, sports vision skill assessment may become a common aspect of patient care.

Similarly, visual performance training procedures need a degree of validation to engender broader acceptance. Some of the same desirable characteristics described for evaluation procedures pertain to training procedures as well. Training programs should attempt to demonstrate vision skill improvement with relevant laboratory and clinical research. The improvement of vision skill performance should also be correlated to a concurrent improvement in sports performance, if possible. However, isolating one area of intervention as being solely responsible for changes in performance is incredibly difficult. This is true for any area of sports training, including strength training, conditioning, speed and agility training, nutritional regimens, and sports psychology. If the improvement of obviously important vision skills is evident from well-controlled research, the transfer to sports performance offers a logical correlation that perhaps would be more readily accepted than only anecdotal reports.

Sports vision specialists have tremendous potential to provide consultation services. The vision factors that influence perception are generally not calculated in the development of sports products. The sports vision specialist is in a unique position to facilitate product innovation in a potentially unique direction. The sports vision specialist can provide scientifically supported advice in areas such as the selection of product colors, the optical properties of performance eyewear, the engineering of performance tints, and the desirable properties of contact lenses for athletes. These potential opportunities could yield fulfilling professional experiences for the practitioner.

The author hopes that, in some small way, this book will help increase the provision of sports vision services to athletic patients and stimulate interest in elevating the professional development of sports vision. Eye care practitioners have the potential to contribute to the performance of their athletic patients; ultimately, sports vision care can contribute to elevating human potential.

REFERENCES

1. Collier B. The eyes lead the body. *Optom Manag.* 1979;15: 73.
2. Coffey B, Reichow AW. Optometric evaluation of the elite athlete. *Prob Optometry.* 1990;2:32.
3. Daland J. Eskimo snow blindness and goggles. *Opt J Rev Optom.* 1917;39:1334.
4. Loran DFC. An overview of sport and vision. In: Loran DFC, MacEwen CJ, eds. *Sports Vision.* Oxford: Butterworth-Heinemann; 1995.
5. Fullerton HS. Why Babe Ruth in the greatest home run hitter: *Popular Science Monthly* tests in the laboratory his brain, eye, ear and muscle — and gets his secret. *Pop Sci Mon.* 1921;99:19.
6. Abel O. Eyes and baseball. *West Opt World.* 1924;12:401.
7. Blodi FC. Some famous persons with visual problems as shown on postage stamps. *Doc Ophthalmol.* 1991;77:295.
8. Voisin A, Elliott DB, Regan D. Babe Ruth: with vision like that, how could he hit the ball? *Optom Vis Sci.* 1997;74:144.
9. Fimreite V, Ciuffreda KJ, Yadav NK. Effect of luminance on the visually-evoked potential in visually-normal individuals and in mTBI/concussion. *Brain Inj.* 2015;29:1199.
10. Ciuffreda KJ, Ludlam DP, Yadav NK, et al. Trumatic brain injury: visual consequences, diagnosis, and treatment. *Adv Ophthalmol Optometry.* 2016;1:307.
11. Ciuffreda KJ, Wang B. Vision training and sports. In: Hung GK, Pallis JM, eds. *Biomedical Engineering Principles in Sports.* New York: Kluwer Academic; 2004:407–433.
12. Appelbaum LG, Erickson G. Sports vision training: a review of the state-of-the-art in digital training techniques. *Int Rev Sport Exerc Psychol.* 2018;11:160.
13. Stringham JM, Hammond BR. Macular pigment and visual performance under glare conditions. *Optom Vis Sci.* 2008; 85:82–88.
14. Hammond BR, Fletcher LM, Roos F, et al. A double-blind, placebo-controlled study on the effects of lutein and zeaxanthin on photostress recovery, glare disability, and chromatic contrast. *Invest Ophthalmol Vis Sci.* 2014;55:8583.
15. Stringham JN, Garcia PV, Smith PA, et al. Macular pigment and visual performance in glare: benefits for photostress recovery, disability glare, and visual discomfort. *Invest Ophthalmol Vis Sci.* 2011;52:7406.
16. Vishwanathan R, Neuringer M, Snodderly DM, et al. Macular lutein and zeaxanthin are related to brain lutein and zeaxanthin in primates. *Nutr Neurosci.* 2013;16:21.
17. Renzi-Hammond LM, Bovier ER, Fletcher LM, et al. Effects of a lutein and zeaxanthin intervention on cognitive function: a randomized, double-masked, placebo-controlled trial of younger healthy adults. *Nutrients.* 2017;9:1246.
18. Bovier ER, Renzi LM, Hammond BR. A double-blind, placebo-controlled study on the effects of lutein and zeaxanthin on neural processing speed and efficiency. *PLoS One.* 2014;9:e108178.
19. Bovier ER, Hammond BR. A randomized placebo-controlled study on the effects of lutein and zeaxanthin on visual processing speed in young healthy subjects. *Arch Biochem Biophys.* 2015;15(572):54.
20. Zieman B, Reichow A, Coffey B. Optometric trends in sports vision: knowledge, utilization, and practitioner role expansion potential. *J Am Optom Assoc.* 1993;64:490.
21. Beatty RM, Bakkum BW, Hitzman SA, Beckerman S. Sports vision screening of Amateur athletic union junior olympic athletes: a ten-year follow-up. *Optom Vis Perf.* 2016;4(3): 97.

CHAPTER 2

Visual Task Analysis in Sports

Vision care for athletes should begin with the identification of visual factors that potentially contribute to peak human performance so that these specific functions can be isolated and measured, if possible. The visual demands critical to success in sports can vary tremendously. For example, a dynamic and reactive sport such as basketball has very different visual demands than the static precision requirements of target shooting. This chapter provides an approach to this task analysis process, which is essential to provide appropriate vision care for athletes in any sport or position.

A practitioner's depth of knowledge concerning a sport activity provides the foundation for delivering the highest quality vision care for the athlete. Personal participation in the sport activity by the practitioner offers the most intimate insights into the visual task demands encountered by the athlete. However, many crucial insights into the visual task demands of a sport activity can be acquired by extensive interaction with the athlete or other experts (e.g., coach, athletic trainer) in the sport. These insights can be further supplemented by observation of the sport activity, which may offer the opportunity for a personal experience. For example, the first time the author worked with a skeet shooter, extensive interaction with the athlete was necessary because the author had no personal experience with this sport. This interaction was followed up with a visit to the shooting range for observation of the activity and personal experience to gain further insights into the visual task demands of skeet shooting.

Many other avenues are available for information concerning the demands of a specific sport activity. The American Optometric Association (AOA) Sports and Performance Vision website offers a collection of detailed insights into the many visual factors involved in a variety of sports in the form of webinars, downloadable documents, and guidebooks.[1] The sport-specific guidebooks were compiled with input from experienced optometric practitioners and are available with membership in the AOA. Information concerning less-common recreational activities can easily be found by searching on the Internet or consulting the many sports periodicals and books available. Consultation with a practitioner who has extensive experience with athletes in the sport activity can provide additional valuable insights for the task analysis process.

GENERAL VISUAL CHARACTERISTICS OF THE SPORT OR ACTIVITY

Visual factors comprise the visual task demands of any sport activity. A series of task subcategories is presented and can be used to develop a profile of the salient features involved in a sport.

Static Versus Nonstatic

Static task demands are those in which the visual information is stationary, allowing for a steady image to be processed. Sport activities with static task demands include archery, target shooting sports, golf, free throw shooting in basketball, and free penalty shots on goal in soccer and hockey. These sport tasks allow the athlete to fine-tune the motor response based on stable visual information.

Nonstatic task demands are those in which the visual information is in motion, necessitating the constant processing of changes in the visual information. Many sport activities have nonstatic demands (Box 2.1). For example, the running back in football does not typically have much time to study the defensive movements of the opponent before choosing a path to run.

Nondynamic Versus Dynamic

Dynamic is used in this chapter to describe the athlete during a sport activity. In many sports the athlete must perform while in motion (Box 2.2). The hockey player must continue to process the action in a game despite being challenged to maintain balance while in motion, with constantly interrupted views of the action.

In nondynamic sports activities the athlete is relatively stationary when performing. Nondynamic sports include the examples listed in Box 2.2. Even though movement occurs in golf during the swing at the ball, the athlete is allowed to analyze the visual information used to guide each stroke while remaining relatively motionless.

BOX 2.1
Sports With Nonstatic Visual Demands

Baseball
Softball
Basketball
Boxing
Cycling
Football
Hockey
Lacrosse
Martial arts
Motor racing
Racquet sports
Sailing
Skating
Skeet and trap shooting
Skiing
Soccer
Surfing
Water polo
Volleyball

BOX 2.2
Dynamic Sports in Which the Athlete Must Perform While in Motion and Nondynamic Sports in Which the Athlete is Relatively Stationary

Dynamic Sports	Nondynamic Sports
Baseball and softball	Archery
Basketball	Golf
Boxing	Motor racing
Football	Shooting sports
Gymnastics	
Hockey	
Lacrosse	
Martial arts	
Motor racing	
Mountaineering	
Racquet sports	
Skating	
Skiing	
Soccer	
Surfing	
Track-and-field events	
Water polo	
Volleyball	

Sustaining Demands

The duration of the competition determines how long the athlete must sustain visual performance. In one study the majority of sports were determined to be completed within 2 h.[2] Therefore many sports require sustained performance longer than 1 h (Box 2.3). In a sport activity such as mountaineering, the ability to sustain a high level of visual information processing over many hours with little rest is not only an asset but also life protecting.

The duration of each individual event in some other sports is short, even though performance levels must be sustained for the length of the competition. These types of sports typically have significant rest intervals during the course of the competition, such as those listed in Box 2.3. The demand on visual information processing is generally intense during the event, such as in alpine skiing, but the athlete is allowed a generous amount of time between events to rest.

Contrast Levels

The judgment of subtle contrast differences is a common visual task in sports. Contrast levels can be affected by changing illumination levels produced by weather,

---

BOX 2.3
Sports With Sustained Performance Demands (More Than 1

Sustained Performance	Short Duration
Baseball and softball	Archery
Basketball	Baseball and softball batting
Boxing	Drag racing
Cycling	Fencing
Football	Gymnastics
Golf	Speed and figure skating
Hockey	Skiing (alpine and jumping)
Lacrosse	Shooting sports
Motor racing	Track-and-field events
Mountaineering	
Racquet sports	
Sailing	
Nordic skiing	
Soccer	
Water polo	
Volleyball	

artificial illumination, shadows, glare, playing surface conditions, and backgrounds. Additionally, the relative contrast of the object is reduced any time the object is in motion, so that fast action sports tend be more demanding on contrast sensitivity. For example, a classic black-and-white patterned soccer ball has high contrast when stationary but significantly reduced contrast when kicked with a large amount of spin. Because the spin of the ball provides vital clues concerning its flight trajectory, the ability to discriminate the contrast of the ball pattern is potentially beneficial to the athlete (Box 2.4). The selection of filters or refractive correction modality may also be affected by the contrast sensitivity demands of a sport (see Chapter 6). For example, the downhill skier must select the filter that provides optimal transmission characteristics to enhance relevant contrast information for the current light conditions.

The judgment of subtle contrast differences does not offer an advantage in some sports, such as archery, target shooting sports, and some track-and-field events.

Target Size

Significant differences may exist in the size of the visual information that must be discriminated in different sport activities. For example, the visual discrimination task for a hockey puck is much more demanding than that for a basketball. For each sport activity, the interaction between the size of the visual target or object and the viewing distances encountered in the sport should

be evaluated to determine the visual discrimination demands. Significant interaction may also exist between visual discrimination level and contrast sensitivity demands. Again with the soccer example, the size of the soccer ball is relatively large, but the judgment of ball spin requires an enhanced level of visual discrimination than the ball size would suggest.

Distance Versus Near

The viewing distance where most of the visual information is received from can be analyzed to determine the vision demands for the athlete. In billiards, for example, the distances that must be clearly focused are fairly predictable. In other sports, such as hockey, the viewing distances may vary considerably during the course of the competition. Most sports have aspects that require clear vision for distances beyond 3 m (Box 2.5). However, there are some sports that have aspects of the activity that involve near- and intermediate-distance focus.

Boundaries

Boundaries for the competition area are established in many sports. In some sports, such as table tennis and billiards, the boundaries are relatively small and can

---

BOX 2.4
Sports With Contrast Judgment Demands

Baseball
Softball
Basketball
Cycling
Football
Golf
Hockey
Lacrosse
Motor racing
Mountaineering
Racquet sports
Sailing
Skating
Skeet and trap shooting
Skiing
Soccer
Surfing
Water polo
Volleyball

BOX 2.5
Sports With Vision Demands at Distances Further Than 3

Far-Distance Demands	Near-Distance Demands
Archery	Billiards
Baseball and softball	Boxing
Basketball	Cycling
Cycling	Martial arts
Football	Motor sports
Golf	Shooting sports
Hockey	Wrestling
Lacrosse	
Motor racing	
Mountaineering	
Racquet sports	
Sailing	
Shooting sports	
Skating	
Skiing	
Soccer	
Surfing	
Track-and-field events	
Water polo	
Volleyball	

easily be seen during the competition. In other sports, such as soccer and football, the competitive boundaries are too large to be seen entirely at all times during competition. The extent of the boundaries establishes the peripheral vision demands for the athlete and may also affect the selection of refractive correction modality.

Visual Space Ranges

The athlete must attempt to control a range of physical space in many sports by constantly processing the visual information in that physical space. The physical space can be relatively confined, as in wrestling, or it may be much larger, as in sailing competitions. This factor also relates to the peripheral vision demands for the athlete.

Figure/Ground Color, Texture, Shade

An analysis of the figure/ground characteristics encountered in a sport can assist in the selection of filters to enhance performance. This aspect relates to contrast sensitivity, but is specific to color contrast demands. For example, a skeet or trap shooter must quickly locate an orange-colored target (sporting clay) against the background of the ground (brown dirt, green grass, brown grass, etc.), any foliage (trees, shrubbery, etc.), and the sky (blue sky, partly cloudy sky, heavily overcast sky, etc.). The selection of the optimal filter for the current light levels and backgrounds is an essential aspect of competitive skeet or trap shooting. Filter selection may offer significant benefits in many sports by sharpening contrast and enhancing critical visual information. Filters also offer a potential benefit by muting distracting visual "noise" from the background. Filter selection is discussed in detail in Chapter 6.

Visual Time

Many sport situations have an established time course of action in which visual processing characteristics can be analyzed. The time course of a Major League Baseball pitch is one situation that has been scrutinized by researchers from a variety of backgrounds.[3,4] Depending on the speed of the pitch, the Major League batter has approximately 400 ms between the release of the pitch and the time the ball arrives at the plate. Because the swing takes approximately 150 ms to complete, the batter has approximately 250 ms to process the visual information from the pitch and decide on the appropriate response. These time characteristics are discussed in greater detail in Chapter 3. However, many other sport situations have time characteristics that unfold in a relatively predictable manner. The serve in many

racquet sports and volleyball, the pitch in cricket, penalty shots on goal in soccer and hockey, the judgment of hurdles in track, the judgment of the approach in high jump and pole vault in field events, the judgment of maneuvers in gymnastics and diving, and the flight of clay pigeons in skeet or trap shooting all have a range of time characteristics that define the visual processing demands for successful performance.

In other sport situations, the time course of the action can be less predictable (e.g., skiing, cycling, boxing, kayaking, motor sports, wrestling), thereby elevating the role of reactive visual information processing skills for success. Some sports have essentially no reactive component to the motor response (e.g., archery, target-shooting sports, golf, billiards). Many sports require development of the ability to modulate attention appropriately for success.

Directional Localization

In some sports the accuracy of directional localization is often critical to success. Directional localization is the ability to determine the exact direction of visual information (e.g., a target, object, opponent, teammate, terrain). For example, the ability to putt in golf requires the athlete to discriminate precisely the subtleties of the terrain for the shot to determine the best path for the putt. This skill requires the athlete, in part, to determine correctly the direction that the shot needs to take to account for the slope of the terrain and distance of the putt. Farnsworth[5] discusses this aspect of golf in detail. Directional localization ability is a crucial feature for success, to varying degrees, in sports such as those listed in Box 2.6.

Depth Discrimination and Spatial Localization

The other aspect of localization involves judgment of distance to other competitors, to a target, or of the trajectory that the target is taking. As in the previous example with directional localization, the golfer must judge the direction that a putt needs to take and also determine the stroke response that will cause the ball to traverse the specific distance to the hole. Therefore as with directional localization, the ability to accurately judge spatial localization is found to varying degrees in almost all sports.

Gaze Angles

Many sports require that the athlete process visual information coming from nonprimary positions of gaze. In volleyball, for example, much of the action takes place above the athletes' heads, requiring an upgaze eye

Archery
Baseball and softball
Basketball
Billiards
Bowling
Boxing
Cycling
Diving
Football
Golf
Gymnastics
Hockey
Kayaking
Lacrosse
Martial arts
Motor racing
Racquet sports
Sailing
Shooting sports
Skating
Skiing
Soccer
Surfing
Track-and-field events
Water polo
Wrestling
Volleyball

position to view the action. Therefore for each sport or position, an appraisal of relevant gaze positions directs the vision evaluation, particularly concerning ocular alignment and stereopsis assessment. Sports such as hockey and skiing require a significant amount of judgments with the eyes in downgaze position. In other sports, such as billiards, cycling, swimming, and volleyball, much of the visual information requires an upgaze eye position. Some sports also require a significant number of judgments while the eyes are in a lateral gaze position, such as baseball or softball batting and golf. Many other sport activities can involve all positions of gaze at any time, such as baseball, softball, basketball, football, lacrosse, racquet sports, soccer, and wrestling.

Body Position and Balance

Precise body position and maintenance of balance can be critical features of sport performance and are often critically considered in sport biomechanics. In a sport such as luge, meticulous attention is devoted to develop optimal body positioning and adjustments. Development of this skill area can produce the difference needed for success in this sport, in which milliseconds matter. Training and enhancement of body position and balance maintenance are essential elements for most sports, and sports in which they are not relevant (e.g., auto racing) are rare.

Stress (Cognitive and Cardiovascular)

A universal aspect of sports is the influence of stress on performance. Most of the stress encountered in sports is cognitive in nature, in which the athlete must control the locus of attention despite a significant amount of potential distractions and pressures inherent in the sports environment. The competitive diver must ignore irrelevant visual and auditory information as well as the knowledge of their previous performances relative to the other competitors. This is typically the territory of the sports psychologist, whose goal is to assist the athlete in controlling attentional focus for optimal sports performance. Many sports also add the factor of cardiovascular stress to cognitive stress during competition. The Olympic biathlete must control breathing and heart rate to shoot accurately while competing in a cross-country skiing race, an example of both cognitive and cardiovascular stress features that must be controlled for optimal performance. This universal feature to sports performance has led many practitioners to evaluate visual performance skills under stress-inducing conditions.

Visual Attention Demands (Central vs. Peripheral vs. Split Attention)

The visual attention demands for an athlete can be primarily central (e.g., target shooting), peripheral (e.g., seeing the release of the clay pigeons in skeet shooting), or split between central and peripheral processing (e.g., the striker in soccer seeing the goal and goalkeeper while simultaneously monitoring the movements of teammates and opponents). Peripheral vision can be argued to be relevant in almost every sport because it is a critical element of balance maintenance. Therefore even in predominantly central processing sports such as target shooting, archery, and baseball and softball batting, peripheral processing is a performance factor. However, in these types of sports situations the attentional focus is predominantly central and processing of extraneous peripheral information can degrade performance. Most of the sports discussed in this chapter compel the athlete to balance attention between the central and peripheral visual information for optimal performance, although aspects of performance may be predominantly central or peripheral in nature.

Dynamic team sports such as basketball, football, hockey, lacrosse, soccer, and water polo involve the simultaneous movement and tracking of teammates and opponents alike. The ability to track and make optimal decisions from complex movement patterns is critical to success in these sports, and previous research has indicated that visual tracking skills are enhanced in expert athletes.[6–8] This aspect of evaluation and training for these sports is commonly referred to as multiple object tracking (MOT) abilities.

E-Sports

E-sports is a rapidly growing industry that warrants the attention of sports vision practitioners. E-sports include organized video game competitions between individuals or teams at the amateur, collegiate, or professional level. Although there is scant research identifying visual performance factors in competitive gaming, research has demonstrated that the gaming experience has an impact on sensorimotor, attentional, and executive brain areas.[9–12] Most of the attention in the eye care literature focuses on the management of computer vision syndrome symptoms, such as eye strain, fatigue, eye irritation/burning, redness, and blurred or double vision.[13,14] A visual task analysis can be performed on specific competitive games to determine the relevant visual skill demands for successful performance. Certainly, many games involve demands on static and dynamic visual acuity, contrast sensitivity, peripheral awareness, oculomotor function, speed of recognition, MOT, and eye-hand reaction speed. Research has demonstrated that action video gaming promotes visual processing,[15–17] contrast sensitivity,[16] oculomotor performance,[18] eye-hand coordination,[19,20] and cognitive attention factors.[21–24]

ENVIRONMENTAL ANALYSIS IN SPORTS AND RECREATION

Participation in sports can occur in many different environmental conditions. These conditions can have detrimental effects on visibility or produce ocular hazards. The presence of ocular hazards should be evaluated, and issues of appropriate ocular, face, or head protection should be thoroughly addressed. The choice of the best protective eyewear should consider the mechanical forces or foreign body potentials encountered in a sport; the optimal designs for protection and visual performance are discussed in detail in Chapter 6.

Sports take place under many types of natural and artificial lighting. Variations in lighting can affect performance when critical visual information is tainted by the altered lighting. Studies have demonstrated that when visibility starts to diminish because of reducing light levels, reaction times also begin to slow in relation to the decreasing light level.[25–30] The effects of glare on visual performance is a particular burden in some sports and should be exhaustively addressed. Although little can be changed about natural lighting conditions outdoors, the use of specific filters and filter densities can be explored to determine maximal benefits for the athlete. This aspect of task analysis is discussed in detail in Chapter 6.

The use of eyewear or contact lenses can be adversely affected by many factors encountered in sports. Eyewear can create visibility problems in conditions of precipitation, water, and mud and are particularly prone to troubles with sweat, dust, and lens fogging. Many of these problems can be alleviated by contact lenses; however, contact lens wear can be complicated by temperature, altitude, wind, and humidity. These issues are addressed in detail in Chapter 6.

VISUAL TASK ANALYSIS EXAMPLES

Many methods exist for evaluating the visual tasks critical for successful sports performance. Many of these visual factors have been briefly discussed in this chapter, and sports can be organized into categories with similar visual task demands. An example of this approach is described in the following. However, meticulous scrutiny of the factors specific to a particular sport activity often yield more profitable information concerning the visual aspects that elevate the potential for peak sports performance.

Dynamic Reactive Sports

Many sports have dynamic visual features that need to be rapidly processed by the athlete to determine the best motor response. These sports often require the athlete to balance attention between the central and peripheral information for optimal performance, especially in team and racing sports. Sports that are dynamic and reactive in nature, and generally require the athlete to balance the central and peripheral visual attention, include those listed in Box 2.7.

In many dynamic sports, judgment of ball spin is a critical element to determine a successful response, such as tennis, soccer, and volleyball. The judgment of ball spin relies on visual resolution ability, dynamic visual acuity, contrast sensitivity, and oculomotor function to provide the best visual information for processing; therefore these visual skills should be evaluated in athletes participating in these sports. In racing

---

BOX 2.7
Dynamic Reactive Sports

Baseball and softball
Basketball
Boxing
Cycling
Diving
Fencing
Football
Gymnastics
Hockey
Kayaking
Lacrosse
Martial arts
Motor racing
Racquet sports
Skating
Skeet and trap shooting
Skiing
Soccer
Surfing
Swimming
Track-and-field events
Water polo
Wrestling
Volleyball

---

sports such as cycling, kayaking, motor (car, motor-cycle) racing, skiing, and swimming, central visual information is often critical for determining the most advantageous path or timing of responses and contrast levels frequently change significantly during competition. Racing sports, however, also entail a significant peripheral vision demand to monitor competitors during the race. These types of dynamic reactive sports can be distinguished from other types of team sports in which central visual information is often less important than peripheral information. Team sports such as basketball, football (certain positions), hockey, lacrosse, soccer, and water polo are examples in which peripheral information for some aspects is often more vital than central details and MOT abilities are advantageous. Performance in combative sports such as boxing, fencing, martial arts, and wrestling relies on responsiveness to peripheral visual information more than resolution thresholds for central vision. Therefore assessment of peripheral awareness, MOT, and reaction factors can be more important than visual acuity measurements.

The judgment of depth is a crucial factor in all the dynamic reactive sports listed, necessitating an assessment of the pertinent visual factors that contribute to accurate depth perception. In addition, an assessment of speed of

recognition is valuable in all these sports because athletes are required to process visual information rapidly to determine the best motor response. Depending on the type of motor responses typically made in competition, visual reaction times to eye-hand, eye-foot, and/or eye-body testing paradigms are indicated for all dynamic reactive sports. Additionally, visual coincidence anticipation can provide valuable information in the evaluation of athletes competing in baseball, softball, football (receivers), hockey, lacrosse, racquet sports, skeet and trap shooting, soccer, and volleyball.

Example: sports vision evaluation for baseball
Case History: Include the supplementary questions listed in Chapter 4

Static Visual Acuity: Landolt rings at 6 m, oculus dexter (OD), oculus sinister (OS), oculus unitas (OU)

Dynamic Visual Acuity: Assessment methods and protocols?

Contrast Sensitivity Function: Vistech or Vector Vision tests

Refractive Status

Ocular Alignment: Cover test in primary gaze and the eight secondary gaze positions

Depth Perception: Howard-Dolman stereopsis at 6 m (threshold and speed)

Accommodative Facility: Haynes Near-Far Facility Test

Oculomotor Skills

Speed of Recognition

Multiple Object Tracking: NeuroTracker or Senaptec Sensory Station

Visual Motor Reaction Time (Eye-Hand and Eye-Foot): MOART (Multi-Operational Apparatus for Reaction Time) system

Eye-Hand Coordination: Binovi Touch Saccadic Fixator

Visual Coincidence Anticipation: Bassin Anticipation Timer

Nondynamic Precision Sports
Nondynamic precision sports are characterized by significant demands placed on central vision to assist in determining exact directional and spatial localization. Sports such as archery, billiards, bowling, golf, and target shooting involve targets that are stationary; therefore no demand is made to react to changing visual information. Although critical demands are placed on the processing of central visual information, balancing that central information with peripheral visual information is a fundamental aspect of performance in all these sports.

The sports vision evaluation for athletes competing in nondynamic precision sports typically emphasizes static visual acuity and refractive status, pertinent elements contributing to accurate depth perception, accommodative function, field dependence or independence, and visualization and imagery.

Example: sports vision evaluation for golf

Case History: Include the supplementary questions listed in Chapter 4

Static Visual Acuity: Landolt rings at 6 m, OD, OS, OU

Contrast Sensitivity Function: Vistech or Vector Vision tests

Refractive Status

Ocular Alignment: Cover test in primary gaze and in putting stance with head tilt; fixation disparity at 6 m in primary gaze and in putting stance with head tilt

Depth Perception: Howard-Dolman stereopsis at 6 m (threshold)

Accommodative Facility: Haynes Near-Far Facility Test

Oculomotor Skills

Field Dependence or Independence: Rod and frame test

REFERENCES

1. https://www.aoa.org/optometrists/tools-and-resources/sports-and-performance-vision/spv-club-kit/pdf-and-protocols, https://www.aoa.org/optometrists/membership/aoa-sections/aoa-sections/sports-vision-section/baseball, https://www.aoa.org/optometrists/membership/aoa-sections/aoa-sections/sports-vision-section/hockey, https://www.aoa.org/optometrists/membership/aoa-sections/aoa-sections/sports-vision-section/motocross, https://www.aoa.org/optometrists/membership/aoa-sections/aoa-sections/sports-vision-section/rugby. Retrieved from 23 June 2020.
2. Obstfeld H, Pope R, Efron N, et al. Sports vision correction. In: Loran DFC, MacEwen CJ, eds. *Sports Vision*. Oxford: Butterworth-Heinemann; 1995:131.
3. Bahill AT, Karnavas WJ. The perception of baseball's rising fastball and breaking curveball. *J Exp Psychol Hum Percept Perform*. 1993;19(3).
4. Adair RK. *The Physics of Baseball*. New York: Perennial; 2002:29−46.
5. Farnsworth CL. *See it and Sink it: Mastering Putting Through Peak Visual Performance*. New York: HarperCollins; 1997.
6. Zhang X, Yan M, Yangang L. Differential performance of Chinese volleyball athletes and nonathletes on a multiple-object tracking task. *Percept Mot Skills*. 2009; 109:747.
7. Faubert J. Professional athletes have extraordinary skills for rapidly learning complex and neutral dynamic visual scenes. *Sci Rep*. 2013;3:1154.
8. Romeas T, Faubert J. Soccer athletes are superior to non-athletes at perceiving soccer-specific and non-sport specific human biological motion. *Front Psychol*. 2015;6:1343.
9. Latham AJ, Patston LLM, Tippett LJ. The virtual brain: 30 years of video-game play and cognitive abilities. *Front Psychol*. 2013;4:629.
10. Boot WR. Video games as tools to achieve insight into cognitive processes. *Front Psychol*. 2015;6:3.
11. Kuhn S, Gallinat J, Mascherek A. Effects of computer gaming on cognition, brain structure, and function: a critical reflection on existing literature. *Dialogues Clin Neurosci*. 2019;21:319−330.
12. Gong D, Ma W, Liu T, et al. Electronic-sports experience related to functional enhancement in central executive and default mode areas. *Neural Plast*. 2019:1940123.
13. Rosenfield M. Computer vision syndrome: a review of ocular causes and potential treatments. *Ophthalmic Physiol Optic*. 2011;31:502−515.
14. Portello JK, Rosenfield M, Bababekova Y, et al. Prevalence of computer vision syndrome (CVS) and dry eye in office workers. *Ophthalmic Physiol Optic*. 2012;32:375−382.
15. Li RW, Ngo C, Nguyen J, Levi DM. Video-game play induces plasticity in the visual system of adults with amblyopia. *PLoS Biol*. 2011;9:e1001135.
16. Li R, Polat U, Makous W, Bavelier D. Enhancing the contrast sensitivity function through action video game training. *Nat Neurosci*. 2009;12:549−551.
17. Green CS, Bavelier D. Action-video-game experience alters the spatial resolution of vision. *Psychol Sci*. 2007;18: 88−94.
18. West GL, al-Aidroos N, Pratt J. Action video game experience affects oculomotor performance. *Acta Psychol*. 2013; 142:38−42.
19. Jones EG, Burton H, Saper CB, Swanson LW. Midbrain, diencephalic and cortical relationships of the basal nucleus of Meynert and associated structures in primates. *J Comp Neurol*. 1976;167:385−419.
20. Kennedy AM, Boyle EM, Traynor O, et al. Video gaming enhances psychomotor skills but not visuospatial and perceptual abilities in surgical trainees. *J Surg Educ*. 2011; 68:414−420.
21. Green CS, Bavelier D. Action video game modifies visual selective attention. *Nature*. 2003;423:534−537.
22. Green CS, Bavelier D. Effect of action video games on the spatial distribution of visuospatial attention. *J Exp Psychol Hum Percept Perform*. 2006;32:1465−1478.
23. Chisholm JD, Hickey C, Theeuwes J, Kingstone A. Reduced attentional capture in action video game players. *Atten Percept Psychophys*. 2010;72:667−671.

24. Cain MS, Landau AN, Shimamura AP. Action video game experience reduces the cost of switching tasks. *Atten Percept Psychophys.* 2012;74:641–647.

25. Appler DV, Quimby CA. The effect of ambient room illumination upon Wayne Saccadic Fixator performance. *J Am Optom Assoc.* 1984;55:818.

26. Campbell FW, Rothwell SE, Perry MJ. Bad light stops play. *Ophthalmic Physiol Optic.* 1987;7:165.

27. Perry MJ, Campbell FW, Rothwell SE. A physiological phenomenon and its implications for lighting design. *Light Res Technol.* 1987;19(1).

28. Rothwell SE, Campbell FW. The physiological basis for the sensation of gloom: quantitative and qualitative aspects. *Ophthalmic Physiol Optic.* 1987;7:161.

29. Beckerman SA, Zost MG. Effect of lighting levels on performance on the Wayne Computerized Saccadic Fixator and Wayne peripheral awareness trainer. *J Behav Optom.* 1994;5(155).

30. Beckerman S, Fornes AM. Effects of changes in lighting level on performance with the AcuVision 1000. *J Am Optom Assoc.* 1997;68:243.

CHAPTER 3

Visual Information Processing in Sports

Discussion, speculation, and research concerning the role of vision and visual information processing in sports have a long history. There is little debate that vision is a critical factor in sports performance or that visual information is the dominant sensory system when performing practically any perceptual motor task such as those tasks encountered in sports.[1-5] The visual physiologic attributes of athletes have been extensively studied and compared with nonathletes, novices, and other athletes of varying skill levels. Some believe that the literature supports the opinion that athletes possess superior visual systems that allow them to see and process critical visual information better than their peers.[5-9] Others contend that the literature does not support the opinion that their visual system physiology is superior but that elite athletes are able to use available visual information more efficiently and effectively than novices.[10-13] The results of research attempting to address these contentions have been equivocal, thereby allowing both sides of the debate to claim support for their assertions.

Many factors influence sport performance, such as biomechanical factors, strength and conditioning factors, visual factors, and cognitive factors. Experts in any of the relevant fields would be expected to find support for the importance of factors in their area of expertise because they evaluate aspects of performance from the perspective of their expertise. Definitive answers to global questions are rarely ascertained by isolating factors without consideration of the complete process. The suggestion that superior visual skills are of little consequence compared with the cognitive processing of the visual information overlooks the role that visual information plays in cognition. This argument would contend that it is not the golfer's ability to see the details of the green that is critical when attempting a putt but rather the ability of the golfer to interpret that visual information in order to select the appropriate direction and distance for the putt. This is certainly a cogent argument when comparing a novice with an expert golfer with similar visual abilities; the two may see the same information, but the experience of the expert allows interpretation of the contours of the green and judgment of the distance to the hole better than the novice.

However, when comparing golfers with similar skills and experience, the golfer with poor contrast sensitivity will be at a disadvantage in reading the contours of the green when compared with the golfer with excellent contrast sensitivity. This visual disadvantage is present notwithstanding any perceptual adaptations that have developed in the golfer with poor contrast sensitivity in order to succeed; the golfer has deficient ability to use contrast information to judge the contours of the green. No matter how well developed the cognitive processing of visual information becomes, poor visual information creates an impediment to peak performance. Peak sports performance cannot be expected without both adequate visual information and the cognitive abilities to use the visual information. Superior capacity in either vision abilities or cognitive proficiency would logically offer an advantage to the athlete over a peer with less-developed skills.

INFORMATION PROCESSING MODEL FOR SPORTS PERFORMANCE

Sports performance generally requires the athlete to process visual information and execute an appropriate motor response. Many elaborate information processing models have been developed to understand the exact nature of the processes occurring in skilled motor performance. A traditional information processing model of skilled motor performance first proposed by Welford,[14] and later modified by others,[4,11,14-18] is presented here because it provides a useful framework for understanding the relevant aspects of sports performance.

The information processing model in Fig. 3.1 proposes that skilled motor performance is the result of three central processing mechanisms: the perceptual mechanism, the decision mechanism, and the effector mechanism. These three mechanisms are proposed to operate sequentially; however, significant consideration is given to the effects of both intrinsic and extrinsic feedback, as well as the contributions of experiential memory. This process is also referred to as the perception-action cycle, with visuomotor integration guiding the process in this discussion.[19-21]

Sports Vision. https://doi.org/10.1016/B978-0-323-75543-6.00010-3

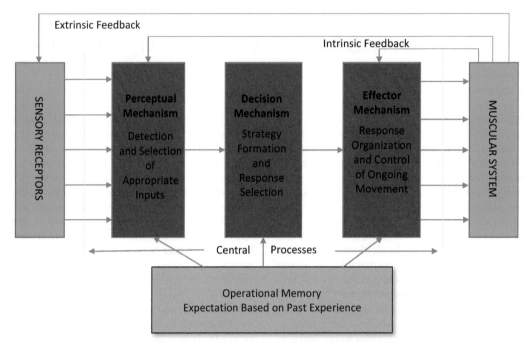

FIG. 3.1 An information processing model of skilled performance. (Modified from Welford AT. The measurement of sensory-motor performance: survey and reappraisal of twelve years progress. *Ergonomics*. 1960;3:189.)

The perceptual mechanism receives an incredible amount of information from a wide variety of sensory receptors (e.g., vision, vestibular, tactile, and auditory receptors). Sensory channel capacity limits the amount of information that can be thoroughly processed, requiring that the current input information be selected for processing that has immediate relevance for executing the required task. This also requires that irrelevant sensory information be filtered out by similar neurologic mechanisms. The athlete's experience and ability to control attention are suggested to guide this selection and filtering process.[14,22] For example, attentional focus and distraction can produce different size estimates, accuracy, and putting errors in golf.[23] The perceptual mechanism is then responsible for organizing and interpreting the processed information in an approach that facilitates optimal performance.

Traditionally, the perceptual mechanism for visual information is conceptualized as a bottom-up process with a neural chain of visual signals from the retina traveling through the lateral geniculate nucleus to the primary visual cortex. From these basic responses, the neural signal is then fed forward through increasing complex visual processing regions that are tuned to respond to specific properties. The visual signals then diverge into two neural streams that provide additional processing of the signals: a dorsal pathway that provides information about spatial properties (called the "where" pathway) and a ventral pathway through the inferior temporal cortex that provides further information about object details and identification. These two neural streams converge in areas of the prefrontal cortex (PFC) and posterior parietal cortex (PPC) providing significant information to assist with decision making. This traditional, bottom-up sequential processing model has been modified to suggest a more dynamic model that also demonstrates top-down processing. In these models of neural processing, prior experience and attentional focus direct a process of "perceptual binding" that selectively processes critically relevant visual information.[24–27] Perceptual binding guides visual processing of important details in order to overcome the neural limitations of processing all the incoming visual information and thereby improves efficiency and shortens reaction time (RT) to visual signals. The PFC and PPC appear to direct this process by the development of predictive models and stimulus-response mapping in order to rapidly identify critical visual information. For disruptive visual information (e.g., the appearance of an immediate threat), the process is primarily bottom-up, whereas goal-directed attention (e.g., looking for specific details such as the release of a pitch in batting) is top-down and directed by the PFC and PPC. A study comparing team handball athletes to athletes in nonteam sports and nonathletes found that sports expertise did not produce differences in basic attention tasks (attentional breadth, tracking performance, and inattentional blindness), suggesting that any differences in attention skills may be task-specific.[28] Studies of gaze behaviors and visual search patterns during skilled sports performance by elite athletes compared to near-elite athletes show that fixations are typically clustered on features that provide a significant amount of information about the task being viewed.[29] More thorough reviews of the role of visual attention in the perception-action cycle and its application in sports are available.[30,31]

The sensory information that has been processed is conveyed to a decision mechanism. The purpose of the decision mechanism is to determine the appropriate motor response strategies for the sensory information, which may also include the repression of a motor response in some sport situations. The athlete's sport knowledge and past experience obviously exert substantial influence on the effectiveness of decision processing.

The motor response selected by the decision mechanism is transmitted to the effector mechanism. The neural commands necessary to produce the desired response at the correct time are organized and sent to the appropriate brain centers for execution of the action. The motor response is both initiated and controlled by the effector mechanism. Both internal and external information is continually processed by the perception and decision mechanisms, allowing both control and adjustment of the motor response to occur when sufficient time exists to alter the response.

This model is both simple and practical for understanding the processes occurring when an athlete must react and respond to sensory information in a sport situation. Comparisons have been made between this model and the functioning of a computer; the computer receives information input, processes that information in the manner that it was programmed, and produces the planned output result. Although this analogy of computer hardware and software has been challenged, and other factors are not clearly revealed by this model, it remains a useful global method for understanding the processes involved in sports performance. The computer analogy also clarifies the importance of both superior hardware and software for achieving peak human performance.

PERCEPTUAL MECHANISM

In the information processing model presented, the perceptual mechanism stage of processing is the most

directly related to the realm of the vision care provider. It is the basic role of the vision care provider to ensure that the sensory receptors for visual information are functioning adequately. A comprehensive vision evaluation should evaluate the patency of the basic functions of the visual apparatus and identify any deficits that may limit performance potential. A secondary level of vision care is the evaluation of visual performance skills that relate to sports performance, yet it has been challenging to develop visual performance evaluation procedures that appropriately measure relevant vision skills that are directly related to sports tasks. Recommendations for procedures to assess visual performance abilities in athletes are discussed in Chapter 4. Four general areas of visual information processing in the perceptual stage have been defined, each of which is richly supported by intrinsic and extrinsic feedback and experience: visual resolution, depth judgment, eye movements, and peripheral vision.

Visual Resolution

The first aspect of the information processing model is sensory reception of the information. The ability to resolve subtle details can be a factor in perceptual processing if the details contain relevant visual information. Static visual acuity has been found to be better in athletes than in nonathletes in some studies,[32–42] whereas some have found no difference.[43–46] The variance in results is most likely a consequence of the visual acuity testing methods used and the differences in the visual task demands of the variety of sports assessed. The ability to resolve detail when movement between the observer and the test object is induced, referred to as dynamic visual acuity (DVA), has arguably more relevance in many sports than static measurements. Most of the research has attempted to determine the relation between DVA and visual task performance; however, studies have compared athletes and nonathletes.[37,45,47–55] Despite significant differences in methods for measuring DVA, all but one study found better DVA in athletes.[50] A significant amount of human and stimulus variables can affect DVA, including the resolving power of the retina, peripheral awareness, oculomotor abilities, target luminance, angular velocity, the time exposure of the target, and psychologic functions that affect interpretation of visual information. In addition to DVA, measurement of contrast sensitivity function (CSF) has been recommended in athletes because athletes often must perform visual discrimination tasks with suboptimal lighting because of environmental variability. The common conclusions from investigations comparing CSF in athletes indicate elevated CSF in athletes.[34,35,38,49,56–63] Therefore the consensus of studies evaluating the resolution capacities of athletes indicates that although athletes can still perform with suboptimal visual acuities, superior visual resolution capabilities are expected.

The resolution of visual details also requires the athlete to be proficient at adjusting focus for a variety of distances. Studies that have evaluated accommodative facility in athletes compared with nonathletes have had mixed results, primarily because of the method of testing used. The use of lenses to manipulate accommodative demand does not simulate the visual task demands encountered in sports, and studies using this method have found no difference in athlete performance.[43,44,64] The use of resolution threshold demand targets at two different distances with fixation being rapidly alternated between the two charts may better represent the accommodative task demands of sport.[34,65,66]

Depth Judgment

Discrimination of distance information and judgments of spatial localization are commonly encountered in sports. The results of research comparing performance on tests of static stereopsis with a variety of testing procedures in athletic populations have had mixed results; some have found better stereopsis[32,35,38,56,65,67-73] and others have found no difference.[43,64,74,75] The lack of athlete differences in many studies has been suggested to be due to several factors, including (1) many stereopsis assessments are conducted at near distances rather than at far viewing conditions encountered in most sports tasks; (2) the maximum level of stereopsis measured (typically between 20 and 40 arc seconds) is not a threshold level for many competitive athletes; (3) the stereopsis assessments simulate depth by artificially creating disparity with filters, which may produce different thresholds and different results than real image/object depth judgments[76]; and (4) the static nature of the testing may not measure depth perception abilities used in sports, and testing of dynamic stereopsis may discriminate sport-related visual abilities better.[77-85] Many studies have used near stereotests because these are commonly used for clinical assessment, and many assert (without evidence) that stereopsis is nonfunctional beyond 1−2 m. A study of stereopsis assessment using separated LED lights at distances of 20 and 40 m and further found the ability to make depth estimates was present under binocular viewing but not monocular.[86] Better ocular alignment can contribute to better depth perception; however, early findings of lower amounts of heterophoria in athletes[32,68] have not been confirmed in recent studies.[43,64] Various evaluation methods for assessing vergence function have been conducted with athletes and all but one study[64] found better performance in athletes than in nonathletes.[34,43,44,65,87]

Although vergence responses are a type of eye movement used for tracking the trajectory of something moving toward or away from the observer, in addition to a compensating system for ocular misalignment, they are considered in this text because of the direct impact of vergence information on depth localization. Again, the consensus of studies evaluating the binocular abilities of athletes indicates that although athletes can still make distance judgments by using the abundance of monocular cues to depth that are often present, superior binocular depth perception and robust vergence function are expected.

Eye Movements

Oculomotor function is another aspect of the perceptual mechanism in information processing and can include evaluation of pursuit eye movements, saccadic eye movements, and steadiness of fixation. The ability to initiate a pursuit eye movement to maintain fixation of a moving object can be a critical aspect for allowing visual processing of crucial information in sports. The ability to initiate an accurate saccadic eye movement to shift fixation from one location to another is also an essential aspect of many sports tasks. Athletes have not demonstrated shorter latencies for the initiation of pursuit or saccadic eye movements[64,75,88-91]; although if a target trajectory is predictable, shorter latency periods can be learned for these eye movements.[89,91-96] The quality of pursuit and saccadic eye movements in athletes, however, has been found to be better than in nonathletes.[43,85,97,98] In precision sports such as target shooting, skilled athletes demonstrate better ability to maintain steady fixation despite distractions, which is a vital aspect of successful performance.[91] The use of fixations and eye movements to search for critical information efficiently and effectively may be a more sensitive discriminator of expert skill than the traditional measurements of eye movements performed by vision care providers.

The visual search patterns of experts compared with novices during specific sports demands have been the focus of many studies. The study paradigms typically used attempt to discriminate differences in the number of fixations to determine the amount of information assessed by the observer and differences in the duration of fixations to determine the amount of time expended to collect the visual information from each specific fixation. Most studies have found that experts have a lower number of fixations for longer durations than do novices during the viewing of specific sport situations, especially when the subjects are required to move while gaze behaviors are recorded.[99-125] Research that has investigated more open-field viewing conditions, or that use photographic or video displays and do not require physical movement by the subjects, has found the opposite—experts have a greater number of fixations on more peripheral aspects of the action.[126–131] Irregardless of the visual search pattern, the accuracy of object localization and motor response depend on the type and accuracy of the eye movements used.[107,132] A universal finding in all studies of visual search patterns is that the fixations are typically clustered on features that provide a significant amount of information about the task being viewed.[29] Additionally, novices are much less skilled at determining these informational locations and distributing their fixations in a manner most efficient for processing the information within the time constraints of the action. Visual search strategies have been found to vary among individuals at all expertise levels, which can affect results and conclusions in the studies, as can the method for determining expert and novice or near-expert status. The distribution of attention to central and peripheral visual information is also not measured by these systems; therefore determining the exact nature of the visual information being processed during a fixation is difficult. The optimal visual search pattern for specific sports tasks has yet to be determined, if such an optimal pattern exists, because of an inability to demonstrate objectively the features containing the premium information and the most advantageous temporal distribution of fixations for attending to those premium features.

The process of visual search patterns during critical sport situations appears to represent continual cycles of the information processing model presented, in which visual fixation information is processed by the perceptual mechanism, the decision mechanism determines the next appropriate eye movement response (based on experience), and the effector mechanism organizes and controls the signals delivered to the extraocular muscles. A considerable amount of perceptual, motor, and cognitive feedback is present in this process, leading to speculations about the relative value of each portion of the process. As previously mentioned, evidence suggests that all aspects of information processing must be operating optimally to potentiate peak performance.

Peripheral Vision
Processing of information from the peripheral visual fields is a universally beneficial element to successful sports performance, whether the task is to monitor teammates and opponents or maintain steady balance. Results indicate that athletes have a larger extent of horizontal and vertical visual fields than nonathletes[21,68–70,133–138] and that athletes have better form recognition at more peripheral

locations.[43,64,134,135] The restriction of peripheral vision has also been found to increase the latency and accuracy of head movements during eye movement localization tasks[139] as well as significantly degrade balance ability.[140] Therefore peripheral sensitivity also appears to be enhanced in athletes.

The evidence concerning visual resolution, depth judgment, eye movements, and peripheral vision supports the role of excellent visual information as a vital element for the function of the perceptual mechanism in the model of information processing for skilled performance. The evidence also converges on the general conclusion that athletes should, and typically do, possess superior visual skills. The results do, however, clearly illuminate the need for visual evaluation procedures sensitive to the visual task demands required in specific situations of sports, especially if these procedures are to be used to predict performance capabilities of an athlete. For example, one study that reported no difference between the visual skills of experts and novices used an accommodative facility test with a +1.00/−1.00 D flipper at 50 cm.[141] Not only has the use of lenses to assess accommodative facility been found to be nondiscriminatory with athletes but also the use of +1.00 and −1.00 D is such a low accommodative demand at 50 cm that virtually all subjects would perform at maximal capacity, generating a superthreshold response that would predictably result in a lack of discrimination between subject categories. Additional consequences result when considering specific visual skills in isolation without the substantial dynamics of both visual skill interaction and other forms of intrinsic and extrinsic feedback essential in the information processing model.

DECISION MECHANISM
The critical role that the decision mechanism performs in the information processing model is undeniable. The ability to rapidly select the stimulus-response choice most compatible with the sport situation provides the biomechanical elements of performance with the opportunity for success. This mechanism requires the athlete to know where crucial visual information exists, be able to direct attention to those crucial elements, select the best information from all that is available, organize and interpret the information in the most appropriate manner based on experience and memory of similar situations and information, and select the most accurate response with consideration of an anticipated action plan.

In many sport situations, this process must occur in a time interval that approaches the limits of human capacity. In some sport situations, the time factors exceed the human capacity to process the important visual information before initiating a motor response, so the motor response must be initiated with the anticipation of the most likely scenario that will unfold. For example, in a penalty shot in hockey, the puck can cross the goal line within approximately 100 ms of being struck.[142] The typical simple visual RT is approximately 150–200 ms; therefore the goaltender cannot wait until the puck has been hit to predict the trajectory of the shot. Use of advance cues for anticipation of sports action has been studied to address this aspect of performance, which can mean the difference between a smooth, efficient response and an embarrassing misplay.

An athletes' ability to process visual information rapidly from a competition situation and structure that information into a useful composition to facilitate performance decisions is a critical ability acquired as expertise improves. Sports researchers have adopted a study paradigm used with chess in which experts were able to recall more structured chess positions from brief exposures than nonexperts.[143–145] However, the experts did not exhibit superior recall when presented with unstructured chess positions, suggesting that the superior recall of experts was the result of task-specific experience rather than exceptional memory abilities. The same results have been found when speed of recognition has been evaluated in athletes using numerical stimuli rather than sport-specific stimuli.[43,146] These same structured versus unstructured recall differences between experts and novices have been found with athletes in various team sports, including basketball,[147,148] field hockey,[10,149] and football.[12] The organization of common sport situations into a knowledge architecture clearly is a common development with sport expertise. This knowledge architecture offers many advantages, including the ability to process larger quantities of information in a short amount of time and the possibility of priming the perceptual and effector mechanisms for subsequent information.

The superior ability to structure and recall sport-related perceptual information should improve an expert's ability to make more accurate decisions in a shorter amount of time or make those decisions earlier in the time course of the action. Study results have been mixed. Expert field hockey players demonstrated better accuracy than lower level players, but the tactical decisions were not made any faster.[149] Studies of soccer,[114,130,150] volleyball,[151] ice hockey,[152] baseball,[66,153] and motorsports[37] found faster decisions with equivalent accuracy. The crux of the difference in expert performance was proposed to be the ability to use advance visual cues to anticipate the location of subsequent critical information and use that information to improve performance.

The common paradigm for assessing the use of advanced cues for anticipation of sport action has been the use of film occlusion. Subjects watch a brief video of a sports situation and the footage is occluded at various intervals. This occlusion requires the subjects to predict the outcome of the interrupted action (e.g., where the tennis ball will land). This is a form of temporal occlusion that indicates how expertise affects the minimal time interval and the type of information that benefits the experienced athlete.

Spatial occlusion has also been used, in which strategic portions of the footage are masked (e.g., the badminton opponent's racquet) to determine which features provide the best information to the athlete. Studies involving badminton, baseball, cricket, field and ice hockey, soccer, squash, tennis, and volleyball have all demonstrated the superior ability of experts to use advance visual cues to anticipate the outcome of the sport action.[114,126,128,149,151,154–166] These studies provide ample empirical evidence that the development of sport expertise produces enhanced ability to identify and use sport-specific visual cues to anticipate action outcomes. Anticipation of forthcoming action allows the athlete to shuffle the most likely scenarios to the top of the stack of possibilities effectively, thereby reducing the time needed to match stimulus-response choices as the action progresses.

The complex visual behavior of advance cue utilization allows the skilled athlete the enviable advantage of shortening visual RTs in sport-specific tasks and also establishes a proactive feedback mechanism in the information processing model. The accurate processing of cues in advance of sport action allows the athlete to direct attention to the correct locations and temporal aspects of critical features of the action, thereby reducing the athletes' uncertainty about the impending action. Modulation of attention has been shown to be another discriminating aspect of sports performance in athletes and is developed in a manner that is task specific. Elite shooters demonstrate narrower attentional focus with less influence from visual field distractions,[91,167] whereas volleyball players have a more expansive attentional focus.[168] The ability to modulate attention appropriately, and often split attention between multiple stimuli,[169] is another valuable aspect of the decision mechanism in the information processing model.

As expertise is developed in a sport, the complex knowledge structures acquired facilitate expanded and enhanced use of mental imagery strategies. Mental rehearsal is the act of constructing mental images of an event, and it is commonly used by elite athletes in preparation for performance.[168−179] Studies have demonstrated that mental imagery may share the same types of neural processes as visual perception, which has significant implications in sports.[180] Mental imagery of motor skill performance shares cognitive processes with physical skill performance,[181−187] and comparable brain activity in the areas of motor preparation and performance has been demonstrated.[188−191] Similar muscles and motor programs are also activated during imagery, and expertise levels influence the amount of muscular response during skill imagery.[182,184,192−196] As the use of mental rehearsal is expanded and enhanced with sport skill development, the possibility of priming the perceptual and effector mechanisms for subsequent information offers significant potential advantages if the advance visual cues are accurately located and interpreted.

The fundamental role of the decision mechanism in achieving peak sports performance is indisputable. The ability of the elite athlete to find and use critical features in sport situations quickly and convert that information rapidly into effective response strategies through anticipation and response priming characterizes the elite athlete as "intelligent."

EFFECTOR MECHANISM

The effector mechanism is responsible for converting information processed by the perceptual mechanisms and decision mechanisms into appropriate motor response signals. The organization and control of the motor response signals must be sufficiently accurate to allow the proper biomechanical action sequence to occur with precise timing for optimal performance. Coordination of hand reactions, foot reactions, body reactions, and balance adjustments must be directed with efficient precision within the time constraints of the specific sport situation. The information from the perceptual and decision mechanisms concerning the space-time behavior of critical factors in fast-action sports should contain the vital information necessary for the motor responses to occur at the proper time and location. For successful performance, the motor responses must also be sufficiently adjustable to allow modification on the basis of continuing input from the perceptual and decision mechanisms as the sport action continues.

Visual-motor RT refers to the amount of time that elapses between the initiation of a visual stimulus and the completion of a motor response to that stimulus. The effector mechanism is responsible for translating the processed information to the neuromuscular system, which sends the information to the muscles that need to be stimulated to make the appropriate motor response. The measure of a simple RT reflex represents the minimal amount of time required to process a visual stimulus presentation and perform a simple motor response to that stimulus. The assessment of simple RT may be the most direct method of evaluating the effector mechanism because the requirements of the perceptual and decision mechanisms are minimal. Several studies have found faster simple RTs in athletes (both eye-hand and eye-foot RTs) in various sports compared with nonathletes, and it has been demonstrated to be a discriminator between expertise levels.[64,70,197−206]

A simple stimulus-response procedure that requires minimal cerebral processing will result in a faster RT than a complex stimulus-response procedure that requires discrimination of visual information.[207,208] Peripheral eye-hand or eye-foot response, also called eye-hand and eye-foot coordination, is a repeated complex RT function for an extended period in which synchronized motor responses with the hands or feet must be made in response to unpredictably changing visual stimuli. The studies designed to provide normative information for athletes using available instrumentation to evaluate peripheral eye-hand response have had mixed results depending on the testing paradigm.[34,43,146,204,209−212] A test paradigm that adds a layer of quick decision-making to the task in order to determine how effectively an athlete can make an uncomplicated decision to either generate a motor response or inhibit it is called Go/No Go.[213,214] A study of baseball players found more variable RTs in a baseball-specific Go/No-Go task based on the level of experience, but this variability was not found in nonathletes or tennis and basketball players.[204,212] In a study of executive functioning, high-level youth soccer players outperformed youth amateur players in suppressing ongoing motor responses and in the ability to attain and maintain an alert state.[215] Eye-body coordination is similar to eye-hand coordination, except that the athlete must make synchronized motor responses to visual stimuli by shifting balance of the whole body. Very limited information is available concerning this type of visual-motor reaction skill in athletes.[34]

The ability to maintain balance while processing complex, fast-action visual information is a task demand fundamental to many sports. The athlete is frequently required to preserve balance while the oculomotor system is engaged in pursuit, saccadic, and/or vergence eye movements. Some normative data have been provided for athletes on the basis of subjective assessment protocols,[34] and a series of investigations found that vision played an important role in dynamic balance skill acquisition in gymnastics.[216–219]

Balance maintenance may also be affected by the athlete's relative field dependence or independence, which refers to the cognitive style of processing information to discern relevant stimuli from an irrelevant stimulus background. The theory implies that field-dependent persons rely more on external cues during information processing and field-independent persons use internal cues more.[219–223] Kane postulated that field independence was an advantage for athletes competing in "closed skill" sports (e.g., diving, gymnastics, track and field) because they tend to rely more on internal physical components such as body orientation when executing motor responses.[224] Field dependence was considered an advantage in "open skill"[225,226] team sports (e.g., basketball, football, hockey) because athletes must make constant adjustments in performance to external factors (teammates, opponents, etc.).[225] Much is still to be discovered concerning the use of visual, vestibular, and other sensory information to make discrete and accurate adjustments in balance during sports.

Complex Interactions Mediating Effector Mechanism Responses

The ability to predict the arrival of an object or stimulus at a designated place can be measured with a motor response and is referred to as visual coincidence anticipation timing (CAT). Excellent perceptual processing combined with exceptional decision processing in fast-action sports can provide a significant advantage in executing the most appropriate motor responses.[227–237] A substantial body of research addresses the many factors that influence the impressive human ability to perform the complex visual-motor tasks encountered in sports. The literature contains extensive information—from the basic physiologic and neuronal mechanisms to global models using physics computations—to explain how human beings can catch or hit a ball. Covering all these factors to the degree that would do justice to the collective contributions is beyond the scope of this chapter; however, some basic information distilled from the research is presented in the context of the information processing model.

To hit or catch a ball successfully, the athlete must judge the spatial information of height, rightward or leftward displacement, and distance of the ball. In addition to these three-dimensional space judgments, the temporal aspects of time to contact must be calculated with exacting precision. Several visual cues are available to assist the athlete in making these judgments, including

retinal image and disparity information. Some neurons in the visual cortex are tuned to binocular retinal image disparity, providing information about the depth position of an object.[238–240] The difference in retinal locations for the ball as seen by the right eye and left eye constitutes binocular disparity, supplying the stereoscopic perception of relative distance.[241–244] Binocular stereopsis judgments can be made at relatively far distances, not just for near distances.[86] In addition, evidence indicates that a system of binocularly driven cortical neurons sensitive to motion in depth is separate from the position in depth system.[240,245–255]

The perception of motion in depth is also produced by a changing retinal image size information system that operates relatively independent of the changing retinal disparity system.[249,256,257] Ample evidence shows that human beings possess cortical neurons that are selectively sensitive to changing image size and that these "looming" detectors provide a significant amount of information for judging time to contact even under monocular viewing conditions.[258–260] Additional monocular visual information about time to contact is also available from the flow pattern of visual information,[249,261–264] and this information also appears to be processed by the changing size system.[249] Regan and Beverly[265] concluded that:

> The relative effectiveness of changing-disparity and changing-size as stimuli for motion-in-depth sensation varies as follows: (a) changing disparity grows relatively more effective as velocity increases (according to a power law); (b) changing disparity grows relatively more effective as inspection time increases; (c) changing disparity grows relatively more effective as the linear horizontal width of the target decreases; (d) the relative effectiveness of changing disparity and changing size shows marked intersubject variability (at least 80:1).

The precision of the motion in depth system is hypothesized to be attributable to a relative excitation mechanism in the stereomotion channels for changing size and changing disparity that acts similar to the opponent-color stage of human color discrimination. Separate stereomotion channels also seem to exist for different directions of motion: one for motion that is approaching the head and one for motion of a receding object.[251]

The retinal information concerning changing disparity and changing size is sufficiently accurate to judge time to contact with a ball; however, it does not provide exact information concerning the actual distance of the ball or its speed.[266,267] Stereoscopic depth perception from calibrations within the vergence system and from motion in depth information provides precise information about relative depth but not about the exact distance location.[268–271] Ocular vergence information is notoriously unstable when the vestibular signals must contend with a freely moving head,[272–274] and changes in vergence angle or changes in absolute disparity do not affect binocular fusion or the perception of motion in depth for images beyond a few meters when independently altered.[271] Binocular viewing offers advantages in catching or hitting a ball[275–277]; however, monocular catching ability can be trained to similar skill levels as binocular viewing.[278] Comparison of binocular and monocular performance of a table tennis hitting task revealed that only stroke consistency was affected under monocular viewing, not accuracy or movement time.[279] A frame of reference to assist the judgment of relative depth has been shown to improve catching and hitting performance,[277,280] and the vergence system demonstrates a rapid ability to recalibrate.[281–283] It also appears that coupling the CAT skills with the typical physical movements used in the activity, such as batting in cricket, significantly improves anticipation accuracy and is less susceptible to the effects of blur.[284,285]

Because the time to contact can be determined by the changing size and changing disparity information available to the visual system from an approaching ball, Lee[286] derived an optical quantity signified by the Greek letter tau (τ) and the τ-margin[287] to describe the calculation of time to contact on the basis of the relative rate of dilation of the ball's optical contours during approach. Many studies have confirmed the use of τ in guiding motor responses during acts requiring spatial and temporal judgments.[229,232,234,287–299] Further studies elaborating the τ-margin found that the rate of constriction of the optical gap separating the moving object from the interception point also provides sensitive information concerning time to contact.[230,236,300]

The actual performance of catching tasks has demonstrated that extensive feedback from the visual and kinesthetic systems constantly updates the time to contact judgments[301,302] and that observer movement improves the judgments.[284,285,303–305] It appears that freedom to intercept a moving target at any location significantly improves the accuracy of the timing of contact and is better in faster moving targets.[305] Visual and kinesthetic feedback during motor task acquisition and performance has been manipulated in many studies, and removal of vision feedback typically produces decrements in performance.[94,306–315] Elaborate models have been constructed (and debated) to explain how baseball fielders select a path and movement speed to intercept a ball in flight[304,316–321] or hit a ball in flight.[266,267,322] Misjudgment of ball velocity can cause

significant perceptual misjudgments concerning the trajectory and appearance of speed changes.[225,267,323] Similarly, studies of gaze behaviors for hitting a bouncing ball, such as in tennis or cricket, show anticipatory saccades are made prior to the bounce in order to expedite ball tracking after the bounce.[324]

The quality of visual input is a critical factor to sports task performance, and extensive feedback from the sensory receptors provides continuous information for performance adjustment. The value of skill repetition and performance experience cannot be underestimated in its role of providing the effector mechanism with the framework for effectively and efficiently using the information from the perceptual mechanism. The gifted athlete's ability to make the correct responses routinely and consistently generates the appearance of effortless "natural" ability, a venerated description in sports society,[325] thereby neglecting to duly recognize the contribution of years of demanding practice and experience.[326]

Collectively, the wealth of research information provides extensive insight into the mechanisms responsible for successful sports performance. The information processing model for skilled performance provides a useful structure for applying this information to specific tasks. An application of the model is presented for batting in baseball, often called "the single hardest act in all of sports."[327,328]

APPLICATION OF THE INFORMATION PROCESSING MODEL TO BATTING IN BASEBALL

The time frame from when the pitcher releases the ball to when it reaches the average point of contact with the bat must first be considered. Simplified calculations have suggested that a 90-mph fastball pitch reaches the bat approximately 400 ms after release and a 75-mph curveball arrives in approximately 480 ms.[267] The type of pitch thrown will have significant consequences on the flight trajectory of the ball because of the properties of aerodynamics; this is discussed in the decision mechanism portion of the information processing model. The batter will have access to visual and cognitive cues to help anticipate the most likely type of pitch to expect, but time must be allocated for completing the mechanics of the swing. Although batters typically complete the swing in 150 ms, some can perform this feat faster.

For the purposes of this application, a 400-ms time frame is presented for the time course between the pitcher's release and the contact with the bat, and

150 ms is used for completion of the swing mechanics. The pitcher is at the moment of release and the clock is ticking.

Perceptual Mechanism

The perceptual mechanism is responsible for organizing, processing, and interpreting the sensory information to facilitate the optimal response to the pitch. The successful batter uses efficient and effective visual search patterns during the pitching motion to analyze any advance cues to the pitch type,[108,127] hopefully narrowing the trajectory probabilities that need to be considered by the decision mechanism. The batter also has access to information about the inclinations of the pitcher, the pitch count, the current situation in the game, and the presence of any base runners to guide attentional focus. At the moment of release, the batter initiates a saccadic eye movement to direct foveal fixation to the release point[108] or pitcher's elbow,[127] while processing spatial information from the arm angle and height and locations of the release. Basic physiology indicates that retinal cell information must be encoded and assembled, a process that takes approximately 25 ms. This retinal information must be conducted to the visual cortex, requiring another 20 ms. The visual cortex must process the retinal information to construct the image; because a substantial amount of memory is available, this process takes approximately 30 ms. Therefore the visual information contained in the pitch release takes approximately 75 ms to process, and the ball is now one-fifth of the distance to the plate. The visual images can be continuously processed with only the 25-ms conduction delay requiring that the batter maintain pursuit eye movements.[329] Electroencephalographic studies demonstrate that fastballs are discriminated at the earliest points in their trajectory, relative to the curveballs or sliders. This is advantageous because less time is afforded on a fastball pitch to make a decision whether to swing or not swing, compared to off-speed pitches.

How good is the visual information being received? Previous studies have demonstrated superior visual resolution skills, contrast sensitivity, and DVA in baseball players.[32,35,48,51,54,57,66] Although enhancing the seams of the baseball has been shown to improve curveball hitting, the sport demands that the visual system use the subtle cues of a traditional ball.[330] Some measures of stereopsis have been found to be superior in baseball players,[35,82,83] as has the visual field size of female softball players.[138] The interaction effect of the dominant eye and dominant hand on batting in baseball has received considerable scrutiny. Although the findings have been somewhat contradictory, the preponderance of evidence indicates no relation between eye dominance patterns and batting performance.[331–338]

Because the use of pursuit eye movements to track a pitch all the way to contact appears to be impossible, the batter must use a complex combination of pursuit and saccadic eye movements, along with rotational head movements, to track the approaching ball.[339–341] Similar eye and head movements have been found in cricket batting.[89,324] One study of pursuit and saccadic eye movement quality found subjectively better performance in those athletes with better batting averages.[97] Anticipatory saccades are common in tracking a pitch, in which the pursuit eye movements fall far enough behind the ball that a saccade is initiated to a location where the trajectory of the ball can be intercepted.[88,342] The mechanism of saccadic suppression prevents the batter from seeing during, and for approximately 20 ms after, the saccadic eye movement.[343,344] Therefore a faster pursuit eye movement system, coupled with rotational head movement, offers an advantage to track a pitch. The vestibuloocular system is used to a small degree to stabilize eye posture during head movements, and vergence eye movements do not appear to be used to track the pitch.[88]

How good is the visual system in providing the information for predicting when the ball will arrive? The visual acuity, CSF, and DVA of the batter must be sufficient to detect the seam rotation of the ball in order to judge the pitch type and ultimately the anticipated speed and trajectory the ball will travel. The retinal image information provided by changing size and changing disparity detectors for motion in depth supplies the capability of judging time to contact (τ) within 2–10 ms.[231,293] For objects subtending less than 1.5° (a baseball further than 10 feet away), cortical neurons are sensitive to changing size characteristics as low as 0.02°.[258] This capability is well above the visual threshold at the moment of release, providing the batter the opportunity to estimate time to contact with an accuracy of better than ±9 ms. A batter must estimate the time to contact to within 7–9 ms[267,329,345] to hit a 90-mph ball close to the center of percussion of the bat; other estimates, however, and estimates from cricket suggest that accuracy may need to be even better than ±9 ms.[266]

How good is the visual system in providing the information for predicting what location the ball will arrive at? The batter needs to judge the vertical height of the ball to within 0.75 inches and the inside-outside location of the pitch with respect to the batter's body to within 3 inches.[346] The batter can estimate the ball's vertical speed from the retinal velocity information combined with the distance to the ball. The range of speeds encountered in pitched balls is within the human capability for accurately judging time to contact within 5%.[347,348] Because the batter can only estimate pitch speed, and the visual system is incapable of providing more than just a relative estimate of distance,[268–271] judgments of ball location are susceptible to significant uncertainty. This may explain why batters are typically better at timing the arrival of the pitch than at judging the location of the ball.

The perceptual mechanism is under significant time constraints to process the critical visual information through the dorsal ("where") and ventral ("when") neural streams to the PFC and PPC. Top-down processing directed by the PFC and PPC based on prior experience and attentional focus direct perceptual binding to selectively process critically relevant visual information regarding the pitch, thereby shortening the processing time needed to make a decision about the batting response.

Decision Mechanism

Because the swing will take approximately 150 ms to initiate to the point of contact, the decision of where and when to swing must be made by 250 ms after the release. If the ball has been followed by head rotations and pursuit eye movements, then a nearly continuous stream of information has been available with information critical to selecting the proper response. As mentioned previously, the batter may also have additional information concerning the idiosyncrasies of the pitcher, the current situation in the game, the status of the pitch count, and the wealth of information stored from previous experience. This additional information, combined with the pitching motion information acquired before the moment of release, provides the potential for preselecting the most likely pitch scenarios for quicker recognition.

Many models have been proposed to explain how cognition occurs in situations such as batting in baseball,[164,349] but a minimum of 50 ms is needed to select the appropriate response and send it to the effector mechanism to begin the action. This means the batter has approximately 200 ms to process the visual information to make an accurate decision; more time than that is a luxury that is not available for a pitch of this speed. This time is not much longer than measurements of simple RT in human beings (approximately 150 ms)[350] and is much shorter than the RTs to complex choice conditions demonstrated by Hick.[351] The batter has many issues of spatial and temporal uncertainty to resolve because of the aerodynamics and Magnus forces produced by the

seam and texture of a baseball and these issues must be resolved rather quickly. A variety of pitch types can be delivered in a manner that can lead a batter to misjudge velocity and trajectory.[352–354] Occlusion studies have demonstrated that the early portion of the pitch provides sufficient information for experienced batters to set accurate probabilities about different types of pitches.[164,349]

The skill of the pitcher can place the batter at the edge of human physiologic capacity. A fastball thrown at 95 mph will arrive approximately 25 ms faster than a 90-mph fastball and arrive at a height approximately 3 inches higher. Considering the human weakness for estimating velocity, a misjudgment of the pitch speed would affect the time to contact assessment as well as the height location of the ball. The loss of 25 ms also needs to be subtracted from some aspect of the visual information processing model. The 25 ms will most likely be sacrificed from the decision mechanism because the perceptual mechanism is crucial for making the spatiotemporal judgments, and the time needed for the effector mechanism is relatively set.

Effector Mechanism

At 225 ms from the moment of release, the initial muscle response for a swing must occur. The first muscles to respond are the back leg muscles, and although approximately 25 ms are required to initiate the response, the movement does not commit the batter to a swing at the pitch.[329] The rest of the swing mechanics takes approximately 150 ms, but further visual processing can provide feedback for adjustments. After the first 50 ms of the swing, the bat is moving at approximately 30% of its final velocity and the swing can be changed substantially (or checked) on the basis of continued visual information processing.[329] By 100 ms into the swing, the bat is moving at approximately 75% of its final speed and cannot be changed because of the time factors to the muscles.[329] Some can execute the swing more rapidly than the time course described, which may allow more time for visual information processing and decision-making. However, studies have not found correlation between simple motor RT and batting skill[355] or a difference during play in cricket batting.[157]

OPTOMETRY/OPHTHALMOLOGY AND VISUAL INFORMATION PROCESSING

Many vision performance evaluations and sports vision training programs attempt to assess and improve overall processing of visual information. Most sports vision training programs attempt to affect the perceptual mechanism by improving the requisite visual skills for successful sports performance. The fundamental goal of sports vision training programs is to focus the athlete to process larger quantities of information in a shorter amount of time while simultaneously priming the perceptual and effector mechanisms for subsequent information. Ultimately, this improves the speed and efficiency of the decision mechanism, which is additionally enhanced by procedures that provide feedback on visual attention and encourage the development and use of mental imagery. Training options that provide natural or simulated sports-related conditions may provide additional benefits to a sports vision training program by assisting in the transfer of improvements to the sport. Although many unanswered questions regarding the role of sports vision training and sports performance still exist, the conclusion that improved visual skills compounded with improved ability to modulate attention and use positive mental imagery should have a salutary effect on overall visual information processing is a logical one.

Chapter 4 discusses the evaluation of visual skills in athletes, and Chapter 8 discusses the development of sports vision training programs that use the framework of the visual information processing model described in this chapter. Many other professionals also affect the visual information processing and motor responses of the athlete. For example, the development of biomechanically advantageous motor performance skills and an optimal mental mindset directly affect the effector and decision mechanisms and also have a salutary effect on the perceptual mechanism. The athlete can potentially reap tremendous benefits from directly addressing all aspects of sports performance.

REFERENCES

1. Colavita FV. Human sensory dominance. *Percept Psychophys.* 1974;16:409.
2. Lee DN, Lishman JR. Visual proprioceptive control of stance. *J Hum Mov Stud.* 1975;1:87.
3. Posner MI, Nissen MJ, Klein RM. Vision dominance: an information processing account of its origins and significance. *Psychol Rev.* 1976;83:157.
4. Abernethy B, Kipper V, Mackinnon LT. *The Biophysical Foundations of Human Movement.* Champaign, IL: Human Kinetics; 1997.
5. Ciuffreda KJ, Wang B. Vision training and sports. In: Hung GK, Pallis JM, eds. *Biomedical Engineering Principles in Sports.* New York: Kluwer Academic/Plenum Publishers; 2004:407–433.
6. Stine CD, Arterburn MR, Stern NS. Vision and sports: a review of the literature. *J Am Optom Assoc.* 1982;53:627.
7. Hitzeman SA, Beckerman SA. What the literature says about sports vision. *Optom Clin.* 1993;3:145.
8. Gregg JR. *Vision and Sports: An Introduction.* Stoneham, MA: Butterworth; 1987:17–32.
9. Hazel CA. The efficacy of sports vision practice and its role in clinical optometry. *Clin Exp Optom.* 1995;78:98.
10. Starkes JL, Deakin J. Perception in sport: a cognitive approach to skilled performance. In: Straub WF, Williams JM, eds. *Cognitive Sport Psychology.* Lansing, NY: Sport Science Association; 1984:115–128.
11. Abernethy B. Enhancing sports performance through clinical and experimental optometry. *Clin Exp Optom.* 1986;69:189.
12. Garland DJ, Barry JR. Sports expertise: the cognitive advantage. *Percept Mot Skills.* 1990;70:1299.
13. Abernethy B, Wann J, Parks S. Training perceptual-motor skills for sport. In: Elliott B, ed. *Training in Sport: Applying Sport Science.* New York: John Wiley & Sons; 1998:1–68.
14. Welford AT. The measurement of sensory-motor performance: survey and reappraisal of twelve years progress. *Ergonomics.* 1960;3:89–230.
15. Whiting HTA. *Acquiring Ball Skill: A Psychological Interpretation.* London: Bell; 1969.
16. Martenink RG. *Information Processing in Motor Skills.* New York: Holt, Rhinehart and Winston; 1976.
17. Stelmach GE. Information-processing framework for understanding motor behavior. In: Kelso JAS, ed. *Human Motor Behavior: An Introduction.* Hillsdale, NJ: Lawrence Erlbaum; 1982:63–91.
18. Abernethy B, Russel DG. Skill in tennis: considerations for talent identification and skill development. *Austr J Sport Sci.* 1983;3(3).
19. Fuster JM. Prefrontal cortex and the bridging of temporal gaps in the perception-action cycle. *Ann NY Acad Sci.* 1990;606:318–329.
20. Fuster JM. Prefrontal neurons and the cognitive foundation of motor action. *Adv Neurol.* 1992;57:351–360.
21. Quintana J, Fuster JM. From perception to action: temporal integrative functions of prefrontal and parietal neurons. *Cerebr Cortex.* 1999;9:213–221.
22. Pashler HE. *The Psychology of Attention.* Cambridge, MA: MIT Press; 1997.
23. Gray R, Canal-Bruland R. Attentional focus, perceived target size, and movement kinematics under performance pressure. *Psychon Bull Rev.* 2015;22:1692–1700.
24. Treisman AM, Gelade G. A feature-integration theory of attention. *Cognit Psychol.* 1980;12:97–136.
25. Wolfe JM, Horowitz TS. What attributes guide the deployment of visual attention and how do they do it? *Nat Rev Neurosci.* 2004;5:495–501.
26. Hardcastle VG. Consciousness and the neurobiology of perceptual binding. *Semin Neurol.* 1997;17:163–170.
27. Singer W. Consciousness and the binding problem. *Ann NY Acad Sci.* 2001;929:123–146.
28. Memmert D, Simons DJ, Grimme T. The relationship between visual attention and expertise in sports. *Psych sport exerc.* 2009;10:146–151.
29. Vickers JN. Origins and current issues in quiet eye research. *Curr Issues Sport Sci.* 2016;1:1–11.

30. Miller BT, Clapp WC. From vision to decision: the role of visual attention in elite sports performance. *Eye Contact Lens.* 2011;37:131−139.
31. Nakata H, Yoshie M, Miura A, Kudo K. Characteristics of the athletes' brain: evidence from neurophysiology and neuroimaging. *Brain Res Rev.* 2010;62:197−211.
32. Winograd S. The relationship of timing and vision to baseball performance. *Res Q Am Assoc Health Phys Educ.* 1942;13:481.
33. Fremion AS, DeMyer WE, Helveston EM, et al. Binocular and monocular visual function in world class tennis players. *Bin Vis.* 1986;1:147.
34. Coffey B, Reichow AW. Optometric evaluation of the elite athlete. *Probl Optom.* 1990;2:32.
35. Laby DM, Rosenbaum AL, Kirschen DG, et al. The visual function of professional baseball players. *Am J Ophthamol.* 1996;122:476.
36. Quintana MS, Roman IR, Calvo AL, Molineuvo JS. Perceptual visual skills in young highly skilled basketball players. *Percept Mot Skills.* 2007;104:547−561.
37. Schneiders AG, John Sullivan S, Rathbone EJ, et al. Visual acuity in young elite motorsport athletes: a preliminary report. *Phys Ther Sport.* 2010;11(2):47−49.
38. Laby DM, Kirschen DG, Pantall P. The visual function of Olympic-level athletes − an initial report. *Eye Contact Lens.* 2011;37:116−122.
39. Beatty RM, Bakkum BW, Hitzman SA, Beckerman S. Sports vision screening of amateur athletic union junior Olympic athletes: a ten-year follow-up. *Optom Vis Perf.* 2016;4(3):97.
40. Roberts JW, Strudwick AJ, Bennett SJ. Visual function of English Premier League soccer players. *Sci Med Football.* 2017;1:178−182.
41. Klemish D, Ramger B, Vittetoe K, et al. Visual abilities distinguish pitchers from hitters in professional baseball. *J Sports Sci.* 2018;36:171−179.
42. Gao Y, Chen L, Yang S, et al. Contributions of visuo-oculomotor abilities to interceptive skills in sports. *Optom Vis Sci.* 2015;92:679−689.
43. Christenson GN, Winkelstein AM. Visual skills of athletes versus nonathletes: development of a sports vision testing battery. *J Am Optom Assoc.* 1988;59:666.
44. Omar R, Kuan YM, Zuhairi NA, et al. Visual efficiency among teenaged athletes and non-athletes. *Int J Ophthalmol.* 2017;10:1460−1464.
45. Jorge J, Fernandes P. Static and dynamic visual acuity and refractive errors in elite football players. *Clin Exp Optom.* 2019;102:51−56.
46. Barrett BT, Flavell JC, Bennett SJ, et al. Vision and visual history in elite/near-elite-level cricketers and rugby-league players. *Sports Med Open.* 2017;3:39.
47. Bailey IL, Sheedy JE, Fleming DP, et al. Dynamic visual acuity: rotational measurement [abstract]. *Invest Ophthalmol Vis Sci.* 1988;29(suppl):78.
48. Rouse MW, DeLand P, Christian R, et al. A comparison study of dynamic visual acuity between athletes and nonathletes. *J Am Optom Assoc.* 1988;59:946.
49. Coffey B, Reichow AW. Athletes vs nonathletes: static visual acuity, contrast sensitivity, dynamic visual acuity [abstract]. *Invest Ophthalmol Vis Sci.* 1989;30(suppl):517.
50. Long G, Rourk D. Training effects on the resolution of moving targets—dynamic visual acuity. *Hum Factors.* 1989;31:443.
51. Ishigaki H, Miyao M. Differences in dynamic visual acuity between athletes and nonathletes. *Percept Mot Skills.* 1993;77:835.
52. Quevedo-Junyent L, Aznar-Casanova JA, Merindano-Encina D. Comparison of dynamic visual acuity between water polo players and sedentary students. *Res Q Exerc Sport.* 2011;82:644−651.
53. Wimshurst ZL, Sowden PT, Cardinale M. Visual skills and playing positions of Olympic field hockey players. *Percept Mot Skills.* 2012;114:204−216.
54. Hoshina K, Tagami Y, Mimura O, et al. A study of static, kinetic, and dynamic visual acuity in 102 Japanese professional baseball players. *Clin Ophthalmol.* 2013;7:627−632.
55. Miskewicz-Zastrow A, Bishop E, Zastrow A, et al. A standardized procedure and normative values for measuring binocular dynamic visual acuity. *Optom Vis Perf.* 2015;3:169−175.
56. Melcher MH, Lund DR. Sports vision and the high school student athlete. *J Am Optom Assoc.* 1992;63:466.
57. Hoffman LG, Polan G, Powell J. The relationship of contrast sensitivity functions to sports vision. *J Am Optom Assoc.* 1984;55:747.
58. Reichow AW, Coffey B. A comparison of contrast sensitivity in elite athletes vs normal population [abstract]. *Am J Optom Physiol Optic.* 1986;63:82P.
59. Kluka DA, Love PA, Allen S. Contrast sensitivity functions of selected collegiate female athletes. *Sports Vis.* 1989;5:18.
60. Kluka D, Love P. Contrast sensitivity in international special Olympics, national invitational volleyball championships, and recreational volleyball players. *Palaestra J.* 1992;8(11).
61. Schneider HG, Kluka DA, Love PA. Contrast sensitivity and sighting dominance in selected professional and collegiate football players. *J Optom Vis Dev.* 1992;23:23.
62. Love PA, Kluka DA. Contrast sensitivity in elite women and men softball players. *Int J Sports Vis.* 1993;1:25.
63. Kluka DA, Love PA, Sanet R, et al. Contrast sensitivity function profiling: by sport and sport ability level. *Int J Sports Vis.* 1995;2(5).
64. Hughes PK, Blundell NL, Walters JM. Visual and psychomotor performance of elite, intermediate and novice table tennis competitors. *Clin Exp Optom.* 1993;76:51.
65. Coffey B, Reichow AW. Athletes vs nonathletes: 6m vergence ranges, accommodative-vergence facility, and 6m speed of stereopsis [abstract]. *Optom Vis Sci.* 1990;67(suppl):81.
66. Burris K, Vittetoe K, Ramger B, et al. Sensorimotor abilities predict on-field performance in professional baseball. *Sci Rep.* 2018;8:116.

67. Banister H, Blackburn JM. An eye factor affecting proficiency at ball games. *Br J Psychol.* 1931;21:382.

68. Montebello RA. *The Role of Stereoscopic Vision in Some Aspects of Baseball Playing Ability* [thesis]. Ohio State University College of Optometry; 1953.

69. Graybiel A, Jokl E, Trapp C. Russian studies of vision in relation to physical activity and sports. *Res Q Am Assoc Health Phys Educ.* 1955;26:480.

70. Olsen EA. Relationship between psychological capacities and success in college athletics. *Res Q Am Assoc Health Phys Educ.* 1956;27:79.

71. Ridini LM. Relationship between psychological functions tests and selected sport skills of boys in junior high. *Res Q Am Assoc Health Phys Educ.* 1968;39:674.

72. Boden LM, Rosengren KJ, Martin DF, Boden SD. A comparison of static near stereo acuity in youth baseball/softball players and non-ball players. *Optometry.* 2009;80:121−125.

73. Hunfalvay M, Orr R, Murray N, Roberts C-M. Evaluation of stereo acuity in professional baseball and LPGA athletes compared to non-athletes. *Vis Dev Rehabil.* 2017;3: 33−41.

74. Clark B, Warren N. Depth perception and interpupillary distance as factors in proficiency in ball games. *Am J Psychol.* 1935;47:485.

75. Deshaies P, Pargman D. Selected visual abilities of college football players. *Percept Mot Skills.* 1976;43:904.

76. Leske DA, Birch EE, Holmes JM. Real depth versus Randot stereotests. *Am J Ophthalmol.* 2006;142:699−701.

77. Weissman S. Sex differences in dynamic stereoacuity. In: *Proceedings of the 80th Annual Convention, American Psychological Association.* Vol. 7. 1972:81.

78. Weissman S, Slonim P. Effects of knowledge of results on dynamic stereo acuity in males and females. *Percept Mot Skills.* 1973;36:964.

79. Slonim PS, Weissman S, Galzer E, et al. Effects of training on dynamic stereo acuity performance by males and females. *Percept Mot Skills.* 1975;40:359.

80. Solomon H, Zinn W. An introduction to dynamic sports vision. *Optom Monthly.* 1983;74:569.

81. Zinn WJ, Solomon H. A comparison of static and dynamic stereoacuity. *J Am Optom Assoc.* 1985;56:712.

82. Soloman H, Zinn HJ, Vacroux R. Dynamic stereoacuity: a test for hitting a baseball? *J Am Optom Assoc.* 1988;59:522.

83. Hofeldt AJ, Hoefle FB. Stereophotometric testing for Pulfrich's phenomenon in professional baseball players. *Percept Mot Skills.* 1993;77:407.

84. Laby DM, Kirschen DG. Dynamic stereoacuity: preliminary results and normative data for a test for the quantitative measurement of motion in depth. *Bin Vis Eye Muscle Surgery Q.* 1995;10:191.

85. Hofeldt AJ, Hoefle FB, Bonafede B. Baseball hitting, binocular vision, and the Pulfrich phenomenon. *Arch Ophthalmol.* 1996;114:1490.

86. Palmisano S, Gillam B, Govan DG, et al. Stereoscopic perception of real depths at large distances. *J Vis.* 2010; 10(6), 19, 1−16.

87. Falkowitz C, Mendel H. The role of visual skills in batting averages. *Optom Wkly.* 1977;68:33.

88. Bahill AT, LaRitz T. Why can't batters keep their eyes on the ball? *Am Sci.* 1984;72:249.

89. Land MF, McLeod P. From eye movements to actions: how batsmen hit the ball. *Nat Neurosci.* 2000;3:1340−1345.

90. Lenoir M, Crevits L, Goethals M, et al. Are better eye movements an advantage in ball games? A study of prosaccadic and antisaccadic eye movements. *Percept Mot Skills.* 2000;91:546−552.

91. Di Russo F, Pitzalis S, Spinelli D. Fixation stability and saccadic latency in elite shooters. *Vis Res.* 2003;43: 1837−1845.

92. Whittaker SG, Eaholtz G. Learning patterns of eye motion for foveal pursuit. *Invest Opthalmol Vis Sci.* 1982;23:393.

93. McHugh DE, Bahill AT. Learning to track predictable target waveforms without a time delay. *Invest Opthalmol Vis Sci.* 1985;26:932.

94. Carnahan H, Hall C, Lee TD. Delayed visual feedback while learning to track a moving target. *Res Q Exerc Sport.* 1996;67:416.

95. Adolphe RM, Vickers JN, Laplante G. The effects of training visual attention on gaze behavior and accuracy: a pilot project. *Int J Sports Vis.* 1997;4:29.

96. Elmurr P, Cornell E, Heard R. Saccadic eye movements (part 2): the effects of practice on saccadic reaction time. *Int J Sports Vis.* 1997;4:13.

97. Trachtman JN. The relationship between ocular motilities and batting average in little leaguers. *Am J Optom Arch Am Acad Optom.* 1973;50:914.

98. Kubitz K, Roberts C-M, Hunfalvey M, Murray N. A comparison of cardinal gaze speed between major league baseball players, amateur prospects, and non-athletes. *J Sport Perform Vis.* 2020;2(1):e17−28.

99. Mourand RR, Rockwell TH. Strategies of visual search by novice and experienced drivers. *Hum Factors.* 1972;14: 225.

100. Bard C, Fleury ML. Analysis of visual search activity during sport problems situations. *J Hum Mov Stud.* 1976;3: 214.

101. Bard C, Fleury M, Carriere L, et al. Analysis of gymnastic judges' visual search. *Res Q Exerc Sport.* 1980;51:267.

102. Tyldesly DA, Bootsma RJ, Bomhoff GT. Skill level and eye movement patterns in a sports oriented reaction time task. In: Rieder H, Mechling H, Reischle K, eds. *Motor Learning and Motor Behaviour: Contribution to Learning in Sports.* Cologne, Germany: Hoffmann; 1982:290−296.

103. Ripoll H, Papin J, Guezennec J, et al. Analysis of visual scanning patterns of pistol performers. *J Sports Sci.* 1985;3:93.

104. Coulibaly Z, Ripoll H. Analysis of visual scanning patterns of volleyball players in problem solving tasks. In: *Contemporary Sports Psychology Proceedings from the VI World Congress in Sport Psychology.* Orebro: VEJE Publishing; 1986:104.

105. Goulet C, Fleury M, Bard C. Analysis of advance visual indices in receiving a tennis serve. *Can J Sport Sci.* 1988; 13:79.

106. Petrakis E. Visual observation patterns of tennis teachers. *Res Q Exerc Sport.* 1986;57:254.

107. Ripoll H, Bard C, Paillard J. Stabilization of the head and eyes on target as a factor in successful basketball shooting. *Hum Mov Sci.* 1986;5:47.

108. Shank MD, Haywood KM. Eye movements while viewing a baseball pitch. *Percept Mot Skills.* 1987;64:1191.

109. Ripoll H. Uncertainty and visual strategies in table tennis. *Percept Mot Skills.* 1989;68:507.

110. Abrams R, Meyer DE, Kornblum S. Eye-hand coordination: oculomotor control in rapid aimed limb movements. *J Exp Psychol Hum Percept Perform.* 1990;16:248.

111. Vickers JN. Gaze control in putting. *Perception.* 1992;21: 117.

112. Helsen W, Pauwels JM. A cognitive approach to visual search in sport. In: Brogan D, Gale A, Carr K, eds. *Visual Search 2.* London: Taylor Francis; 1993:379−388.

113. McMorris T, Copeman R, Corcoran D, et al. Anticipation of soccer goalkeepers facing penalty kicks. In: Reilly T, Clarys J, Stibbe A, eds. *Science and Football II.* London: E&FN Spon; 1993:250−254.

114. Williams AM, Burwitz L. Advance cue utilisation in soccer. In: Reilly T, Clarys J, Stibbe A, eds. *Science and Football II.* London: E&FN, Spon; 1993:239−244.

115. Vickers JN. Control of visual attention during the basketball free throw. *Am J Sports Med.* 1996;24:S93.

116. Vickers JN. Visual control when aiming at a far target. *J Exp Psychol Hum Percept Perform.* 1996;22:342.

117. Vickers JN, Adolphe RM. Gaze behavior during a ball tracking and aiming skill. *Int J Sports Vis.* 1997;4:18.

118. Singer RN, Williams AM, Frehlich SG, et al. New frontiers in visual search: an exploratory study in live tennis situations. *Res Q Exerc Sport.* 1998;69:290.

119. Kato T, Fukuda T. Visual search strategies of baseball batters: eye movements during the preparatory phase of batting. *Percept Mot Skills.* 2002:380.

120. Moreno FJ, Reina R, Luis V, et al. Visual search strategies in experienced and inexperienced gymnastic coaches. *Percept Mot Skills.* 2002;95:901.

121. Land MF. Vision, eye movements, and natural behavior. *Vis Neurosci.* 2009;26:51−62.

122. Piras A, Lobietti R, Squatrito S. A study of saccadic eye movement dynamics in volleyball: comparison between athletes and non-athletes. *J Sports Med Phys Fit.* 2010; 50:99−108.

123. Piras A, Vickers JN. The effect of fixation transitions on quiet eye duration and performance in the soccer penalty kick: instep versus inside kicks. *Cognit Process.* 2011;12: 245−255.

124. Timmis MA, Turner K, van Paridon KN. Visual search strategies of soccer players executing a power vs. placement penalty kick. *PLoS One.* 2014;9(12):e115179.

125. Wilson M, Causer J, Vickers J. Aiming for excellence: the quiet eye as a characteristic of expertise. In: Baker J, Farrow D, eds. *Handbook of Sport Expertise.* London: Routledge/Taylor and Francis; 2015:22−37.

126. Abernethy B, Russell DG. Expert-novice differences in an applied selective attention task. *J Sport Psychol.* 1987;9: 326.

127. Goulet C, Bard M, Fleury M. Expertise differences in preparing to returns a tennis serve: a visual information processing approach. *J Sport Psychol.* 1989;11:382.

128. Abernethy B. Expertise, visual search, and information pick-up in squash. *Perception.* 1990;19:63.

129. Ripoll H, Kerlirzin Y, Stein JF, et al. Analysis of information processing, decision making, and visual strategies in complex problem solving sport situations. *Hum Mov Sci.* 1995;14:335.

130. Williams AM, Davids K, Burwitz L, et al. Visual search strategies in experienced and inexperienced soccer players. *Res Q Exerc Sport.* 1994;65:127.

131. Williams AM, Davids K. Anxiety, expertise and visual search strategies in karate. *J Sport Exerc Psychol.* 1999;21: 362.

132. Honda H. Spatial localization in saccade and pursuit eye movement conditions: a comparison of perceptual and motor measures. *Percept Psychophys.* 1985;38(41).

133. Hobson R, Henderson MT. A preliminary study of the visual field in athletics. *Proc Iowa Acad Sci.* 1941;48: 331.

134. Johnson WG. *Peripheral Perception of Athletes and Non-athletes, and the Effect of Practice* [thesis]. University of Illinois; 1952.

135. Buchellew WF. *Peripheral Perception and Reaction Time of Athletes and Non-athletes* [thesis]. University of Illinois; 1954.

136. Stroup F. Relationship between measurements of field of motion perception and basketball ability in college men. *Res Q Am Assoc Health Phys Educ.* 1957;28:72.

137. Williams JM, Thirer J. Vertical and horizontal peripheral vision in male and female athletes and non-athletes. *Res Q Am Assoc Health Phys Educ.* 1976;46:200.

138. Berg WP, Killian SM. Size of the visual field in collegiate fast-pitch softball players and nonathletes. *Percept Mot Skills.* 1995;81:1307.

139. Semmelow J. Identification of peripheral visual images in a laterally restricted gaze field. *Percept Mot Skills.* 1990;70: 175.

140. Loopeker K, Rowley B. *The Effects of Reduced Ski Goggle Field and Tint on Stability and Balance* [thesis]. Pacific University; 2002.

141. Tyldesley DA. Motion prediction and movement control in fast ball games. In: Cockerill IM, MacGilivary WW, eds. *Vision in Sport.* Cheltenham, England: Stanley Thomas; 1981:91−115.

142. de Groot AD. Perception and memory versus thought: some old ideas and recent findings. In: Kleinmuntz B, ed. *Problem Solving: Research, Method and Theory.* New York: Wiley; 1966:19−50.

143. Chase WG, Simon HA. Perception in chess. *Cognit Psychol.* 1973;4:55.

144. Chase WG, Simon HA. The mind's eye in chess. In: Chase WG, ed. *Visual Information Processing.* New York: Academic Press; 1973:404−427.

145. Allard F, Graham S, Paarsalu ME. Perception in sport: basketball. *J Sport Psychol.* 1980;2:14.

146. Milne DC, Lewis RV. Sports vision screening of varsity athletes. *Sports Vis.* 1993;1:8.

147. Allard F, Burnett N. Skill in sport. *Can J Psychol*. 1985;39: 294.

148. Starkes JL. Skill in field hockey: the nature of the cognitive advantage. *J Sport Psychol*. 1987;9:146.

149. Helsen W, Pauwels JM. The use of a simulator in the evaluation and training of tactical skills in football. In: Reilly T, Lees A, Davids K, et al., eds. *Science and Football*. London: E&FN Spon; 1987:493–497.

150. Allard F, Starkes JL. Perception in sport: volleyball. *J Sport Psychol*. 1980;2(22).

151. Thiffault C. *Tachistoscopic training and its effect upon perceptual speed of ice hockey players [thesis]*. Los Angeles, CA: University of Southern California; 1974.

152. Jones CM, Miles TR. Use of advanced cues in predicting the flight of a lawn tennis ball. *J Hum Mov Stud*. 1978;4: 231.

153. Reichow AW, Garchow KE, Baird RY. Do scores on a tachistoscope test correlate with baseball batting average? *Eye Contact Lens*. 2011;37:123–126.

154. Salmela JH, Fiorito P. Visual cues in ice-hockey goal tending. *Can J Appl Sport Sci*. 1979;4:56.

155. Isaacs LD, Finch AE. Anticipatory timing of beginning and intermediate tennis players. *Percept Mot Skills*. 1983; 57:451.

156. Abernethy B, Russell DG. Advanced cue utilisation by skilled cricket batsmen. *Aust J Sci Med Sport*. 1984;16(2).

157. McLeod P. Visual reaction time and high-speed ball games. *Perception*. 1987;16(49).

158. Milgram P. A spectacle-mounted liquid crystal tachistoscope. *Behav Res Methods Instrum Comput*. 1987;19:449.

159. Abernethy B. Visual search in sport and ergonomics: its relationship to selective attention and performer expertise. *Hum Perform*. 1988;1:205.

160. Abernethy B. The effects of age and expertise upon perceptual skill development in a racquet sport. *Res Q Exerc Sport*. 1988;59:210.

161. Wright DL, Pleasants F, Gomez-Meza M. Use of advanced visual cue sources in volleyball. *J Sport Excerc Psychol*. 1990;12:406.

162. Houlston DR, Lowes R. Anticipatory cue utilisation processes amongst expert and non-expert wicket keepers in cricket. *Int J Sport Psychol*. 1993;24:59.

163. Starkes JL. A new technology and field test of advance cue usage in volleyball. *Res Q Exerc Sport*. 1995;66:162.

164. Paull G, Glencross D. Expert perception and decision making in baseball. *Int J Sport Psychol*. 1997;28:35.

165. Tremayne P, Barry RJ. Elite pistol shooters: physiological patterning of best vs. worst shots. *Int J Psychophysiol*. 2001; 41:19.

166. Miyoshi S, Mori S, Hirose N. Effects of advance visual cue utilization on anticipation of ball direction. *Shinrigaku Kenkyu*. 2012;83:202–210 (Japanese).

167. Pesce-Anzander C, Bosel R. Modulation of the spatial extent of the attentional focus in high-level volleyball players. *Eur J Cognit Psychol*. 1995;10:247.

168. Mahoney M, Avener J. Psychology of the elite athlete: an exploratory study. *Cog Ther Res*. 1997;1:135.

169. Bjurwell C. Perceptual-motor behavior in sport: the double reaction. *Percept Mot Skills*. 1991;72:137.

170. Meyers AW, Cooke CJ, Cullen J, et al. Psychological aspects of athletic competitors: a replication across sports. *Cog Ther Res*. 1979;3:361.

171. Greenspan MJ, Feltz DL. Psychological interventions with athletes in competitive situations: a review. *Sport Psychol*. 1989;3:219.

172. Davis H. Cognitive style and nonsport imagery in elite ice hockey performance. *Percept Mot Skills*. 1990;71:795.

173. Cumming J, Hall C. Athletes' use of imagery in the off-season. *Sport Psychol*. 2002;16:160–172.

174. Callow N, Hardy L. Types of imagery associated with sport confidence in net ball players of varying skill levels. *J Appl Sport Psychol*. 2001;13:1–7.

175. Olsson CJ, Jonsson B, Nyberg L. Internal imagery training in active high jumpers. *Scand J Psychol*. 2008;49: 133–140.

176. Guillot A, Nadrowska E, Collet C. Using motor imagery to learn tactical movements in basketball. *J Sport Behav*. 2009;32:189–206.

177. Weinberg R, Butt J, Knight B, et al. The relationship between the use and effectiveness of imagery: an exploratory investigation. *J Appl Sport Psychol*. 2003;15:26–40.

178. Arvinen-Barrow M, Weigand DA, Thomas S, et al. Elite and novice athletes' imagery use in open and closed sports. *J Appl Sport Psychol*. 2007;19:93–104.

179. White A, Hardy L. An in-depth analysis of the uses of imagery by high-level slalom canoeists and artistic gymnasts. *Sport Psychol*. 1998;12:387–403.

180. Finke RA. Mental imagery and the visual system. *Sci Am*. 1986;254:88.

181. MacKay DG. The problem of rehearsal or mental practice. *J Mot Behav*. 1981;13:274.

182. Hale BD. The effects of internal and external imagery on muscular and ocular concomitants. *J Sport Psychol*. 1982; 4:374.

183. Feltz DL, Landers DM. The effects of mental practice on motor skill learning and performance: a meta-analysis. *J Sport Psychol*. 1983;5:25.

184. Kohl RM, Roenker DL. Mechanism involvement during skill imagery. *J Mot Behav*. 1983;15:179.

185. Feltz DL, Landers DM, Becker BJ. *A Revised Meta-Analysis of the Mental Practice Literature on Motor Skill Learning*. Washington, DC: National Academy Press; 1988.

186. Requin J. Neural basis of movement representations. In: Requin J, Stelmach GE, eds. *Tutorials in Motor Neurosciences*. Dordrecht, The Netherlands: Kluwer; 1991:333–345.

187. Jeannerod M. The representing brain: neural correlates of motor intention and imagery. *Brain Behav Sci*. 1994;17:187.

188. Roland PE, Larsen B, Lassen NA, et al. Supplementary motor area and other cortical areas in organization of voluntary movement in man. *J Neurophysiol*. 1980;43:118.

189. Decety J, Ingvar DH. Brain structures participating in mental stimulation of motor behavior: a neuropsychological interpretation. *Acta Psychol*. 1990;73(13).

190. Decety J, Kawashima R, Gulyas B, et al. Preparation for reaching: a PET study of the participating structures in the human brain. *Neuroreport*. 1992:761.

191. Decety J. Do imagined and executed actions share the same neural substrate? *Cognit Brain Res*. 1993;3:87.

192. Jacobson E. Electrophysiology of mental activities. *Am J Psychol*. 1932;44:676.

193. Ulich E. Some experiments on the function of mental training in the acquisition of motor skills. *Ergonomics*. 1967;10:411.

194. McGuigan FJ. Covert oral behavior during the silent performance of language tasks. *Psychol Bull*. 1970;74:309.

195. Harris DV, Robinson WJ. The effects of skill level on EMG activity during internal and external imagery. *J Sport Psychol*. 1986;8:105.

196. Decety J, Michel F. Comparative analysis of actual and mental movements times in two graphic tasks. *Brain Cognit*. 1989;11:87.

197. Knapp BN. Simple reaction times of selected top-class sportsmen and research students. *Restor Q*. 1961;32:409.

198. Whiting HTA, Sanderson FH. Dynamic visual acuity and performance in a catching task. *J Mot Behav*. 1974;6:87.

199. Blundell NL. Critical visual-perceptual attributes of championship level tennis players. In: Howell ML, Wilson BD, eds. *Kinesiological Sciences: Proceedings of the VII Commonwealth and International Conference on Sport, Physical Education, Recreation and Dance*. Brisbane, Australia: University of Queensland; 1984:51−59.

200. Kioumourtzoglou E, Kourtessis T, Michalopoulou M, et al. Differences in several perceptual abilities between experts and novices in basketball, volleyball, and waterpolo. *Percept Mot Skills*. 1998;86:899.

201. Harbin G, Durst L, Harbin D. Evaluation of oculomotor response in relationship to sports performance. *Med Sci Sports Exerc*. 1989;21:258.

202. Montes-Mico R, Bueno I, Candel J, et al. Eye-hand and eye-foot visual reaction times of young soccer players. *Optometry*. 2000;71:775.

203. Ando S, Kida N, Oda S. Central and peripheral visual reaction time of soccer players and nonathletes. *Percept Mot Skills*. 2001;92:786−794.

204. Nakamoto H, Mori S. Sport-specific decision-making in a Go/NoGo reaction task: difference among nonathletes and baseball and basketball players. *Percept Mot Skills*. 2008;106:163−170.

205. Dogan B. Multiple-choice reaction and visual perception in female and male elite athletes. *J Sports Med Phys Fit*. 2009;49:91−96.

206. E A, Kocak S. Coincidence-anticipation timing and reaction time in youth tennis and table tennis players. *Percept Mot Skills*. 2010;110(3 Pt 1):879−887.

207. Henry M. Stimulus complexity, movement, age, and sex in relation to reaction latency and speed in limb movements. *Res Q Sports Med*. 1961;32:353.

208. Keele S. Motor control. In: Boff K, Kaufman L, Thomas J, eds. *Handbook of Perception and Human Performance*. New York: John Wiley & Sons; 1986:30−60.

209. Sherman A. A method for evaluating eye-hand coordination and visual reaction time in athletes. *J Am Optom Assoc*. 1983;54:801.

210. Mitchell JA, Nicholson DW, Maples WC. Standardization of the Wayne Saccadic fixator. *J Behav Optom*. 1990;1:199.

211. Vogel GL, Hale RE. Initial norms using the Wayne Saccadic fixator for eye-hand coordination and visual reaction times. *J Behav Optom*. 1990;1:206.

212. Kida N, Oda S, Matsumura M. Intensive baseball practice improves Go/NoGo reaction time, but not the simple reaction time. *Brain Res Cogn Brain Res*. 2005;22:257−264.

213. Erickson GB, Citek K, Cove M, et al. Reliability of a computer-based system for measuring visual performance skills. *Optometry*. 2011;82:528−542.

214. Willms A, Dalton KN. Establishment of standard methods for the measurement of eye-hand visual-motor reaction time. *Optom Vis Perf*. 2017;5(2):49−56.

215. Verburgh L, Scherder EJA, van Lange PAM, Oosterlaan J. Executive functioning in highly talented soccer players. *PLoS One*. 2014;9(3):e91254.

216. Robertson S, Collins J, Elliott D, et al. The influence of skill and intermittent vision on dynamic balance. *J Mot Behav*. 1994;26:333.

217. Robertson S, Elliott D. The influence of skill in gymnastics and vision on dynamic balance. *Int J Sport Psychol*. 1996;27:361.

218. Robertson S, Elliott D. Specificity of learning and dynamic balance. *Res Q Exerc Sport*. 1996;67:69.

219. Croix G, Chollet D, Thouvarecq R. Effect of expertise level on the perceptual characteristics of gymnasts. *J Strength Condit Res*. 2010;24:1458−1463.

220. Witkin HA, Dyk RB, Paterson HF, et al. *Psychological Differentiation*. New York: Wiley; 1982.

221. Witkin HA, Lewis HB, Hertzman M, et al. *Personality through Perception*. Westport, CT: Greenwood; 1972.

222. Hodgson CI, Christian E, McMorris T. Performance on the portable rod and frame test predicts variation in learning the kayak roll. *Percept Mot Skills*. 2010;110:479−487.

223. Counil L. Field dependence and orientation of upside-down posture in water. *Percept Mot Skills*. 2015;120:15−24.

224. Kane JE. Personality, body concept and performance. In: Kane JE, ed. *Psychological Aspects of Physical Education and Sport*. London: Western Printing Services; 1972:91−127.

225. Knapp B. *Skill in Sport*. London: Routledge & Kegan Paul; 1964.

226. Jones MG. Perceptual studies: perceptual characteristics and athletic performance. In: Whiting HTA, ed. *Sports Psychology*. London: Kimpton; 1972:96−115.

227. Sharp RH, Whiting HTA. Information processing and eye-movement behavior in a ball catching skill. *J Hum Mov Stud*. 1975;1:124.

228. Franks IM, Weicker D, Robertson DGE. The kinematics, movement phasing and timing of a skilled action in response to varying conditions of uncertainty. *Hum Mov Sci*. 1985;4:91.

229. Bootsma RJ, van Wieringen PCW. Visual control of an attacking forehand drive. In: Meijer OG, Roth K, eds. *Complex Movement Behavior: The Motor-Action Controversy.* Amsterdam: North-Holland; 1988:189–199.

230. Bootsma RJ. *The Timing of Rapid Interceptive Actions: Perception-Action Coupling in the Control and Acquisition of Skill.* Amsterdam: Free University Press; 1988.

231. Bootsma RJ. Accuracy of perceptual processes subserving different perception-action systems. *Q J Exp Psychol.* 1989; 41A:489.

232. Bootsma RJ, van Wieringen PCW. Timing an attacking forehand drive in table tennis. *J Exp Psychol Hum Percept Perform.* 1990;16:21.

233. Bootsma RJ. Predictive information and the control of action. *Int J Sport Psychol.* 1991;22:271.

234. Savelsbergh GJP, Whiting HTA, Bootsma RJ. "Grasping" tau. *J Exp Psychol Hum Percept Perform.* 1991;17:315.

235. Bootsma RJ, Peper CE. Predictive visual information sources for the regulation of action with special emphasis on catching and hitting. In: Proteau L, Elliott D, eds. *Vision and Motor Control.* Amsterdam: North-Holland; 1992:285–314.

236. Bootsma RJ, Oudejans RRD. Visual information about time-to-collision between two objects. *J Exp Psychol Hum Percept Perform.* 1993;19:1041.

237. Siegel D. Response velocity, range of movement, and timing accuracy. *Percept Mot Skills.* 1994;79:216.

238. Barlow H, Blakemore CB, Pettigrew JD. The neural mechanism of binocular depth perception. *J Physiol.* 1967;193:327.

239. Pettigrew JD, Nikara T, Bishop PO. Binocular interaction on single units in cat striate cortex: simultaneous stimulation by single moving slit with receptive fields in correspondence. *Exp Brain Res.* 1968;6:391.

240. Cyander M, Regan D. Neurons in cat parastriate cortex sensitive to the direction of motion in three-dimensional space. *J Physiol.* 1978;274:549.

241. Wheatstone C. Contributions to the physiology of vision. Part the first. On some remarkable and hitherto unobserved, phenomena of binocular vision. *Phil Trans Roy Soc Lond.* 1838;128:371.

242. Ogle KN. The optical space sense. In: Davson H, ed. *The Eye.* Vol. 4. New York: Academic Press; 1962.

243. Julesz B. *Foundations of Cyclopean Perception.* Chicago: University of Chicago Press; 1971.

244. Regan D, ed. *Binocular Vision.* London: Macmillan; 1991.

245. Beverley KI, Regan D. Evidence for the existence of neural mechanisms selectively sensitive to the direction of motion in space. *J Physiol.* 1973;235:17.

246. Richards W, Regan D. A stereo field map with implications for disparity processing. *Invest Ophthalmol Vis Sci.* 1973;12:904.

247. Beverly KI, Regan D. The relation between discrimination and sensitivity in the perception of motion in depth. *J Physiol.* 1975;249:387.

248. Regan D, Beverley KI, Cyander M. Stereoscopic subsystems for position in depth and for motion in depth. *Proc R Soc Lond Ser B.* 1979;204:485.

249. Regan D, Beverly KI, Cyander M. The visual perception of motion in depth. *Sci Am.* 1979;241:136.

250. Poggio GF, Talbot WH. Mechanisms of static and dynamic stereopsis in foveal cortex of rhesus monkey. *J Physiol.* 1981;315:469.

251. Cyander M, Regan D. Neurons in cat visual cortex tuned to the direction of motion in depth: effect of positional disparity. *Vis Res.* 1982;22:967.

252. Regan D, Cyander M. Neurons in cat visual cortex tuned to the direction of motion in depth: effect of stimulus speed. *Investig Ophthalmol Vis Sci.* 1982;22:535.

253. Regan D, Erkelens CJ, Collewijn H. Visual field defects for vergence eye movements and for stereo motion perception. *Invest Ophthalmol Vis Sci.* 1986;27:806.

254. Hong X, Regan D. Visual field defects for unidirectional and oscillatory motion in depth. *Vis Res.* 1989;29:809.

255. Spileers W, Orban GA, Gulyan B, et al. Selectivity of cat area 18 neurons for direction and speed in depth. *J Neurophysiol.* 1990;63:936.

256. Regan D, Beverley KI. Illusory motion in depth: aftereffect of adaptation to changing size. *Vis Res.* 1978;18:209.

257. Beverley KI, Regan D. Separable aftereffects of changing-size and motion-in-depth: different neural mechanisms? *Vis Res.* 1979;19:727.

258. Regan D, Beverley KI. Looming detectors in the human visual pathway. *Vis Res.* 1978;18:415.

259. Regan D, Cyander M. Neurons in area 18 cat visual cortex selectively sensitive to changing size: non-linear interactions between responses to two edges. *Vis Res.* 1979;19: 699.

260. Regan D, Gray R. Binocular processing of motion: some unresolved questions. *Spatial Vis.* 2009;22:1–43.

261. Gibson JJ. *The Perception of the Visual World.* Boston: Houghton Mifflin; 1950.

262. Gordon DA. Static and dynamic fields in human space perception. *J Opt Soc Am.* 1965;55:1296.

263. Koenderink JJ, van Doorn AJ. Local structure of movement parallax of the plane. *J Opt Soc Am.* 1976;66:717.

264. Regan D, Beverley KI. Visually-guided locomotion: psychophysical evidence for a neural mechanism sensitive to flow patterns. *Science.* 1979;205:311.

265. Regan D, Beverley KI. Binocular and monocular stimuli for motion in depth: changing-disparity and changing-size feed the same motion-in-depth stage. *Vis Res.* 1979; 19:1331.

266. Regan D. Visual judgments and misjudgments in cricket, and the art of flight. *Perception.* 1992;21:91.

267. Bahill AT, Karnavas WJ. The perception of baseball's rising fastball and breaking curveball. *J Exp Psychol Hum Percept Perform.* 1993;19:3.

268. Gogel WC. Convergence as a cue to absolute distance. *J Psychol.* 1961;52:287.

269. Foley JM, Richards W. Effects of voluntary eye movement and convergence on the binocular appreciation of depth. *Percept Psychophys.* 1972;11:423.

270. von Hofsten C. The role of convergence in visual space perception. *Vis Res.* 1976;16:193.

271. Regan D, Erkelens CJ, Collewijn H. Necessary conditions for the perception of motion in depth. *Investig Ophthalmol Vis Sci*. 1986;27:584.

272. Steinman RM, Collewijn H. Binocular retinal image motion during active head rotation. *Vis Res*. 1980;20:415.

273. Steinman RM, Cushman WB, Martins AJ. The precision of gaze: a review. *Hum Neurobiol*. 1982;1:97.

274. Steinman RM, Levinson JZ, Collewijn H, et al. Vision in the presence of known natural retinal image motion. *J Opt Soc Am*. 1985;2:226.

275. McLeod P, McLaughlin C, Nimmo-Smith I. Information encapsulation and automaticity: evidence from the visual control of finely timed actions. In: *Attention and Performance XI*. Hillsdale, NJ: Erlbaum; 1985:391−400.

276. Judge SJ, Bradford CM. Adaptation to telestereoscopic viewing measured by one-handed ball-catching performance. *Perception*. 1988;17:783.

277. von Hofsten C, Rosengren K, Pick HL, et al. The role of binocular information in ball catching. *J Mot Behav*. 1992;24:329.

278. Savelsbergh GJP, Whiting HTA. The acquisition of catching under monocular and binocular conditions. *J Mot Behav*. 1992;24:320.

279. Graydon J, Bawden M, Holder T, et al. The effects of binocular and monocular vision on a table tennis striking task under conditions of spatio-temporal uncertainty. *Int J Sports Vis*. 1996;3:35.

280. Rosengren K, Pick HL, von Hofsten C. Role of visual information in ball catching. *J Mot Behav*. 1988;20:150.

281. von Hofsten C. Recalibration of the convergence system. *Perception*. 1979;8:37.

282. Redding GM, Rader SD, Lucas DR. Cognitive load and prism adaptation. *J Mot Behav*. 1992;24:238.

283. Redding GM, Wallace B. Effects of pointing rate and availability of visual feedback on visual and proprioceptive components of prism adaptation. *J Mot Behav*. 1992;24:226.

284. Mann DL, Abernethy B, Farrow D. Visual information underpinning skilled anticipation: the effect of blur on a coupled and uncoupled in situ anticipatory response. *Atten Percept Psychophys*. 2010;72:1317−1326.

285. Mann DL, Abernethy B, Farrow D. Action specificity increases anticipatory performance and the expert advantage in natural interceptive tasks. *Acta Psychol*. 2010;135:17−23.

286. Lee DN. A theory of visual control of braking based on information about time-to-collision. *Perception*. 1976;5:437.

287. Lee DN, Young DS. Visual timing in interceptive actions. In: Ingle DJ, Jeannerod M, Lee DN, eds. *Brain Mechanisms and Spatial Vision*. Dordrecht, The Netherlands: Martinus Nijhoff; 1985:1−30.

288. Lee DN. Visuo-motor coordination in space-time. In: Stelmach G, Requin J, eds. *Tutorials in Motor Behavior*. Amsterdam: North-Holland; 1980:281−293.

289. Lee DN, Reddish PE. Plummeting gannets: a paradigm of ecological optics. *Nature*. 1981;293:293.

290. Todd JT. Visual information about moving objects. *J Exp Psychol Hum Percept Perform*. 1981;7:795.

291. Lee DN, Lishman JR, Thomson JA. Visual regulation of gait in long jumping. *J Exp Psychol Hum Percept Perform*. 1982;8:448.

292. Wagner H. Flow-field variables triggering landing in flies. *Nature*. 1982;297:147.

293. Lee DN, Young DS, Reddish PE, et al. Visual timing in hitting an accelerating ball. *Q J Exp Psychol*. 1983;35A:333.

294. Warren WH, Young DS, Lee DN. Visual control of step length during running over irregular terrain. *J Exp Psychol Hum Percept Perform*. 1986;12:259.

295. Laurent M, Dinh Phung R, Ripoll H. What visual information is used by riders in jumping. *Hum Mov Sci*. 1989;8:481.

296. Stoffregen TA, Riccio GE. Responses to optical looming in the retinal center and periphery. *Ecol Psychol*. 1990;2:251.

297. Van der Horst ARA. *A Time-Based Analysis of Road User Behaviour in Normal and Critical Encounters*. Soest, The Netherlands: Practicum Drukkerij; 1990.

298. Laurent M. Visual cues and processes involved in goal-directed locomotion. In: Patla AE, ed. *Adaptability of Human Gait: Implications for the Control of Locomotion*. Amsterdam: North-Holland; 1991:99−123.

299. Lee DN, Young DS, Rewt D. How do somersaulters land on their feet? *J Exp Psychol Hum Percept Perform*. 1993;18:1195.

300. Tresilian JR. Perceptual information for the timing of interceptive action. *Perception*. 1990;19:223.

301. Diggles VA, Grabiner MD, Garhammer J. Skill level and efficacy of effector visual feedback in ball catching. *Percept Mot Skills*. 1987;64:987.

302. Peper L, Bootsma RJ, Mestre DR, et al. Catching balls: how to get the hand to the right place at the right time. *J Exp Psychol Hum Percept Perform*. 1994;20:591.

303. Oudejans RRD, Michaels CF, Bakker FC, et al. The relevance of action in perceiving affordances: perception of catchableness of fly balls. *J Exp Psychol Hum Percept Perform*. 1996;22:879.

304. Fink PW, Foo PS, Warren WH. Catching fly balls in virtual reality: a critical test of the outfielder problem. *J Vis*. 2009;9(13):14.

305. Brenner E, Smeets JBJ. How people achieve their amazing temporal precision in interception. *J Vis*. 2015;15(3), 8, 1−21.

306. Cicciarella CF. Effects of loss of visual feedback in performance of two swimming strokes. *Percept Mot Skills*. 1982;55:735.

307. Mount J. Effectiveness of visual vs kinesthetic instruction for learning a gross motor skill. *Percept Mot Skills*. 1987;65:715.

308. Williams JG. Visual demonstration and movement production: effects of motoric mediation during observation of a model. *Percept Mot Skills*. 1987;65:825.

309. Miller G, Gabbard C. Effects of visual aids on acquisition of selected tennis skills. *Percept Mot Skills*. 1988;67:603.

310. Sewell LP, Reeve TG, Day RA. Effect of concurrent visual feedback on acquisition of a weightlifting skill. *Percept Mot Skills.* 1988;67:715.

311. Williams JG. Effects of kinetically enhanced video-modeling on improvement of form in a gymnastic skill. *Percept Mot Skills.* 1989;69:473.

312. Smith TL, Eason RL. Effects of verbal and visual cues on performance of a complex ballistic task. *Percept Mot Skills.* 1990;70:1163.

313. Bennett S, Davids K. The manipulation of vision during the powerlift squat: exploring the boundaries of the specificity of learning hypothesis. *Res Q Exerc Sport.* 1995;66:210.

314. Magill RA, Schoenfelder-Zohdi B. A visual model and knowledge of performance as sources of information for learning a rhythmic gymnastics skill. *Int J Sport Psychol.* 1996;27:7.

315. Layton C, Avenell L. Differences in kata performance time and distance from a marker for experienced shotokan karateka under normal sighted and blindfolded conditions. *Percept Mot Skills.* 2002;95:47.

316. Dienes Z, McLeod P. How to catch a cricket ball. *Perception.* 1993;22:1427.

317. McBeath MK, Shaffer DM, Kaiser MK. How baseball outfielders determine where to run to catch fly balls. *Science.* 1995;268:569.

318. Letters. *Science.* 1995;268:1681.

319. Technical comments on catching fly balls. *Science.* 1995;273:256.

320. McLeod P, Dienes Z. Do fielders know where to go to catch the ball or only how to get there? *J Exp Psychol Hum Percept Perform.* 1996;22:531.

321. Adair RK. Running, fielding, and throwing. In: *The Physics of Baseball.* New York: Perennial; 2002:145–162.

322. Sim M, Shaw RE, Turvey MT. Intrinsic and required dynamics of a simple bat-ball skill. *J Exp Psychol Hum Percept Perform.* 1997;23:101.

323. Gyulai E. Perceptual inequality between two physically equal constant velocities. *Percept Mot Skills.* 1990;71:235.

324. Mann DL, Nakamoto H, Logt N, et al. Predictive eye movements when hitting a bouncing ball. *J Vis.* 2019; 19(14):28.

325. Malamud B. *The Natural.* New York: Noonday Press; 1952.

326. Ciborowski T. "Headiness" or "intelligence" for baseball in the collegiate athlete. *Percept Mot Skills.* 1995;81:795.

327. Kindel S. The hardest single act in all of sports. *Forbes.* 1983;132:180.

328. Williams T, Underwood J. *The Science of Hitting.* New York: Simon-Schuster; 1986.

329. Adair RK. The swing of the bat. In: *The Physics of Baseball.* New York: Perennial; 2002:29–46.

330. Osborne K, Rudrud E, Zezoney F. Improved curveball hitting through the enhancement of visual cues. *J Appl Behav Anal.* 1990;23:371.

331. Adams GL. Effect of eye dominance in baseball batting. *Res Q Am Assoc Health Phys Educ.* 1965;36(3).

332. Tieg D. *Major League Baseball Research Project.* Ridgefield, CT: Institute for Sports Vision; 1980:1–9.

333. Portal JM, Romano PE. Patterns of eye-hand dominance in baseball players. *N Engl J Med.* 1988;319:655.

334. Dunham P. Coincidence-anticipation performance of adolescent baseball players and nonplayers. *Percept Mot Skills.* 1989;68:1151.

335. Milne C, Buckolz E, Cardenas M. Relationship of eye dominance and batting performance in baseball players. *Int J Sports Vis.* 1995;2:17.

336. Classe JG, Daum KM, Semes LP, et al. Association between eye and hand dominance and hitting, fielding and pitching skill among players of the Southern Baseball League. *J Am Optom Assoc.* 1996;67:81.

337. Goss DA. The relationship of eye dominance and baseball batting: a critical literature review. *J Behav Optom.* 1998;9:87.

338. Laby DM, Kirschen DG, Rosenbaum AL, et al. The effect of ocular dominance on the performance of professional baseball players. *Ophthalmol Times.* 1998;105:864.

339. Hubbard WA, Seng CN. Visual movements of batters. *Res Q Am Assoc Health Phys Educ.* 1954;25:42.

340. Fogt NF, Zimmerman AB. A method to monitor eye and head tracking movements in college baseball players. *Optom Vis Sci.* 2014;91:200–211.

341. Fogt N, Persson TW. A pilot study of horizontal head and eye rotations in baseball batting. *Optom Vis Sci.* 2017;94: 789–796.

342. Ripoll H, Fleurance P. What does keeping one's eye on the ball mean? *Ergonomics.* 1988;31:1647.

343. Stark L, Michael JA, Zuber BL. Saccadic suppression: a product of the saccadic anticipatory signal. In: Evans CR, Mulholland TB, eds. *Attention in neurophysiology: an international conference.* London: Butterworths; 1969:281–303.

344. Matin E. Saccadic suppressions and the dual mechanism theory of direction constancy. *Vis Res.* 1982;22:335.

345. Messier SP, Owen MG. Bat dynamics of female fast pitch softball batters. *Res Q Exerc Sport.* 1984;55:141.

346. Adair RK. Properties of bats. In: *The Physics of Baseball.* New York: Perennial; 2002:112–144.

347. McKee SP. A local mechanism for differential velocity discrimination. *Vis Res.* 1981;21:491.

348. Orban GA, De Wolf J, Maes H. Factors influencing velocity coding in the human visual system. *Vis Res.* 1984;24: 33.

349. Sherwin J, Muraskin J, Sajda P. You can't think and hit at the same time: neural correlates of baseball pitch classification. *Front Neurosci.* 2012;6:177.

350. Glencross DJ, Cibich BJ. A decision analysis of games skills. *Austr J Sports Med.* 1977;9:72.

351. Hick WE. On the rate of gain of information. *Q J Exp Psychol.* 1952;4(11).

352. Watts RG, Sawyer E. Aerodynamics of a knuckleball. *Am J Phys*. 1975;43:960.

353. McBeath MK. The rising fastball, baseball's impossible pitch. *Perception*. 1990;19:545.

354. Adair RK. Pitching. In: *The Physics of Baseball*. New York: Perennial; 2002:47−78.

355. Classe JG, Semes LP, Daum KM, et al. Association between visual reaction time and batting, fielding, and earned run averages among players of the Southern Baseball League. *J Am Optom Assoc*. 1997;68:43.

CHAPTER 4

Visual Performance Evaluation

The search for the association between visual abilities and sports performance has a long and rich history. Many researchers and clinicians have sought to reveal the vision skills that correlate to success in sports and to refine the procedures to assess the quality of those vision skills. In a 1982 literature review, the authors concluded that ample evidence supported the contention that athletes typically have better visual abilities than nonathletes and that top athletes benefit from visual abilities that often are superior to lower level athletes.[1] In another extensive review of the literature in 1993, the authors agreed with these contentions but cautioned that the visual skills related to successful athletic performance are specific to the sport being investigated.[2] The authors further cautioned that attributes such as size, speed, quickness, psychologic status, experience level, and influence of coaches confound the ability to predict performance quality solely based on an evaluation of visual skills. Further caution is warranted because a small percentage of top athletes demonstrate poor performance on some aspects of vision skills.

The quest for understanding all the elements that play a role in athletic success is being conducted globally across many disciplines. Each discipline seeks to identify factors that contribute to peak human performance by isolating and measuring specific functions, and most sports vision evaluations attempt the same approach.[3–5] The sports vision practitioner must identify the vision factors thought to be essential to performance of the visual tasks critical for success in the sport and evaluate the quality of those skills in the most appropriate, accurate, and repeatable manner. Chapters 2 and 3 provide an approach to the task analysis process, a process that is essential to provide a suitable evaluation for each sport and position. The three central processing mechanisms proposed in the modified Welford model described in Chapter 2 are used to categorize the common assessments that comprise many sports vision evaluations.[6] This chapter provides an evidence-based description of common assessment areas and the relative value of each assessment area in an evaluation. Appendix A provides testing protocols and normative information compiled by the American Optometric Association Sports Vision Section.

CASE HISTORY

The case history can be the most important part of any patient visit, and successful practitioners maximize the potential inherent in this opportunity. Every patient should be asked about sports activities because a vision issue related to recreational or sports performance is an uncommon reason for seeking vision care. Providing vision care services that encompass all areas of a patient's activities is an excellent method for demonstrating an understanding of the patient's needs.

A working knowledge of the visual task demands for sports and recreational activities allows the practitioner to ask pertinent questions and better understand the responses provided by the athlete. The information in Chapters 2 and 3 should assist the practitioner in developing a list of relevant questions to address the specific visual needs of athletes in a wide variety of sports. Information concerning less common recreational activities can easily be found by searching the Internet or consulting the many sports periodicals and books available.

The case history for an athlete should start with the basic elements of a history for a comprehensive vision examination, including questions regarding main concerns, secondary vision concerns, personal and family eye history, and personal and family medical history. Of special concern to the athlete are symptoms of blur, diplopia, or visual discomfort. Athletes report difficulty seeing more commonly than expected.[7] A preexamination checklist that the patient fills out before starting the examination is an effective tool to help the patient mentally prepare for the case history and for the doctor to identify areas to explore in greater depth.[8] The preexamination history is also a means of educating the patient about the implications of sports performance issues not commonly associated with eyes. A sample sports vision case history preexamination form can be found in Appendix A.

Vision correction and eye protection are crucial elements to investigate in the athlete's history, including

Sports Vision. https://doi.org/10.1016/B978-0-323-75543-6.00008-5

history of vision correction. If the athlete is wearing spectacles during sport participation, the eye care practitioner is obligated to determine the type of frame and lenses used and warn the athlete of the risk of injury posed by ophthalmic materials that have limited impact resistance.[9] Similarly, the practitioner should assess the suitability of any protective eyewear used during sports. The practitioner should specifically probe for any eye injuries sustained during sports or recreational activities and ascertain any long-term effects of an injury. An understanding of how any ocular injuries were evaluated and managed can help determine whether additional health procedures are indicated. Refractive correction with contact lenses should also be explored to determine the effectiveness of the lenses for the specific visual demands of the sport. The visual results from refractive surgery are important to determine in athletes, especially in those with critical vision demands. Chapter 6 discusses the issues with types of vision correction and protection used in sports, and Appendix A has sample questions to include on the case history preexamination form.

An evaluation of the environmental conditions encountered during sports participation is useful in determining the most effective vision correction and protection for the athlete. The practitioner should question the athlete regarding any ocular hazards encountered, including dust and foreign body potential. Factors of humidity, wind, temperature, altitude, sweat, precipitation, and environmental variability can produce profound effects on the type of vision correction used. Additional environmental issues with natural and artificial lighting, glare, and variable target contrast should also be considered when determining the optimal vision prescription.

The case history is also an excellent opportunity to identify vision symptoms related to traumatic brain injury, also known as concussion. In the recent years, there has been a significant interest in identifying and managing sport-related concussion (see Chapter 7). A fundamental aspect of identifying concussion is symptom assessment, and this is a core element of most concussion screening and diagnosis instruments. The Brain Injury Vision Symptom Survey (BIVSS) is a 28-item questionnaire designed to survey vision symptoms following mild-to-moderate brain injury and has been validated in adult subjects.[10,11] While the BIVSS is available online, any athlete can self-identify common oculomotor and visual symptoms found with traumatic brain injury, including[12,13]

- avoidance of near tasks
- oculomotor-based reading difficulties

- eye-tracking problems
- eye-focusing problems
- eye strain
- diplopia
- dizziness
- vertigo
- vision-derived nausea
- increased sensitivity to visual motion
- visual inattention and distractibility
- short-term visual memory loss
- difficulty judging distances (relative and absolute)
- difficulty with global scanning
- difficulty with personal grooming, especially involving the face
- inability to interact/cope visually in a complex social situation (e.g., minimal eye contact)
- inability to tolerate complex visual environments (e.g., grocery store aisles and highly patterned floors)

Supplementary questions can yield information concerning the athlete's visual performance during sports, such as the following[3,4,7,14–17]:

- Do you ever feel that your vision compromises your athletic performance?
- Do you notice inconsistency in your performance during a game or an event?
  - Is that inconsistency noticed early or late in the competition?
  - Is that inconsistency noticed during critical competition situations?
  - Is that inconsistency noticed during day or night competition?
- Do you experience loss of concentration during sports performance?
- Do you ever have difficulty keeping your eyes on a moving object (ball, puck, etc.)?
- Do you have difficulty judging ball rotation?
- Do you ever notice difficulty with depth perception?
- Do you ever have difficulty knowing where the ball or other players are?
- Do you ever notice decreased peripheral vision during sports performance?
- Do you ever notice sensitivity to lights or difficulty recovering vision after looking into bright lights?
- Do you show little improvement in sports performance, even with dedicated practice and coaching?
- Do you make the same mistake time and time again in competition?
- Do you use visualization or imagery techniques?

These questions naturally lead the clinician to follow up with sport-specific performance details related to the expressed symptoms. The most common symptoms reported by Amateur Athletic Union Junior Olympic

Games participants in a review of 10 years of screenings were difficulty seeing, headaches, and sensitivity to lights.[18] Additional areas to probe in the case history are the goals and motivation of the athlete to determine potential receptiveness to the variety of possible intervention modes. The ultimate goal of the patient history is to raise the index of suspicion for vision inefficiencies that may interfere with peak performance. An effective case history can help select appropriate visual performance assessment procedures for the sports vision evaluation and ensure that visual problems are not interfering with maximal athletic performance.

PERCEPTUAL MECHANISM

Static Visual Acuity

Static visual acuity (SVA) is "the ability to see a nonmoving target at a fixed distance."[5] SVA is commonly measured at far (6 m) or simulated distance viewing and is a standard part of the vision evaluation of athletes.[3–5,17–48] SVA has been measured in athletes both monocularly and binocularly with the Keystone telebinocular (www.keystoneview.com), standard Snellen charts, logMAR charts, and tumbling E and Landolt C optotypes. The author prefers to measure both monocular and binocular SVAs with Landolt C optotypes or a logMAR chart (Bailey-Lovie or ETDRS [Early Treatment Diabetic Retinopathy Study])[49,50] at a distance of 3 m or further.

The athlete should be evaluated with the habitual correction used for sports participation. Interestingly, a large percentage of athletes have been reported to have a significant uncorrected refractive error; those athletes who do wear refractive correction either do not wear that correction for sports or they are undercorrected.[7,44,51] A measurement of SVA should also be performed with the best optical correction in place to assess any change in visual acuity produced by that correction. Recommendations for the use of, or change in, vision correction during sports participation are discussed in Chapter 6.

The measurement of SVA is an essential element of any vision evaluation because degraded visual acuity can have a detrimental effect on many other aspects of visual performance. Reduced visual acuity has been shown to affect dynamic visual acuity (DVA),[52] depth perception,[53,54] and accommodative accuracy.[55] Some studies have found better SVA in athletes than in nonathletes[3,18,32,42,43,46,47,56–60] and some have found no difference.[31,45,48,61] Some athletes may perform at a high level despite having deficient visual acuity.[18–20,22,57,58,62] Several studies in which visual acuity was degraded with plus addition lenses did not find a detrimental effect of defocus.[63–65] However, review of the study protocols reveals that subjects were assessed on predictable, repetitive motor tasks.

The expected level of visual acuity most likely depends on the visual task demands of each sport situation because studies of different athlete populations have found differing visual acuity results. For example, the average visual acuity of professional baseball players has been found to be significantly better than the general population average,[47,56] whereas this has not consistently been found in soccer.[46,48,58] The method used to measure visual acuity also has an influence on the research results. When SVA is assessed using chart systems with 20/20 (6/6) as the best acuity measurable, there is no statistically significant difference between the visual ability of athletes and that of nonathletes.[7,31] Even when a best acuity demand of 20/15 (6/4.5) is presented, Laby et al.[56] found that 81% of professional baseball players could achieve that level. Laby et al. subsequently modified their assessment method to achieve acuity demands down to 20/7.5, reporting overall mean SVAs of approximately 20/13, with several athletes attaining SVAs of 20/9.2 or better.[56] Considering all these differences, mixed results, and the demands of the sport, it is suggested that for many athletes an SVA of at least 20/15 (6/4.5) OD (oculus dexter), OS (oculus sinister), and OU (oculus unitas) is a desired standard for competitive athletes.[3]

Dynamic Visual Acuity

Many of the visual demands in sports require discrimination of information that is moving, such as judging the speed and trajectory of a tennis serve. Traditional SVA measurements do not fully address the visual demands encountered in some types of sports, especially those in which judgments about rapidly moving objects are important. A significant amount of early research investigated the physiologic parameters of resolving visual targets in motion, referred to as *dynamic visual acuity* (DVA).[52,66–87] Ludvigh and Miller[68,70–73] were the first to use the term DVA, and DVA has been defined as the ability to resolve detail when relative movement exists between the observer and the test object.[88]

Many variables in the stimulus parameters can affect DVA, including target luminance, angular velocity, and the time exposure of the target.[52,66–87] Human attributes that can affect DVA include the resolving power of the retina, peripheral awareness, oculomotor abilities, and psychologic functions that affect interpretation of visual information.[52,66–87,89] From the research, several conclusions have been made concerning DVA:

(1) visual acuity for a moving target is reduced compared with that of a stationary target, and acuity becomes progressively more reduced with increasing velocity of the target; (2) the correlation between SVA and DVA decreases with increasing target velocity; (3) a progressive decline in acuity occurs with advancing age that accelerates in older age groups and is more pronounced with DVA than SVA; and (4) males, in general, perform consistently better than females on DVA tasks.[79,81,82,90] Enhancement of either the target parameters or physiologic abilities of the subject can improve DVA abilities.[78,79,89]

DVA research was stimulated by the theory that, for many activities, discrimination of moving objects (or stationary objects while the person is in motion) is a critical element of human performance.[82] This concept applies to sport situations as well as common daily tasks such as driving.[75,78,79,82] Several attempts have been made to determine the relation between DVA and visual task performance; however, further investigation is necessary to correlate clinical measurements of DVA with visual task performance.[a] Most of these studies have found that athletes demonstrate superior DVA abilities than nonathletes and that elite athletes have better DVA than do amateur or nonelite athletes.[a] This finding suggests that there is an important link between elite athletes and DVA ability. On the other hand, Ward and Williams reported no significant differences in performance on a DVA test between elite and subelite youth soccer players.[91] However, their use of a predictable rotator device to measure this function may not have been ecologically appropriate to simulate the visual task demands of a large-field, dynamic sport such as soccer.

DVA is a widely recommended visual function to evaluate in athletes.[b] Despite the significant amount of research conducted with DVA parameters and the many applications of DVA features to daily activities, limited resources are available to assess this ability. Significant variations in the clinical measurement of DVA have been used with the type of target, the size of the target, the direction of the stimulus movement (or subject movement), and the amount of time that the stimulus is exposed. This variability in measurement parameters has led to several different recommendations for normative performance in athletes as well as different performance characteristics for athletes compared with nonathletes.[3,5,17,35–37,48,51,59,92–103]

Studies have found that football (soccer) goalkeepers have significantly better DVA than forwards,[48] and that DVA (Target Capture on the Nike Sensory Station and Senaptec Sensory Station) is associated with lower strikeout rates in professional baseball.[104] A study with professional baseball players in Japan did not find differences in DVA by competitive level but it did find a significant difference when measuring kinetic visual acuity (measurement using an object moving from a distant point toward the subject).[98] The use of kinetic visual acuity has shown that athletes in interceptive sports have better DVA in the dominant eye compared with nonathletes.[60]

Few DVA measurement systems are currently available, and older methods use a predictable rotator device, with some adding a portable laser (Fig. 4.1).[99,105] Rotators are available from Bernell (www.bernell.com) and JW Engineering (www.jtac.com) as well as other retailers. There are formal and informal assessments of DVA advocated for assessment of vestibuloocular response in brain injury, but these assessments are not suitable for differentiation of performance in athletes. The instruments used to measure DVA and kinetic visual acuity are available from Kowa (Tokyo, Japan) as the dynamic vision analyzer HI-10 and kinetic visual acuity meter AS-4, respectively. The

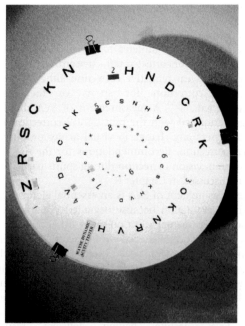

FIG. 4.1 Bernell Rotator with visual acuity chart for dynamic visual acuity testing.

---

[a]References: 23–27,48,58,59,68,70–73,75,78,79,82,90,91, 111–115
[b]References: 3–6,17,23–27,30,31,34–37,39,40,56,58,89, 92–94,116–118.

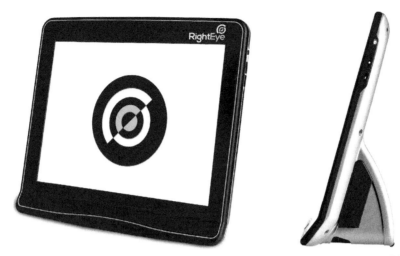

FIG. 4.2 RightEye system to assess dynamic visual acuity. (Courtesy RightEye, LLC.)

inVision package from NeuroCom was a system that showed promise as an effective diagnostic tool in a study to establish preliminary normative data[106] and demonstrated acceptable test-retest reliability, but it is no longer commercially available.[107] More recently, computer software has been designed by Centro de Optometria Internacional (COI-SV at www.coi-sl.es) and DynVA (also referred to as DinVA 3.0) to assess DVA,[48,95,96] and the DinVA 3.0 has been shown to be a valid and reliable measure of DVA.[96] The Nike SPARQ Sensory Station included a test of DVA called Target Capture that demonstrated good test-retest reliability and is currently available from Senaptec (www.senaptec.com).[108] The RightEye Dynamic Visual Acuity Tests (www.righteye.com; see Fig. 4.2) include measures of DVA with head still while the object is moving, head moving while the object is still, and both head and object moving. All three measures of DVA with RightEye have shown good test-retest reliability and have the added benefit of incorporating information collected from a remote eye tracker.[109] A study of collegiate baseball players in Japan found significantly better DVA compared with nonathletes when subjects were allowed to track the target rather than hold steady fixation.[110] The authors of this study suggested that the better DVA of athletes was primarily due to an improved ability to track moving targets with their eyes rather than due to improved perception of moving images on the retina.

Contrast Sensitivity

Contrast sensitivity measures the visual system's ability to process spatial or temporal information about objects and their backgrounds under varying lighting conditions.[88] Measurement of contrast sensitivity function (CSF) has been recommended in athletes because many sports involve visual discrimination tasks in suboptimal lighting due to environmental variability.[2,3,5] Snellen-type visual acuity measurements may not be sensitive to the subtle visual discrimination tasks inherent in many sports because the acuity task is usually performed only under high-contrast conditions. Consider the decreased contrast effect of a white, cloudy sky as a background when judging the trajectory of a fly ball in baseball when the ball is also predominantly white. Ginsburg[119,120] has suggested that lower spatial frequencies provide spatial localization information about objects and that higher spatial frequencies are the first to be affected by illumination, movement, and increased viewing distance. In sports that require the athlete to process visual information from an object in motion (e.g., a baseball pitch), evaluation of CSF at high spatial frequencies may provide vital diagnostic information.

Several investigations have compared CSF in athletes by using gratings of varying spatial frequency.[3,35,43,56,60,121−129] The general results from these studies demonstrate elevated CSF across all spatial frequencies for athletes, and a study of Olympic athletes in a variety of sports demonstrated some differences by sport.[43] Specifically, softball athletes performed significantly better than track-and-field athletes on both Landolt C and grating acuity at 18 cycles per degree.[43] Athletes may have a positive benefit in CSF with aerobic excercise.[130] Contrast sensitivity also may be degraded in contact lens wearers if the lenses are not optimal,

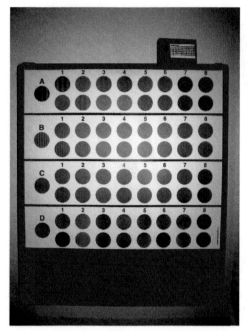

FIG. 4.3 The CSV-1000E contrast sensitivity chart.

even when visual acuity appears acceptable.[131−134] Interestingly, reducing CSF seemed to affect rifle shooting performance more than reducing visual acuity in a study to determine minimum impairment criteria for vision-impaired shooting.[135] Therefore contrast sensitivity measurement is an essential part of the evaluation of athletes who wear contact lenses during sports participation.

Many systems are commercially available to measure CSF. Most use grating patterns that vary in spatial frequency and contrast level; however, fixed-chart and computer-generated symbols of varying contrast levels are also available. Contrast sensitivity measurements usually involve detection of a threshold contrast level at each spatial frequency, with the resultant CSF plotted on a graph.[136] The principal instruments used to measure CSF in athletes are the Vistech Contrast Test System (www.vistechconsultants.com) and Vector Vision contrast sensitivity test (www.vectorvision.com). These systems were primarily chosen for the speed of test administration and portability of the tests.[3−5,17,35,37,56,123−132,134] The Vistech system is externally lit and requires a light meter to calibrate, whereas the Vector Vision test is internally illuminated and somewhat self-calibrating (Fig. 4.3). Major concerns have been reported regarding the reliability and repeatability of the Vistech Contrast Test System for measuring CSF, although other studies have demonstrated adequate reliability and repeatability.[137−140] Letter-based CSF charts, such as the Pelli-Robson chart or Mars Letter Contrast Sensitivity Test, have shown better repeatability,[141,142] while the Mars charts may be more practical for sports vision use due to better portability and durability.[143] Computer-based measures of CSF have become widely available as computer-based acuity chart systems have become ubiquitous, offering CSF assessment using a variety of optotpyes or grating patterns. The Nike SPARQ Sensory Station, and the similar Senaptec Sensory Station, use a concentric ring pattern rather than a vertically oriented grating to assess CSF.[108] The use of a concentric ring target is thought to minimize the influence on astigmatism on CSF and has been found to have good test-retest reliability. Both the Pelli-Robson and Senaptec Sensory Station measure CSF at the height of the CSF (approximately 6 cycles/degree) and the high spatial frequency cutoff (typically 18 cycles/degree).

Whatever CSF test system is chosen, evaluation is often recommended for athletes and should be performed binocularly with habitual sports correction in place.[c] If contact lenses are used in sports, or if more than a one-line difference in monocular SVAs exists, CSF testing should also be performed monocularly. CSF measurement should also be performed with the best optical correction in place to assess any change in CSF produced by that correction and with any performance tints used during sports participation (e.g., ski goggles).[144] The practitioner is encouraged to assess filter performance in natural sunlight because light levels are much more intense outdoors than under artificial lighting. Recommendations for the use of, or change in, vision correction or contact lenses used during sports participation are discussed in Chapter 6.

Refractive Status

Assessment of refractive status is an essential element of the visual evaluation of the athlete. Interestingly, it is such a basic element of a vision evaluation that it is rarely directly discussed in the literature describing evaluation procedures for athletes. Ample data are available concerning visual acuity performance, which has obvious implications for uncorrected refractive errors, but refractive status of the athletes is presented infrequently.[d] Therefore limited information is available concerning the percentage of athletes who have significant uncorrected refractive errors.[7,146]

Only a few reports in the literature concern the percentage of athletes who use vision correction (spectacles

[c]References: 3−6,17,34,35,37,43,56,93,117,118,145
[d]References: 7,15,19−21,30,32,34,37,40,43,45,48,98,145,147

or contact lenses).[7,19,21,30] Studies of athletes participating in the Amateur Athletic Union Junior Olympic Games found that approximately 20%−35% of athletes had refractive error greater than ±0.75 D.[7,18] The incidence of refractive error (myopia, hyperopia, and astigmatism) found in these studies is similar to that found in the general population, dispelling the perception that athletes have a lower incidence of refractive error. A similar study of teenaged athletes found a similar range and mean refractive error in teenaged athletes as in age-matched nonathletes.[45] A study of professional football (soccer) players found that approximately 16% were myopic and 20% were hyperopic, while only 25% used vision correction.[48] Interestingly, a study found a higher rate of refractive error in professional baseball players than in the general population.[148] In contrast, professional baseball players were not found to have a less high-order aberrations compared with a control population; the lower amounts of trefoil were considered clinically insignificant.[149]

Standardized examination procedures to evaluate refractive status are recommended for athletes, and prescribing recommendations are addressed in Chapter 6. The need for cycloplegic examination is left to the discretion of the practitioner and is usually based on concerns regarding latent hyperopia in the athlete. Of note, most young athletes are also students and vision conditions that can affect school performance should be addressed as well. A study found that the SVOne autorefractor provides an acceptable measure of refractive error in baseball players.[148]

Eye/Hand/Foot Preference

The phenomenon of ocular dominance was first described by Giovanni Battista della Porta in 1593,[150] and interest in the relation between ocular dominance and performance has been active ever since. Dominance has been defined as any sort of physiologic preeminence, priority, or preference by one member of any bilateral pair of structures in the body when performing various tasks.[151] Many studies have attempted to determine the best method for assessing the types of eye dominance[152−172] but tests of sighting preference are the most frequently used. Tests that allow binocular viewing under more natural viewing conditions than a traditional sighting test, which forces the athlete to choose one eye over the other, may provide more useful information for sports applications.[173,174]

Many studies have investigated the relation between hand and foot preference and eye preference.[155,156,163,169,175−179] The preferred eye does not always correspond to the preferred hand or foot,

and when they are different the condition is referred to as crossed dominance. Duke-Elder[176] reported that 33% of right-hand dominant people are left-eye dominant, 50% of left-hand dominant people are right-eye dominant, and an estimated 20%−40% of the general population is crossed eye and hand dominant. Athlete populations appear to have a similar distribution of crossed and uncrossed eye-hand preference as found in the general population.[18,42,151,170,174,180,181] Entangled in the issue of testing methods to determine eye preference are reports of dominance switching with hand used when sighting and issues of central dominance in which neither eye is aligned with the sighted target (also sometimes referred to as ambiocular).[35,170,182−184]

Many theories have proposed advantages or disadvantages of having crossed eye and hand dominance in sports performance.[32,42,147,151,170,173,174,180,182−203] These speculations were further inspired by the findings of Coren and Porac,[168] who found that information from the dominant eye is processed approximately 14 ms faster than information from the nondominant eye. Functional magnetic resonance imaging studies further demonstrate a larger activation area in the primary visual cortex of the dominant eye.[204] The effect of the dominant eye on batting in baseball has received considerable scrutiny. Although the findings have been somewhat contradictory, the preponderance of evidence indicates no relation between eye preference patterns and batting performance.[151,182,183,188,190,192,199,200] In a study with golfers, ocular dominance in putting stance was found to be different than in primary gaze; however, the magnitude of dominance in putting stance was not associated with increased putting success.[174] The only sports in which eye dominance appears to be important are "sighting" sports such as target shooting.[186,187,189,191,193,194,196,198] In these sports, ipsilateral (same side) dominance offers advantages to acquiring the skills required for success.[198]

Although the role of ocular preference in sports success is inconclusive, evaluation of a preferred eye, hand, and/or foot has been included in many sports vision evaluations.[4,6,17,18,32−35,37,145,147,192] When assessment of ocular preference in athletes is important, a pointing test paradigm that preserves natural binocular viewing conditions is recommended. Preference can be qualified as strong, partial, none, or mixed.[147,171,182−184]

Ocular Alignment

The precise alignment of the two eyes, triggered by retinal image disparity, is responsible for providing a significant amount of information regarding object location.[205] The amount of innervation exerted by each of the six extraocular muscles in each eye to align on a target or object provides some of the information necessary to judge depth and is logically a critical feature of sports performance when precise depth judgments are necessary for success. Studies have demonstrated that extraocular muscle tonus changes produced by altering the amount of heterophoria result in changes in perceived distance.[206–210] If a shift occurs in a relatively esophoric direction, perceived distances are increased; exophoric shifts induce a shortening of perceived distances. Athletes are commonly agreed to have better ocular alignment, especially when viewing at a far distance, than nonathletes; however, results of studies comparing athletes with nonathletes have not been conclusive.[31,36,45,57,211] Early studies suggested that athletes have lower amounts of heterophoria[57,211] but more recent studies have not confirmed these results.[31,36,60] Because changes in heterophoria produce changes in perceived distance, stability of vergence posture may be a more critical factor in spatial localization than the amount of heterophoria.

The measurement of ocular alignment is a common aspect of a sports vision evaluation; however, the methods used to assess this function vary considerably.[e] The cover test is arguably the standard for the assessment of ocular alignment, although the telebinocular, Maddox Rod, Brock String, and von Graefe phorometry have all been recommended. It should be noted that when using a Brock String to assess fixation disparity at distances further than 2 m, athletes will consistently report the strings crossing in front of the bead because of the relative enlargement of Panum's fusional area. This effect makes the Brock String an inaccurate tool for the assessment of alignment at far distances. Measurements of fixation disparity have been suggested to be more rewarding in sports that require precise spatial localization because it is assessed without dissociation and can potentially evaluate the accuracy and stability of eye alignment.[34,212–214] The AO Vectographic slide or similar apparatus can assess distance fixation disparity characteristics. Whatever methods are chosen, the alignment should be measured in the pertinent gaze positions for the particular sport or position in addition to measurements in primary gaze. Ocular gaze and head position have been reported to influence fixation disparity and heterophoria.[215–217] Coffey et al.[218] found that instability of binocular visual alignment is related to errors in golf putting alignment. Therefore

the measurements should be assessed at fixation distances relevant to the sport demands. Most sports require the athlete to fixate on objects or people at a relatively far distance and judge the relative depth for decisions regarding performance; therefore far alignment should be assessed, with near alignment assessed when a relevant sport demand is present.

Depth Perception

The perception of depth has generated a considerable amount of interest relative to visual performance. Wheatstone[219] was the first to describe and demonstrate the illusion of depth by inducing retinal image disparity, and the psychophysical mechanisms and parameters of stereoscopic vision have been scrutinized extensively. Early research studied static stereoscopic vision,[220–222] whereas later research investigated the perception of depth in motion (dynamic stereopsis).[223–244] These factors are discussed more extensively in Chapter 3.

The relation between depth perception abilities and athletic performance was a logical correlation to explore because many sport tasks require judgments of spatial localization. Several studies have demonstrated that binocular vision can improve performance on certain tasks compared with performance by individuals using only one eye.[242,243,245–251] However, the research comparing performance on tests of static stereopsis with athletic populations have had mixed results.[f] A study of Olympic athletes found that competitors in fencing, softball, soccer, and speed skating exhibited better contour and random dot stereopsis at 20 feet compared to those in track-and-field and archery.[43] In contrast, a study of collegiate baseball players found no correlation between distance stereopsis and any pitching or batting statistics.[252] Similarly, there was no correlation found between stereopsis and batting statistics in youth baseball players, or when comparing athletes in interceptive sports with nonathletes, although the stereopsis testing was performed at 40 cm rather than at a far distance in these studies.[60,253] Studies conducting stereopsis testing at 40 cm have found better stereopsis in youth and professional baseball/softball players compared with nonballplayers and in elite cricket players compared with near-elite or general population data.[61,254,255] The differences in study findings may be the result of the variety of testing distances and procedures used, which have included tests with a telebinocular, Howard-Dolman devices, real-space

---

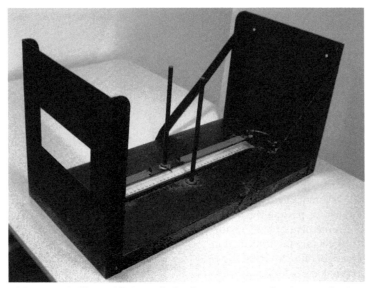

FIG. 4.4 A homemade Howard-Dolman device for assessment of real-space depth perception.

distance judgments, Mentor BVAT computerized system, and vectographic images. It has also been suggested that the lack of correlation in many studies is due to the static nature of the testing and that testing of dynamic stereopsis may yield differential performance and discriminate sport-related visual abilities better.[256-264]

An assessment of depth perception is an almost universal element to a sports vision evaluation.[8] There are several systems that include an assessment of stereopsis, including the Senaptec Sensory Station, M&S Technologies Sports Vision Performance package, and sports vision software available from Centro de Optometria Internacional. The author recommends an evaluation of stereopsis at a distance of 3 m or further, and it is preferable to include an assessment of the speed of stereopsis for dynamic reactive sports. A procedure that measures real depth at a far distance rather than simulated depth at a near distance is also preferred; this can be accomplished with a Howard-Dolman type of device (Fig. 4.4) and has been found to be better in athletes than in nonathletes.[271] It can be valuable to assess stereopsis in nonprimary gaze positions if that is a relevant visual demand for the sport; studies have found differing performance in nonprimary gazes compared with primary gazes.[272,273] A procedure to evaluate dynamic stereopsis is desirable; however, no commercially available instrument is currently available to measure this function with validity and reliability.

Vergence Function

An assessment of vergence subsystem function is frequently recommended for athletes.[3-6,15,17,30,31,34-37,40,44] The underlying premise is that strength and flexibility in vergence function provide better stability of visual information to the athlete, particularly when the athlete must deal with excessive fatigue and psychologic stress. A correlation between stability of vergence information and spatial judgment consistency has been assumed.[3]

Only three studies have reported on vergence range measurements in athletes. Coffey and Reichow[3] reported narrower vergence range findings at 6 m compared with published norms and discussed speculation that narrower vergence ranges relate to more precise spatial judgment ability. Hughes et al.[37] found no statistically significant difference between the vergence ranges at 6 m on elite, intermediate, and novice table tennis competitors. Omar et al.[45] found better vergence break values in teenaged nonathletes compared with athletes for both base-in and base-out ranges at 6 m, but only significantly better on recovery values in the base-in direction. Therefore, measurement of vergence ranges at 6 m may only be valuable as an assessment of motor compensation ability when an athlete has a large heterophoria at 6 m.

An assessment of the near point of convergence (NPC) has been studied as a visual factor in athletes.

---

[8]References: 1,3−6,15,17−20,24,25,28−40,51,56−58,93,116, 117,145,212

Christenson and Winkelstein[32] found athletes performed better on the NPC test than did nonathletes, whereas other studies found better performance in nonathletes.[45,60] The theory is that NPC testing is a dynamic procedure that requires simultaneous performance of oculomotor skills and vergence function and therefore it may assess vergence function more globally than other procedures that isolate aspects of vergence function. Falkowitz and Mendel[190] found that the better batters in a cohort of baseball players had better NPC findings than those whose batting performance was poorest. However, Hughes et al.[37] found no statistically significant difference between athletes at different skill levels and 27% of Junior Olympic athletes did not meet minimum criteria for passing this test.[44] These results suggest that measurement of NPC in athletes may not provide clinically useful information regarding sports performance because the test does not directly simulate the visual tasks found in most sports.

An evaluation of vergence facility has been recommended because the visual demands of many sports involve the ability to adjust vergence posture rapidly.[3] Two methods have been used to measure vergence facility in athletes: the use of prisms to alter the vergence demands at a fixed distance[31,36,37] and the use of charts at two different distances, with fixation being rapidly alternated between the two charts.[3] Christenson and Winkelstein[32] found athletes performed better on a vergence facility test using 8^Δ base out and 4^Δ base in at 6 m than nonathletes, and Omar et al.[45] also found better performance using 12^Δ base out and 3^Δ base in. However, Hughes et al. did not find significant differences among elite, intermediate, and novice table tennis competitors using 10^Δ base out and 4^Δ base in.[37] Coffey and Reichow[3] advocate use of the Haynes distance rock test[529,530] (Fig. 4.5), theorizing that it more closely simulates real-world accommodative-vergence facility. Most athletes need to look between far, intermediate, and near distances quickly, requiring rapid accommodative-vergence responses. When a prism is introduced, the vergence system must adjust ocular alignment to regain image fusion; however, the accommodative system must remain focused close to the plane of the target. This separation of accommodation and vergence is a standard method to assess relative vergence facility at near in patients with asthenopia during near work,[274] but it is generally not a factor in the visual task demands of sports. Therefore use of a near-to-far alternating fixation procedure is recommended for assessing vergence facility in athletes. The performance results of a procedure such as the Haynes distance rock test are influenced by limitations in visual acuity,

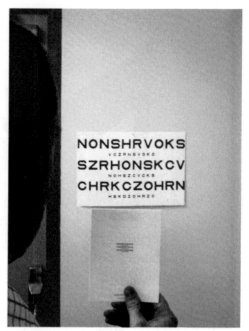

FIG. 4.5 The Haynes distance rock test.

accommodative skills, and oculomotor skills (fixation and saccadic eye movements), and the procedure will not reveal suppression tendencies. Near-Far Quickness on the Nike Sensory Station and Senaptec Sensory Station has been associated with better ability at avoiding strikeouts in professional baseball.[104]

Accommodative Function

An assessment of accommodation subsystem function is frequently recommended for athletes.[h] The underlying premise is that strength and flexibility in focusing ability provide better stability of visual information to the athlete, particularly when the athlete must deal with excessive fatigue and psychologic stress. A correlation between rapid focusing and the visual judgments typically required in rapid-action sports has been assumed.

The earliest study reporting accommodative function in athletes was part of a series of Russian studies. Normal accommodative amplitudes were found in 100 "well-trained" athletes.[211] A study found statistically better performance on amplitude of accommodation in teenaged athletes compared to nonathletes, although the difference may not be clinically significant.[45] Although accommodative amplitude is a

[h]References: 3–6,14,15,17,29–31,33–38,40,116–118

common procedure for assessing accommodative function, the task of clearing letters at a very near distance does not reproduce the typical visual task demands encountered in sports. The approximately 0.6-s latency of the accommodative response has been suggested to preclude it as a factor in many rapid reactive sports.[54]

More recent studies have evaluated accommodative facility to more closely simulate the visual demands of many sports that involve the ability to adjust focus rapidly for a variety of distances. Two methods have been used to measure accommodative facility in athletes: lenses to alter the accommodative demands at a fixed distance[31,36] and charts at two different distances, with fixation rapidly alternated between the two charts.[3] Three studies that used lenses (at near and far distances) to assess accommodative facility in athletes found no significant difference in performance compared to nonathletes.[31,36,45] However, accommodative facility using lenses was found to be better in intermediate and advanced volleyball players compared to beginners and nonplayers.[275] The study using the Haynes distance rock test presented normative data for a population of elite athletes and therefore did not compare performance with that of nonathletes.[3] A study of athletes in interceptive sports found slightly better performance on a near-far accommodative facility test in the athletes.[60] When a lens is introduced, the accommodative system must adjust ciliary muscle tonus to regain image clarity; however, the vergence system must remain aligned with the plane of the target to prevent diplopia. This separation of accommodation and vergence is a standard method to assess relative accommodative facility binocularly at near in patients with asthenopia during near work,[274] but it is not generally a factor in the visual task demands of sports. Therefore the use of an alternating near-to-far fixation procedure is recommended for assessing accommodative facility in athletes. The performance results of a procedure such as the Haynes distance rock test are influenced by limitations in visual acuity, vergence skills, and oculomotor skills (fixation and saccadic eye movements) and the procedure will not reveal suppression tendencies. Near-Far Quickness on the Nike Sensory Station and Senaptec Sensory Station has been associated with better ability at avoiding strikeouts in professional baseball.[104]

Oculomotor Function

One of the most commonly heard coaching imperatives is "keep your eyes on the ball (puck, opponent, target, etc.)." The ability to maintain fixation of a rapidly moving object is frequently a critical aspect for allowing visual processing of crucial information in sports. The ability to change fixation from one location to another rapidly and accurately is also an essential aspect of many sports tasks. In nondynamic sports such as precision target shooting, the ability to maintain steady fixation is a vital aspect of successful performance.[276] Therefore the assessment of oculomotor function can include evaluation of pursuit eye movements, saccadic eye movements, and steadiness of fixation.[277–279] Another aspect of oculomotor function is searching eye movements, as discussed in Chapter 3. However, this function is much more difficult to assess in clinical practice.

An important aspect of oculomotor function is the physiologic time required for initiation of the requisite eye movement for the visual task. The average latency for initiation of a pursuit eye movement is typically 125 ms, and the average latency for initiation of a saccadic eye movement is 200 ms.[280] Studies have found mixed results when comparing pursuit and saccadic eye movement latencies; some have not shown that athletes have shorter latencies for the initiation of pursuit or saccadic eye movements,[32,36,281] whereas some have.[276,282–286] However, if a target trajectory is predictable, reduction of the latency period for pursuit or saccadic eye movements can be learned.[276,283,287–291]

A study of racquet-sport athletes found quicker saccadic responses to positive positional errors compared with nonathletes.[285] Elite shooters have shorter saccadic latencies on both simple reaction to a sudden target appearance and discrimination between targets and distractors,[276,292] and shorter latencies for the first saccade were found to distinguish good from poor cricket batsmen.[283] Further study found elite cricket batsmen used two predictive saccades to anticipate a pitch: one to the location of the ball bounce and then to the location of the bat-ball contact point.[293] These predictive saccades were coupled with head movements to help maintain pursuit eye movement of the ball. Studies with college and professional baseball players found similar head tracking of pitches from a ball machine or live pitcher that assist the maintenance of gaze position close to the ball.[294–297] A study comparing saccade speeds into cardinal gaze positions using RightEye measurements found the professional baseball players had significantly faster speeds in several directions than amateur prospects and nonathletes.[298] Similar differences in head movement have been noted with tennis strokes between experienced and inexperienced players.[299] Positive positional errors are created by displacing the saccadic target in the same direction as the saccadic movement after initiation of the saccade. These results open questions of innate skill versus motor learning through experience and the modulation of attention with eye movement performance. Interestingly, in a study comparing experts in ball sports to controls, athletes did not show shorter latencies in the prosaccade condition (eye movements toward a suddenly appearing stimulus), whereas antisaccades (eye movements away from a suddenly appearing stimulus) showed significantly shorter latencies.[284] Saccade accuracy has been found to be better in fencers and tennis players compared with other athletes and nonathletes.[286]

Pursuit eye movements have the capacity to follow targets at speeds of up to 40 degrees/second (or faster if the trajectory is predictable), and saccadic eye movements have the capacity for speeds up to 1000 degrees/second.[280] Studies comparing the speed of pursuit eye movements in athletes and nonathletes have found mixed results, depending on the sports studied.[281,282,286] Pursuit eye movements have been shown to correlate to expertise in gymnasts of different levels and better performance compared to nonathletes.[300] Accuracy of smooth pursuit eye movements has also been correlated with better batting performance in professional baseball.[301]

The quality of pursuit and saccadic eye movements has been studied with clinical assessment procedures and results suggest that athletes have better eye movement skills.[31,190,302] The quality of eye movement skills has been correlated to batting performance in two studies; however, the subjectivity of the eye movement assessments brings the reliability and validity of these studies into question.[190,302] One study evaluated the quality of saccadic eye movements objectively at 3 m by projecting the King-Devick Test (a test designed for clinical assessment of saccadic fixation eye movement at 40 cm) on a screen; even though results indicated superior performance by athletes compared with nonathletes,[31] the test does not control for visual-verbal automaticity differences. Similarly, measurement of saccadic eye movement speed using optotype naming at 6 m found better performance in intermediate and advanced volleyball players than in beginners and nonplayers.[275]

An assessment of oculomotor function is a common element in a sports vision evaluation.[i] For clinical practice, a subjective assessment of pursuit and saccadic eye movement function using an observational method (e.g., Northeastern State University College of Optometry Oculomotor Test)[303] may be an acceptable screening procedure, but it may not be sensitive to the level of oculomotor function that is diagnostic in

athletes. An objective assessment of saccadic function with a projected King-Devick Test is no longer appropriate because the test design has flaws that have been eliminated with the Developmental Eye Movement Test.[304] A projected Developmental Eye Movement Test is a suitable replacement for the King-Devick Test, but it only assesses saccadic eye movement skills in a simulated reading pattern; therefore it also may not be sensitive to oculomotor functions that are diagnostic for the visual tasks in sports.

The gaze patterns of expert athletes have become an important area of study in the field of sports vision. This area has been largely ignored in clinical practice because these systems are generally prohibitively expensive[305,306]; however, the advent of lightweight portable eye tracking technology has allowed for evaluation and feedback of eye movements in sporting activities that are carried out in natural settings. These systems typically consist of two cameras mounted on an eyeglass-type frame: one to monitor eye position and one to monitor the scene (point-of-view) with an external camera that is positioned to monitor motor performance characteristics. The data collected by the mobile eye tracker is then synchronized with elements of motor performance using software programs that can operate in real time. Studies with such mobile eye trackers have typically found that experts have a lower number of fixations that occur for longer durations than do novices during the viewing of specific sport situations, especially when the subjects are required to move while gaze behaviors are recorded.[307–311] Across a variety of aiming and interceptive tasks, experts typically demonstrate longer fixation durations before initiation of the motor performance. Similarly, these patterns are also found on successful, relative to unsuccessful trials. This long-duration fixation that occurs just prior to motor response has been called the quiet eye (QE) period.[312] The exact neural mechanisms that direct gaze behavior during QE are still under investigation; however, it appears to show an advantageous period of cognitive processing allowing for computation of force, direction, and velocity that guide and fine-tune the motor response.[313]

There are several companies that market complete mobile eye tracking systems for use with sport applications, such as SensoMotoric Instruments (www.smivision.com/en/gaze-and-eye-tracking-systems/applications/sports-professional-training-education.html), Tobii Pro (www.tobiipro.com/fields-of-use/human-performance/), and Arrington Research (www.arringtonresearch.com), but these systems tend to be quite expensive. There are also some recent eye tracking systems that are monitor-based rather than eyeglass-based, such as

---

[i]References: 4,6,16−18,29,32−35,39,43,92,115,116

RightEye (www.righteye.com/sport), Tobii EyeX (www.tobii.com/xperience/products/), and the Eye Tribe Tracker Pro (www.theeyetribe.com/), and offer more affordable options. RightEye includes a monitor-based assessment of pursuit and saccadic eye movements that provides a performance score for sports applications (see Fig. 4.2). These platforms, however, limit the natural environment applications of eyeglass-based systems and have not typically been used for sport-related research.

Peripheral Awareness

The visual field is the entire extent of the external world that can be seen without a change in fixation.[314] In many sports situations, especially team sports, processing of information from the peripheral visual fields is a beneficial element to successful performance. The factors involved in assessment of peripheral vision include the extent of the visual fields, the sensitivity of the visual fields, the visual response speed to peripheral information, and spatial localization accuracy of peripheral stimuli.

Early studies investigated the extent of visual fields in athletes compared with nonathletes. Results indicate that athletes have a larger extent of horizontal and vertical visual fields than do nonathletes[42,211,268,270,315-320] and that athletes have better form recognition at more peripheral locations.[31,36,316,317] One study found no difference in the extent of visual field between varsity and junior varsity college football players, so it may not be a sensitive discriminator of skill level.[269] Some studies have found increases in the extent of visual fields with exercise[211,321-323]; however, these findings have been challenged more recently as being caused by the differences in visual field techniques, limited sample size, and lack of a control group in earlier studies.[324] Recently some studies have assessed the synchronoptical ability: the ability to assess visual information occurring at two different locations simultaneously. For example, the judgment of a foot fault in tennis requires the line judge to determine if the server's foot crossed the line before contact with the ball during the serve. This may be a relevant testing paradigm for sports in which the athlete must process both peripheral and central information simultaneously for optimal performance. Study results demonstrate that synchronoptical differentiation is difficult without support from audition[325] but that the skill appears trainable.[326] A study of basketball players found that skilled players showed significantly higher response accuracy and faster response times than less skilled players in three video-based viewing conditions of basketball scenarios, demonstrating superiority in information

extraction when presented in either central or peripheral vision.[327] Physical activity does not appear to increase peripheral perception performance, but it does improve central perceptual performance.[328] Therefore the search for visual field defects in routine vision testing has a low yield in athletes yet it should be performed as part of the vision examination for sports participation for general health purposes.

Sports vision practitioners have attempted to evaluate peripheral response speed with the Wayne Peripheral Awareness Trainer (PAT) (www.wayneengineering.com) and some normative data have been published.[3,329] The PAT is no longer commercially available; however, it was composed of a central circular module that contained a central fixation light with eight clear rods extending from it with red light-emitting diodes (LEDs) at each end (Fig. 4.6). The athlete holds a joystick, fixates centrally, and moves the joystick in the direction of an LED when it is perceived in peripheral vision. This system only assesses peripheral response speed, not accuracy, and fixation is not monitored in a controlled manner. The level of ambient room lighting affects performance on the Wayne PAT; performance on the instrument significantly improves as room illumination is decreased.[329] The Vienna Test System (www.schuhfried.com) contains several measures of peripheral perception and has been used to evaluate performance in athlete populations.[60,330-334] Moderate to good reliability has been found with the peripheral perception subtests, indicating reasonable applications for assessment in sports.[335] Other systems designed to assess peripheral eye-hand response, discussed later in this chapter, may also provide useful information about peripheral vision performance in athletes. Even though assessment of peripheral vision is recommended as part of a sports vision evaluation, further development is necessary to more closely simulate the visual task demands of sports.[j]

Ocular Health Status

A complete assessment of ocular health is an obligatory portion of a sports vision evaluation.[3-5,17,19,20,52] A complete assessment generally includes evaluation of the external adnexa, anterior segment of the eye with biomicroscopy, pupillary responses, intraocular pressure, posterior segment through a dilated pupil, and the visual fields of each eye. The presence of any ocular abnormality should be fully charted and photographed if possible and the consequences of the abnormality

---

[j]References:
3-6,14,15,17,19,20,25,31,33-37,39,40,93,116,117,336

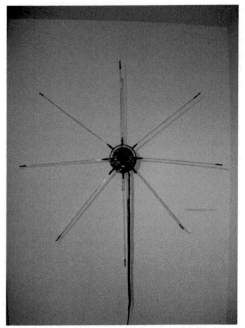

FIG. 4.6 The Wayne Peripheral Awareness trainer. (Courtesy Alan Berman, OD, Ridgefield, Connecticut.)

explained in detail to the athlete. The potential risks of any abnormality to sports participation should be fully addressed and appropriate recommendations discussed for protection of the athlete. Chapters 6 and 7 cover these issues in detail.

DECISION MECHANISM
Speed of Recognition

The ability to process visual information rapidly has been considered an essential element for success in fast-action sports. Athletes must analyze available temporal and spatial information during sports situations relatively quickly to make accurate decisions concerning performance responses. Visual processing speed can be measured psychophysically and has been referred to as inspection time (IT).[337,338] Shorter ITs allow accurate decisions to be made from shorter stimulus durations than from longer ITs. Tachistoscopic procedures to evaluate speed and span of recognition have been used in research for many years.[268,339]

IT measurements have been shown to have a development pattern characteristic of many physical abilities, have good test-retest reliability, and correlate with measures of cognitive abilities.[340,341] Evoked potential findings suggest that IT may be an index of the speed of transfer of information from sensory registers to short-term memory.[342] IT measures may provide a valid and reliable method for evaluating speed of recognition abilities in athletes.[343]

Several studies have investigated speed of recognition abilities in athletes. Most studies have found that experienced athletes can evaluate information more rapidly than inexperienced observers; sport situations studied include baseball, cricket, volleyball, tennis, motorsports, and "fast ball" sports.[59,104,343–350] McLeod,[351] however, did not find faster processing speeds in professional cricketers using film footage of cricket bowlers stopped at stages of the ball delivery, although the study was criticized for a small sample size and no statistical analysis. In addition, the study design only evaluated one of a number of important aspects concerning the movement of a ball in flight.[343] An in-depth analysis of 252 professional baseball players using a series of Bayesian hierarchic latent variable models found that the Perception Span assessment on the Nike Sensory Station had strong associations with on-base percentage and strikeout rate.[104]

Other studies have investigated both speed and span of recognition by evaluating the ability to recall a sequence of numbers presented tachistoscopically for 1/50 of a second and found no difference in athletes compared with nonathletes.[31,37,60] However, another study did find a significant difference in performance both for span of recognition and speed of recognition, even when distraction factors were added to the task to simulate competition conditions.[35] Despite these differences in research results, the author concludes that the use of numerical stimuli may be the confounding factor in the assessment of speed of recognition in athletes; use of target parameters that more closely simulate the visual information processed in sport situations may yield better discrimination of IT abilities that correlate with sports performance.[3,31] For example, the projection of photographs of baseball pitchers shown at the moment of ball release may better assess how rapidly a baseball player can identify the type of pitch being thrown.[350] A study using a metric combining variables of target size, contrast, and presentation time was shown to correlate with several plate discipline metrics in baseball (InzoneSwingPct, inzoneFbSwingPct, ChasePct, FbChasePct, BBperPa).[352] Similarly, oculomotor processing speed has also been correlated with better batting performance metrics in professional baseball.[301] The Perception Span assessment on the Nike Sensory Station and Senaptec Sensory Station uses a grid pattern composed of up to 30 circles (see Fig. 4.7) with a pattern of yellow-green dots flashed simultaneously for 100 ms within the grid.[108] Athletes

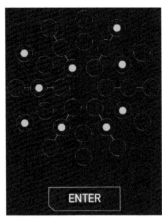

FIG. 4.7 A sample pattern briefly flashed (100 ms) during the Perception Span assessment on the Nike and Senaptec Sensory Stations.

touch the screen to recreate the pattern of dots and the grid pattern increases in size with an increasing number of dots. The use of tachistoscopic testing for speed of visual processing is frequently recommended as part of the vision assessment of athletes.[2,6,15,29,35,39,44,117]

Multiple Object Tracking

In many dynamic, reactive team sports, athletes must track teammates and opponents while simultaneously moving in response to the game. These sports require athletes to extract the crucial visual information from a dynamically changing environment in order to make the best decision on how to respond appropriately. These visual abilities that are critical to success in many sports have been called multiple object tracking (MOT), first described by Pylyshyn and Storm.[353] Research has demonstrated that this form of visuospatial cognition is enhanced in expert athletes.[354–361] Professional athletes have been found to have better MOT scores than high-level amateur athletes and nonathletes,[359] and a study of NBA players found that MOT motion speed thresholds measured in the preseason correlated with a number of in-game statistics, including assists, steals, and assist-to-turnover ratios, during the following season.[360] This preliminary evidence suggests that MOT abilities are fundamental properties for optimal sports performance.

Assessment of MOT is available with the CogniSens NeuroTracker (https://neurotracker.net) and Senaptec Sensory Station. These platforms show a set of identical targets with a random subset of the targets initially identified at the start of a trial to be tracked. At the conclusion of each trial the targets stop and the athlete is asked to identify the targets that were to be tracked. The assessment increases the demand for the athletes by modifying the number of targets to be tracked and the speed at which the objects move. Performance in the MOT task, therefore, is often limited by the number of targets an athlete can follow. As the number of targets increases, limitations in attentional resources lead to diminished performance.[362] In a study of basketball players, elite athletes displayed better tracking performance than the intermediate-level athletes or nonathletes when tracking three or four targets; however, no differences were observed among the three groups when tracking two targets.[363]

Visualization and Imagery

Visualization, or mental imagery, is the act of constructing mental images of an object or event that resemble the actual appearance of the object or event. Studies have suggested that mental imagery may share the same types of neural processes as visual perception, which has significant implications in sports.[364] Some studies have evaluated the differences between visual imagery and motor imagery and suggest they reflect different aspects of mental imagery.[365–368] Elite athletes have been repeatedly shown to use imagery strategies in preparation for performance.[369–377]

Many studies have suggested that mental imagery of motor skill performance shares cognitive processes with the actual performance of motor tasks.[378–385] Neuroimaging studies of subjects performing motor imagery demonstrate brain activity in the areas of motor preparation and performance.[365,386–388] Studies using electromyographic recordings show that mental imagery of a motor activity produces low-level motor effects that correspond to patterns of physical action; similar muscles and motor programs are activated.[379,381,389–393] Motion imagery has also been shown to correspond to attention for visuospatial imformation.[394] Expertise levels influence the amount of muscular response during skill imagery, in which higher levels of expertise produce increased electromyographic activity.[392] Task difficulty and expertise level have also been shown to affect the time required for mental imagery more than that for physical performance.[393,395–400] Athletes with lower skill levels require more time to execute the mental imagery of a physical performance than the actual time required to perform the physical act.

Suin[401–405] first described methods involving mental imagery and relaxation as a psychologic intervention to affect motor performance favorably. The use of mental imagery has become a significant factor for athletes, coaches, sports psychologists, and some sports vision specialists.[371,382,385,406-409] Relatively few studies have investigated the effectiveness of mental imagery in actual competition; most investigate the effect on skill acquisition.[371,410] The results of studies in skill acquisition or skill improvement have been contradictory, although the athlete skill level and length of intervention have been confounding variables for study comparison.[380,411] Sports in which visual motor tasks have been studied include basketball,[412-415] tennis,[416-418] karate,[419-422] swimming,[423] gymnastics,[424] racquetball,[425] archery,[410] golf,[426-429] high jumping,[430] and volleyball.[431]

Although the value of visualization and mental imagery in sports performance has been acclaimed, no objective assessment of individual ability exists. Many subjective assessment procedures are used by sports psychologists, such as the Sport Imagery Ability Questionnaire (SIAQ), which have demonstrated good validity, internal and temporal reliability, invariance across gender, and an ability to distinguish among athletes of different competitive levels.[432] However, use of these, or other, procedures to assess visualization skills is recommended, but they are rarely used by sports vision practitioners.[5,6,40,116,336,531-533]

EFFECTOR MECHANISM
Motor Response Time
The motor response time, also referred to as the motor reaction time (RT), has been defined as the actual time required to complete a simple, predetermined motor movement.[3] Visual motor RT is the total time required by the visual system to process a stimulus plus the time needed to complete the motor response. Motor response time is a measure of the neuromuscular processing portion of the RT reflex, separate from the visual processing portion of RT.

Little has been published concerning the measurement of motor response time. One study used the motor RT program on the Wayne Saccadic Fixator (www.wayneengineering.com) and found significantly faster times in athletes than in nonathletes.[31] Another study presented normative information from a population of elite athletes using a different device.[3] Devices for measuring motor response time are available from Lafayette Instrument (www.lafayetteinstrument.com), and measuring the eye-hand and eye-foot response time is a recommended procedure by some as part of a visual evaluation of athletes.[3,4,31,34]

Central Visual Motor Reaction Time
Visual motor RT, also referred to as psychomotor speed, refers to the amount of time that elapses between the

initiation of a visual stimulus and the completion of a motor response to the stimulus. This is the full completion of the RT reflex, including the period required for the retinal cells to detect the stimulus, the time necessary for the transmission of the retinal cell information to the visual cortex, and the time required for the neuromuscular system to send the information to the muscles that need to be stimulated to make the appropriate motor response. The time interval between the onset of the stimulus and the initiation of the response has been referred to as the reaction or premotor element of the overall RT and the rest of the response is referred to as the motor element.[3,433] Soccer players have shown shorter premotor RTs compared with nonathletes, although the sample was small in this study.[433] The neurophysiologic parameters of RT are discussed extensively in Chapter 3. Many sport situations require the athlete to make a specific motor response to visual information; therefore the speed of visual and neuromuscular processing is considered by many to be a valuable attribute for an athlete.[3,5,7,35,36,270,433-438]

The measure of a simple RT reflex represents the minimal amount of time required to process a visual stimulus presentation and perform a simple motor response to that stimulus. Several studies have found faster simple RTs in athletes (both eye-hand and eye-foot RTs) in various sports compared with nonathletes or as a discriminator between types of sports and expertise levels.[36,112,204,270,438-445] However, other studies have not found this correlation.[35,436,437] Visual RTs have been shown to be impaired by factors such as reduced IQ,[340,341,446] cold,[447] fatigue,[448,449] exercise,[450] and restriction of peripheral visual fields with protective eyewear.[451,452] Gender differences have also been reported, with men achieving faster times than women on average,[3] but other studies have not found this difference.[42,453] Performance on complex visual motor tasks is discussed in the Speed of Recognition and Peripheral Eye-Hand Response sections of this chapter.

The Binovi Touch Saccadic Fixator (www.binovitouch.com), Dynavision D2 (www.info.dynavision international.com), Senaptec Sensory Station, RightEye, Cognivue Advanced (www.cognivue.com), and the Multi-Operational Apparatus for Reaction Time (MOART) system (www.lafayetteinstrument.com) are commercially available devices for measuring visual motor response time; measuring the eye-hand and eye-foot response time is a recommended procedure by some as part of a visual evaluation of athletes.[3-5,34-36,117] The Dynavision D2, Senaptec Sensory Station, and RightEye have demonstrated reliability to assess eye-hand RT.[108,453,454] Options for assessment of eye-foot RT include the MOART system using the foot switch, the

RT-2S Simple Reaction Time Tester (www.atpwork.com), and the Quick Board (www.thequickboard.com).

Peripheral Eye-Hand Response

Peripheral eye-hand response assessment, also sometimes called eye-hand coordination, is the ability to make synchronized motor responses with the hands to visual stimuli. Many sports require the athlete to react with hand movements to rapidly changing visual information, such as in baseball, tennis, hockey, and football. This skill area is a repeated complex RT function for an extended period. A simple stimulus-response procedure that requires minimal cerebral processing results in a faster RT than a complex stimulus/response procedure that requires discrimination of visual information.[455,456]

Studies have been designed to provide normative information for athletes with available instrumentation to evaluate peripheral eye-hand response.[3,31,37,457–459] The instrumentation designed for evaluating peripheral eye-hand response has usually been a two-dimensional panel mounted on a wall with an array of lights. The athlete is required to press a randomly lit button as rapidly as possible with one hand; then another button is lit in a random position on the instrument and the RT reflex cycle is repeated for the established period. The instruments are programmed to test in two primary modes: (1) visual proaction time refers to a self-paced mode for a set period in which each light stays lit until the button is pressed, then the next random light is lit and (2) visual reaction refers to an instrument-paced stimulus presentation in which each light stays lit for a preset amount of time (typically 0.75 s) before automatically switching to another light whether the button is pressed or not. A third option has been referred to as a Go/No-Go task.[108,459] The test setup is similar to other visual RT measures of peripheral eye-hand response; however, the light is either a "go" stimulus (e.g., green) or a "no-go" stimulus (e.g., red). Athletes are instructed to hit the "go" stimulus lights and to not hit the "no-go" stimulus lights. This test paradigm adds a layer of quick decision-making to the task in order to determine how effectively an athlete can make an uncomplicated decision to either generate a motor response or inhibit it. A study of baseball players found more variable RTs in a baseball-specific Go/No-Go task based on the level of experience, but this variability was not found in nonathletes or tennis and basketball players.[443,460] A subsequent study found that Go/No-Go RT is affected by sport-specific stimuli.[461] A study of professional baseball players found that better eye-hand peripheral response correlated with better plate discipline batting metrics (e.g., fewer at bats before gaining a walk, swinging less often at pitches outside the strike zone, the ability to gain a walk), as well as longer playing time and increased likelihood of competing at the major-league level.[462]

One study found better visual proaction times in youth athletes than in nonathletes[463]; however, another study found no difference in visual proaction time between adult athletes and nonathletes.[31] Visual reaction has only been compared in athletes and nonathletes in one study; athletes performed better on the visual reaction setting with the Wayne Saccadic Fixator than did nonathletes.[31] The level of ambient room lighting affects performance on the Wayne Saccadic Fixator and the AcuVision 1000 instruments; performance on the instruments significantly improves as room illumination is decreased.[329,464,465] Peripheral eye-hand response performance was shown to remain stable with perceived fatigue factors.[466] Artificially reducing the depth perception has been shown to diminish peripheral eye-hand response accuracy in the hitting stroke of elite-level table tennis athletes.[467] Gender differences have also been reported that are most likely related to differences in visual RTs, with men achieving faster times than women on average.[3,468]

The Wayne Saccadic Fixator was the original instrument developed for this type of assessment, and although it is no longer commercially available, there are many similar instruments. The Binovi Touch Saccadic Fixator, Dynavision D2, SVT (www.sportsvision.com.au), Vision Coach (www.visioncoachtrainer.com), BATAK Pro (www.batak.com), FitLight (www.fitlighttraining.com), Senaptec Sensory Station, Reflexion (www.reflexion.co), Sanet Vision Integrator (www.svivision.com), and the MOART system are commercially available devices for measuring peripheral eye-hand response; measuring peripheral eye-hand response is a recommended procedure by some as part of visual evaluation of athletes.[3–6,31,34,37–40,44,93,108,116,117,454,469] FitLight is unique in that it employs wireless LED powered lights that are controlled by a computer and can be flexibly placed at distances up to 50 yards from the controller, rather than embedded in a fixed board (see Fig. 4.8). The Senaptec Sensory Station, SVT, and Dynavision D2 have demonstrated reliability and standards for assessing peripheral eye-hand response.[108,454,469] The Vienna Test System contains several measures in the peripheral perception subtests that include RT measurements to peripheral targets and may provide useful information to complement other measures of peripheral eye-hand response.

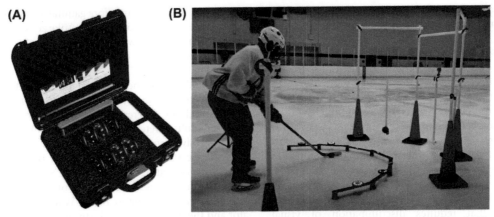

FIG. 4.8 The FitLight system (A) in a portable storage case and (B) set up in a hockey training facility. (Courtesy Amanda Nanasy OD, Florida Institute of Sports Vision, Pembroke Pines, Florida.)

Eye-Body Response

Eye-body response is the ability to make synchronized motor responses with the body to visual stimuli. The procedure is similar to peripheral eye-hand response testing, with the difference being that, with some instruments, the athlete is standing on a square board with a small square fulcrum underneath. The athlete must establish balance on the board and then shift the center of balance of the body in response to the direction of the light stimulus on the wall-mounted panel. The stimulus lights are randomly alternated among the top, bottom, left, and right sides of the panel, and the athlete must shift the center of balance forward, backward, leftward, or rightward, respectively, to engage the switch that extinguishes the light stimulus. Evaluation of eye-body response usually involves performance of the task for an established period and the number of correct body responses is tabulated. An alternative to this paradigm is the use of the Quick Board (see Fig. 4.9) to generate visual patterns to be replicated on the floor mat with the feet; however, there have been no normative or comparative studies published with this instrument.

Only one published study has evaluated this skill in athletes and it provided normative data on a population of elite athletes.[3] Gender differences were reported that are most likely related to differences in visual RT, with men achieving higher scores than women on average.[3] No studies have compared performance between athletes and nonathletes or correlated performance on this procedure with athletic skills. The Wayne Saccadic Fixator was the only commercially available device for measuring eye-body response using a balance board, but it is no longer available. The Quick Board is commercially available, and although it does not currently have standardized procedures for evaluation, it has been used as an evaluation instrument in studies.[470,471] Measuring eye-body response is a recommended procedure by some as part of a visual evaluation of athletes.[3–6,38,39,117]

Coincidence Anticipation Timing

Coincidence anticipation timing (CAT) is the ability to predict the arrival of an object or stimulus at a designated place and is usually measured with a motor response. Theoretically, CAT contributes to the attempt to catch or hit an approaching ball in sports. Predictive visual information concerning the space-time behavior of critical factors in fast-action sports can provide a significant advantage in determining and executing the most appropriate motor responses.[115,472–484]

The Bassin Anticipation Timer (www.lafayetteinstrument.com) is the apparatus most often used to assess CAT in laboratory experiments under the assumption that the task simulates actual anticipation tasks.[445,483,485–492] The Bassin Anticipation Timer consists of tracks of LEDs that can be fit together to make a "runway" of various lengths (Fig. 4.10). The LEDs are sequentially illuminated down the runway in rapid succession to simulate the apparent motion of the stimulus lights traveling at velocities of 1–500 mph. The task requires the athlete to anticipate when the target light will be illuminated as the LEDs are sequentially illuminated along the z-axis approaching the athlete and to make a motor response that coincides with the illumination of the target light. The velocity of the stimulus lights can be calibrated to simulate the action speeds encountered in the athletes' sport, in

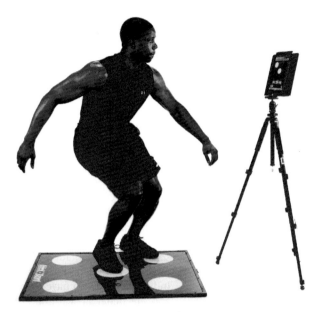

FIG. 4.9 The Quick Board.

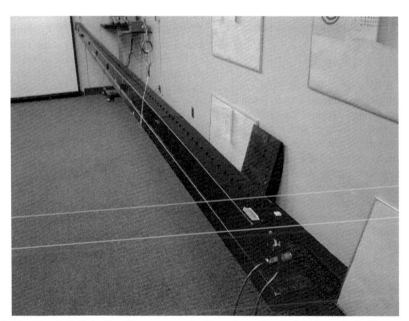

FIG. 4.10 The Bassin Anticipation Timer suspended from the ceiling (height is controlled by a garage door opener).

effect simulating the stimulus parameters experienced by the athlete (e.g., the pitch speeds in baseball batting).

Research results have suggested that timing accuracy improves with increasing velocity and decreasing range of movement response[483,493–495] and that the terminating light chosen and length of the runway affect the accuracy of CAT.[488,491] No differences in CAT performance response accuracy were found when comparing binocular and monocular viewing conditions with the Bassin Anticipation Timer.[496] Studies investigating the results of performance on the Bassin Anticipation Timer to batting performance in baseball and softball have found that the two do not correlate.[487,490] CAT has been shown to be independent of visual acuity skills[113] but heavily influenced by direction of motion in depth.[484] Physiologic arousal, exercise, and caffeine ingestion all appear to sustain CAT performance accuracy.[497,498,534] The superior CAT found in tennis players has been suspected to be influenced by better DVA skills and sport-specific experience,[476] but this correlation has not been corroborated.[115,492] Studies of racket sports, including tennis, badminton, and table tennis, have found differing CAT abilities based on each sport that correspond to the speed of the ball/shuttlecock.[445,499] Several studies have reported sex differences with CAT, and a review of the literature concluded that absolute error on CAT is better, on average, in men than in women.[500]

The Bassin Anticipation Timer is a commercially available device for measuring visual coincidence anticipation; measuring visual coincidence anticipation is not a frequently recommended procedure as part of a visual evaluation of athletes.[4] This procedure is more commonly used for vision skill training and enhancement of visual concentration.

Vision and Balance

The ability to maintain balance while processing complex, fast-action visual information is a task demand fundamental to many dynamic sports. The athlete is frequently required to preserve balance while the oculomotor system is engaged in pursuit and/or saccadic eye movements. The vision and balance test sequence was developed by Coffey and Reichow[3] to evaluate systematically some of the many types of vision and balance demands encountered by the competitive athlete. The sequence involves performance of several different tasks while the subject is either standing or moving on a balance rail secured to the floor. Maintenance of balance is subjectively rated during each task with a scale that defines levels of performance quality. Only one published study has investigated the vision and balance skills described by Coffey and Reichow,[3] and the purpose of the study was to provide normative data on a population of elite athletes. Investigations have evaluated the role of vision on dynamic balance in gymnastics, reporting that vision played an important role in skills acquisition.[501-504] It is not commonly recommended as part of a sports vision evaluation.[4,24] The visual skills involved in the assessment appear relevant; however, test validity and reliability are significant concerns.

Field Dependence and Independence

Field dependence and independence refer to the cognitive style of processing information to discern relevant stimuli from an irrelevant stimulus background. While the theory has many applications, in sports, it implies that field-dependent persons rely more on external cues during information processing and field-independent persons use internal cues more.[505,506] Kane postulated that field dependence was an advantage in "open skill"[507,508] team sports (e.g., basketball, football, hockey) because athletes must make constant adjustments in performance to external factors (teammates, opponents, etc.).[509] Athletes competing in "closed skill"[507,508] sports (e.g., diving, gymnastics, synchronized swimmers, kayaking, track and field) tend to rely more on internal physical components such as body orientation.[504,509-511]

Many studies have concluded that field-independent individuals tend to have higher levels of athletic skills and are better at learning athletic skills.[512-524] Field independence has been determined to be related to fewer injuries in football,[525] and sports training results in increased field independence on certain tests.[526,527] However, some studies have found equivocal or contradictory results; the difference in results has been suggested to be a result of the large variety of tests used in the research.[522] Tests that require subjects to respond to paper-and-pencil tasks (e.g., embedded figures test and group hidden figures test) yield different results than procedures that require the comparison of visual and vestibular information (e.g., rod and frame test). The rod and frame test (Fig. 4.11) appears to be a more reliable method for assessing athletes' relative preferences for visual or proprioceptive stimuli in a conflicting environment. With this test paradigm, athletes participating in closed-skill sports are more field independent than those competing in open-skill sports and higher level athletes are more field independent than lower level athletes.[504,510,511,522,524] The rod and frame test is not routinely used or recommended by eye care providers.

DEVELOPING A SPORTS VISION EVALUATION

Most sports vision evaluations do not assess all the areas described in this chapter for all athletes. The practitioner's mission is to identify those areas that appear to be critical for success in performing the visual tasks required of the athlete as well as those areas that are beneficial to overall performance. The contents of this chapter should show that the visual skills that correlate

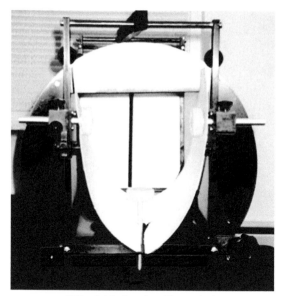

FIG. 4.11 A rod and frame test.

with successful sports performance have not yet been definitively identified. The procedures that yield the most relevant assessment of critical visual skills have yet to be identified definitively as well. However, the critical and beneficial visual skill areas should be included in the evaluation of the athlete by using the best available protocols, when possible. Those areas not identified as critical or beneficial to performance may not require assessment. As the practitioner gains experience with a variety of sports, sport-specific evaluations can be formulated for use with subsequent evaluations of athletes involved in these sports. The assessment areas and procedures used can be modified as needed on the basis of the results of research and the clinician's own experience.

The results of the evaluation should be summarized for the patient, and a performance profile is recommended to highlight areas of strength or weakness. The development of a performance profile and strategies for reporting results and recommendations are presented in Chapter 5. Computerized assessment and training instruments, such as the Senaptec Sensory Station, Sports Vision Performance from M&S, Vizual Edge Performance Trainer (VEPT) (http://vizualedge.com), RightEye Sports Vision EyeQ, and the sports vision software available from Centro de Optometria Internacional, have been developed to provide a testing battery to evaluate several visual, cognitive, and sensorimotor skills in order to generate a performance profile.

The Senaptec Sensory Station (see Fig. 4.12) is a successor to the Sensory Station device originally developed by Nike Inc. The evaluation battery includes 10 sensorimotor tasks (9 in the original Nike device with an MOT task added to the Senaptec device) that have been identified as important for sports performance.[2] These tasks include visual clarity (akin to SVA), contrast sensitivity, depth perception, and MOT, as well as tasks that rely on ocular motor coordination such as near-far quickness, target capture (akin to DVA), perception span, eye-hand coordination (akin to peripheral eye-hand response), go/no-go and eye-hand RT. Evaluation results are registered in a central database to provide feedback for each individual about his or her performance relative to any sports peer group by competition level, as well as to compare to previous individual assessments. Research with the Nike iteration of this system has demonstrated that many tasks in the battery are reliable and cross-validated.[108,528]

Sports Vision Performance by M&S Technologies provides a digital assessment of several visual factors, including visual acuity, contrast sensitivity, eye alignment, depth perception, fusional ability, and developmental eye movement. Subscribers have the ability to compare performance to an established database of athletes. There is no research evidence regarding the reliability or validity of this system; however, many of these measures employ standard psychophysical protocols, so it is reasonable to expect reliability of the measurements.

The VEPT is designed to assess six visual skills: eye alignment, depth perception, convergence, divergence, visual recognition, and visual tracking. VEPT provides quantitative scores for each skill and a combined performance score for the complete battery. There is no research evidence regarding the reliability or validity of this system.

RightEye's Sports Vision EyeQ includes a remote eye tracker for assessments of dynamic visual focus, smooth visual pursuit, eye movement speed, simple RT, choice RT, discriminate RT, binocular vision skills, visual concentration, and contrast sensitivity. A report is generated detailing relative performance in each category. The only research regarding reliability of this system is with the three measures of DVA, which have shown good test-retest reliability.[109]

The sports vision software available from Centro de Optometria Internacional includes several assessments of visual acuity, contrast sensitivity, horizontal and vertical fixation disparity, vergence ranges, Hess Lancaster extraocular muscle function, stereopsis at far, eye-hand coordination, visualization, minimum perception time, and "central-peripheral care." The only research

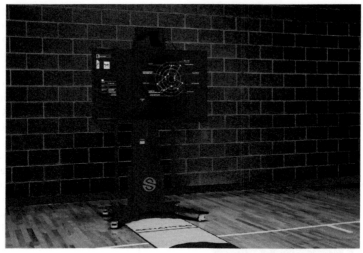

FIG. 4.12 The Senaptec Sensory Station. (Courtesy Senaptec LLC.)

on reliability found that the DinVA 3.0 is a valid and reliable measure of DVA.[96]

These computer-based assessment systems provide a useful platform for measuring important component sensorimotor and cognitive vision skills in athletes by providing a standardized evaluation. Use of this type of system provides a consistent platform for measurements so that athletes can be compared to other athletes in a dataset, or with their own previous performance. These systems also offer the benefit of requiring less physical space than the use of several different instruments to complete a test battery. Of course, not all assessment options are offered in any one system, so supplemental assessment may still need to be completed, as needed. Ultimately, the sports vision practitioner must identify the vision factors thought to be essential to the performance of the visual tasks critical for success in the sport and then determine the most appropriate, valid, and reliable methods for assessment.

REFERENCES

1. Stine CD, Arterburn MR, Stern NS. Vision and sports: a review of the literature. *J Am Optom Assoc.* 1982;53:627.
2. Hitzeman SA, Beckerman SA. What the literature says about sports vision. *Optom Clin.* 1993;3:145.
3. Coffey B, Reichow AW. Optometric evaluation of the elite athlete. *Probl Optom.* 1990;2:32.
4. Berman AM. Clinical evaluation of the athlete. *Optom Clin.* 1993;3(1).
5. Gardner JJ, Sherman A. Vision requirements in sport. In: Loran DFC, MacEwen CJ, eds. *Sports Vision.* Oxford: Butterworth-Heinemann; 1995.
6. Welford AT. The measurement of sensory-motor performance: survey and reappraisal of twelve years progress. *Ergonomics.* 1960;3:189.
7. Beckerman SA, Hitzeman S. The ocular and visual characteristics of an athletic population. *Optometry.* 2001;72:498.
8. Ettinger ER. *Professional Communications in Eye Care.* Boston: Butterworth-Heinemann; 1994.
9. Classe JG. Sports related ocular trauma: a preventable epidemic. *J Am Optom Assoc.* 1996;67:96.
10. Laukkanen H, Scheiman M, Hayes JR. Brain injury vision symptom survey (BIVSS) questionnaire. *Optom Vis Sci.* 2017;94:43–50.
11. Weimer A, Jensen C, Laukkanen H, Hauyes J, Saxerud M. Test-retest reliability of the brain injury vision symptom survey. *Vis Dev Rehabil.* 2018;4(4):177–185.
12. Ciuffreda KJ, Ludlam DP, Kapoor N. Clinical oculomotor training in traumatic brain injury. *Optom Vis Dev.* 2009; 40:16.
13. Ciuffreda KJ, Ludlam DP, Yadav NK, Thiagarajan P. Traumatic brain injury. *Adv Ophthalmol Optom.* 2016;1(1): 307–333.
14. Etting GL. An optometrist's vision of sports. *Calif Optom.* 1977;3:25.
15. Getz DJ. Vision and sports. *J Am Optom Assoc.* 1978;49: 385.
16. Gregg JR. *Vision and Sports: An Introduction.* Stoneham, MA: Butterworth Publishers; 1987:103–104.
17. Berman AM. Sports vision for the primary care practitioner. *Eye Quest Mag.* 1994;4:46.
18. Beatty RM, Bakkum BW, Hitzman SA, Beckerman S. Sports vision screening of amateur athletic union junior Olympic athletes: a ten-year follow-up. *Optom Vis Perf.* 2016;4(3):97.
19. Tussing L. The effect of football and basketball on vision. *Res Q Am Assoc Health Phys Educ.* 1940;11:16.

20. Martin WF. A research study on athletes' vision. *Contacto*. 1963;7:5.
21. Bauscher WA. Vision and the athlete. *Optom Wkly*. 1968; 59:21.
22. Garner AI. What a practitioner should know about an athlete's vision. *Contacto*. 1976;20:24.
23. Garner AI. An overlooked problem: athletes' visual needs. *Phys Sportsmed*. 1977;5:75.
24. Beals RP, Mayyasi AM, Templeton AE, et al. The relationship between basketball shooting performance and certain visual attributes. *Am J Optom Arch Am Acad Optom*. 1971;48:585.
25. Pitts DG. The role of vision in sports and recreational activities. *South J Optom*. 1974;16:11.
26. Runninger J. Vision requirements of competitive sports. *South J Optom*. 1975;17:13.
27. Morris GS, Kreighbaum E. Dynamic visual acuity of varsity women volleyball and basketball players. *Res Q Am Assoc Health Phys Educ*. 1977;48:480.
28. White VW. Visual acuity versus visual skill in athletic performance. *Calif Optom*. 1977;3:22.
29. Erenstone R, Miller NP, Silagy ZS. Optometry at the 1980 Winter Olympics. *J Am Optom Assoc*. 1981;52:647.
30. Harris PA, Blum DS. AOA Sports Vision Section screening of basketball officials. *J Am Optom Assoc*. 1984;55:130.
31. Gregg JR. *Vision and Sports: An Introduction*. Stoneham, MA: Butterworth Publishers; 1987:61−72.
32. Christenson GN, Winkelstein AM. Visual skills of athletes versus nonathletes: development of a sports vision testing battery. *J Am Optom Assoc*. 1988;59:666.
33. Fremion AS, DeMyer WE, Helveston EM, et al. Binocular and monocular visual function in world class tennis players. *Bin Vis*. 1986;1:147.
34. Wachs H. Sports vision. *Behav Optom*. 1991;3:215.
35. Sports vision gets gold at the Barcelona Olympics. *Calif Optom*. 1992;18:6.
36. Melcher MH, Lund DR. Sports vision and the high school student athlete. *J Am Optom Assoc*. 1992;63:466.
37. Hughes PK, Blundell NL, Walters JM. Visual and psychomotor performance of elite, intermediate and novice table tennis competitors. *Clin Exp Optom*. 1993;76:51.
38. Milne DC, Lewis RV. Sports vision screening of varsity athletes. *Sports Vis*. 1993;1:8.
39. Goldsmid MA. Visual fitness and performance in tennis athletes. *Eye Quest Mag*. 1994;38.
40. Berman AM. Sports performance vision testing. *Optom Today*. 1996;4:28.
41. Wilson TA, Falkel J. *Sports Vision Training for Better Performance*. Champaign, IL: Human Kinetics; 2004:1−13.
42. Quintana MS, Roman IR, Calvo AL, Molineuvo JS. Perceptual visual skills in young highly skilled basketball players. *Percept Mot Skills*. 2007;104:547−561.
43. Laby DM, Kirschen DG, Pantall P. The visual function of Olympic-level athletes − an initial report. *Eye Contact Lens*. 2011;37:116−122.
44. Sanghera NK, Baas EA, Bakkum BW, et al. Sports vision evaluation findings in an elite athlete population. *Optom Vis Perf*. 2016;4:107−111.
45. Omar R, Kuan YM, Zuhairi NA, et al. Visual efficiency among teenaged athletes and non-athletes. *Int J Ophthalmol*. 2017;10:1460−1464.
46. Roberts JW, Strudwick AJ, Bennett SJ. Visual function of English Premier League soccer players. *Sci Med Football*. 2017;1:178−182.
47. Klemish D, Ramger B, Vittetoe K, et al. Visual abilities distinguish pitchers from hitters in professional baseball. *J Sports Sci*. 2018;36:171−179.
48. Jorge J, Fernandes P. Static and dynamic visual acuity and refractive errors in elite football players. *Clin Exp Optom*. 2019;102:51−56.
49. Bailey IL, Lovie JE. New design principles for visual acuity letter charts. *Am J Optom Physiol Opt*. 1976;53:740−745.
50. Ferris III FL, Kassoff A, Bresnick GH, et al. New visual acuity charts for clinical research. *Am J Ophthalmol*. 1982;94: 91−96.
51. Jendrusch G, Bornemann R, Froschauer M, et al. Visual performance profile of top skiers. In: International Society for Ski Trauma and Safety, ed. *14th International Symposium on Ski Trauma & Skiing Safety, August 5−10, 2001, Queenstown, New Zealand*. 2001:78.
52. Elkin EH. *The Effect of Target Velocity, Exposure Time and Anticipatory Tracking Time on Dynamic Visual Acuity* [dissertation]. Medford, MA: Tufts University; 1961.
53. Berry RN. Quantitative relations among vernier, real depth and stereoscopic depth acuities. *J Exp Psychol*. 1948;38:708.
54. Coffey B, Reichow AW, Johnson T, et al. Visual performance differences among professional, amateur, and senior amateur golfers. In: Cochran AJ, ed. *Science and Golf II*. London: E&FN Spon; 1994.
55. Moses RA. Accommodation. In: Moses RA, Hart WM, eds. *Adler's Physiology of the Eye. Clinical Application*. St Louis: CV Mosby; 1987.
56. Laby DM, Rosenbaum AL, Kirschen DG, et al. The visual function of professional baseball players. *Am J Ophthalmol*. 1996;122:476.
57. Winograd S. The relationship of timing and vision to baseball performance. *Res Q Am Assoc Health Phys Educ*. 1942;13:481.
58. Jendrusch G, Kaczmarek L, Lange P, et al. Visual requirements and visual performance profile in soccer. *Med Sci Sports Exerc*. 2006;38:446.
59. Schneiders AG, John Sullivan S, Rathbone EJ, et al. Visual acuity in young elite motorsport athletes: a preliminary report. *Phys Ther Sport*. 2010;11(2):47−49.
60. Gao Y, Chen L, Yang S, et al. Contributions of visuo-oculomotor abilities to interceptive skills in sports. *Optom Vis Sci*. 2015;92:679−689.
61. Barrett BT, Flavell JC, Bennett SJ, et al. Vision and visual history in elite/near-elite-level cricketers and rugby-league players. *Sport Med Open*. 2017;3:39.
62. Banister H, Blackburn JM. An eye factor affecting proficiency at ball games. *Br J Psychol*. 1931;21:382.
63. Applegate RA, Applegate RA. Set shot shooting performance and visual acuity in basketball. *Optom Vis Sci*. 1992;69:765−768.

64. Bulson RC, Ciuffreda KJ, Hung GK. The effect of retinal defocus on golf putting. *Ophthalmic Physiol Optic*. 2008; 28:334−344.

65. Mann DL, Abernethy B, Farrow D. The resilience of natural interceptive actions to refractive blur. *Hum Mov Sci*. 2010;29:386−400.

66. Blackburn RH. Perception of movement. *Am J Optom*. 1937;14:365.

67. Graham CH, Cook C. Visual acuity as a function of intensity and exposure time. *Am J Psychol*. 1937;49:654.

68. Ludvigh EJ. The gradient of retinal illumination and its practical significance. *Am J Ophthalmol*. 1937;20:260.

69. Langmuir I. The speed of the deer fly. *Science*. 1938;87: 233.

70. Ludvigh E. Extrafoveal visual acuity as measured with Snellen test-letters. *Am J Ophthalmol*. 1941;24:303.

71. Ludvigh E. Visibility of the deer fly in flight. *Science*. 1947; 105:176.

72. Ludvigh E. The visibility of moving objects. *Science*. 1948; 108:63.

73. Ludvigh EJ. Visual acuity while one of viewing a moving object. *Arch Ophthalmol*. 1949;42:14.

74. Westheimer G. Eye movement responses to a horizontally moving visual stimulus. *AMA Arch Ophthalmol*. 1954; 52:932.

75. Hulbert SF, Burg A, Knoll HA, et al. A preliminary study of dynamic visual acuity and its effects in motorist's vision. *J Am Optom Assoc*. 1958;29:359.

76. Ludvigh EJ, Miller JW. Study of visual acuity during the ocular pursuit of moving test objects. I. Introduction. *J Opt Soc Am*. 1958;48:799.

77. Miller JW. Study of visual acuity during the ocular pursuit of moving test objects. II. Effects of direction of movement, relative movement, and illumination. *J Opt Soc Am*. 1958;48:803.

78. Burg A, Hulbert SF. Dynamic visual acuity and other measures of vision. *Percept Mot Skills*. 1959;9:334.

79. Burg A, Hulbert S. Dynamic visual acuity as related to age, sex and static acuity. *J Appl Psychol*. 1961;45:111.

80. Miller JW, Ludvigh E. The effect of relative motion on visual acuity. *Service Ophthalmol*. 1962;7:83.

81. Weissman S, Freeburne CM. Relationship between static and dynamic visual acuity. *J Exp Psychol*. 1965;69:141.

82. Burg A. Visual acuity as measured by dynamic and static tests: a comparative evaluation. *J Appl Psychol*. 1966;50: 460.

83. Kirshner AJ. Dynamic acuity a quantitative measure of eye movements. *J Am Optom Assoc*. 1967;38:460.

84. Barmack NH. Dynamic visual acuity as an index of eye movement control. *Vis Res*. 1970;10:1377.

85. Brown B. Resolution thresholds for moving targets at the fovea and in the peripheral retina. *Vis Res*. 1972;12:293.

86. Brown B. Dynamic visual acuity, eye movements and peripheral acuity for moving targets. *Vis Res*. 1972;12:305.

87. Brown B. The effect of target contrast variation on dynamic visual acuity and eye movement. *Vis Res*. 1972; 12:1213.

88. Cline D, Hoffstetter HW, Griffin JR. Dictionary of Visual Science. In: Radnor PA, ed. 3rd ed. Chilton; 1980.

89. Hoffman LG, Rouse M, Ryan JB. Dynamic visual acuity: a review. *J Am Optom Assoc*. 1981;52:883.

90. Jendrusch G, Wenzel V, Heck H. The significance of dynamic visual acuity as a performance-influencing parameter in tennis, abstract. *Int J Sports Med*. 1998;19(suppl):46.

91. Ward P, Williams AM. Perceptual and cognitive skill development in soccer: the multidimensional nature of expert performance. *J Sport Exerc Psychol*. 2003;25: 93−111.

92. Rouse MW, DeLand P, Christian R, et al. A comparison study of dynamic visual acuity between athletes and nonathletes. *J Am Optom Assoc*. 1988;59:946.

93. Sherman A. Sports vision testing and enhancement: implications for winter sports. In: Casey M, Foster C, Hixson E, eds. *Winter Sports Medicine*. Philadelphia: FA Davis; 1990:78−84.

94. Ishigaki H, Miyao M. Differences in dynamic visual acuity between athletes and nonathletes. *Percept Mot Skills*. 1993;77:835.

95. Quevedo-Junyent L, Aznar-Casanova JA, Merindano-Encina D. Comparison of dynamic visual acuity between water polo players and sedentary students. *Res Q Exerc Sport*. 2011;82:644−651.

96. Quevedo L, Aznar-Casanova JA, Merindano-Encina D, et al. A novel computer software for the evaluation of dynamic visual acuity. *J Optom*. 2012;5:131−138.

97. Wimshurst ZL, Sowden PT, Cardinale M. Visual skills and playing positions of Olympic field hockey players. *Percept Mot Skills*. 2012;114:204−216.

98. Hoshina K, Tagami Y, Mimura O, et al. A study of static, kinetic, and dynamic visual acuity in 102 Japanese professional baseball players. *Clin Ophthalmol*. 2013;7:627−632.

99. Miskewicz-Zastrow A, Bishop E, Zastrow A, et al. A standardized procedure and normative values for measuring binocular dynamic visual acuity. *Optom Vis Perf*. 2015;3:169−175.

100. Long GM, Penn DL. Dynamic visual acuity: normative functions and practical applications. *Bull Psychonomic Soc*. 1987;25:253.

101. Long GM, Garvey PM. The effects of target wavelength on dynamic visual acuity under photopic and scotopic viewing. *Hum Factors*. 1988;30:3.

102. Coffey B, Reichow AW. Athletes vs. non-athletes: static visual acuity, contrast sensitivity, dynamic visual acuity, abstract. *Invest Ophthalmol Vis Sci*. 1989;30:517.

103. Long GM, Riggs C. Training effects on dynamic visual acuity with free head viewing. *Perception*. 1991;20:363.

104. Burris K, Vittetoe K, Ramger B, et al. Sensorimotor abilities predict on-field performance in professional baseball. *Sci Rep*. 2018;8:116.

105. Smither JA, Kennedy RS. A portable device for the assessment of dynamic visual acuity. *Appl Ergon*. 2010;41: 266−273.

106. Coffey B, Richards L, Olmschenk S, et al. Preliminary normative data for a new device to measure dynamic

visual acuity, abstract. *Optom Vis Sci.* 2004;81(suppl): 127.

107. Coffey B, Buchholz J, Miller K, et al. Test-retest reliability for a new device to measure dynamic visual acuity, abstract. *Optom Vis Sci.* 2005;82. E-abstract 055184.

108. Erickson GB, Citek K, Cove M, et al. Reliability of a computer-based system for measuring visual performance skills. *Optometry.* 2011;82:528–542.

109. Murray N, Hunfalvey M, Roberts CM, Lange B. Reliability and normative data of computerized dynamic visual acuity tests. *Vis Dev Rehabil.* 2017;3:23–32.

110. Uchida Y, Kudoh D, Murakami A, et al. Origins of superior dynamic visual acuity in baseball players: superior eye movements or superior image processing. *PLoS One.* 2012;7(2):e31530.

111. Dippner R. The relation between basketball ability and visual acuity in the unicorn. *Am J Optom Arch Am Acad Optom.* 1973;50:656.

112. Whiting HTA, Sanderson FH. Dynamic visual acuity and performance in a catching task. *J Mot Behav.* 1974;6:87.

113. Sanderson FH, Whiting HTA. Dynamic visual acuity, a factor in catching performance. *J Mot Behav.* 1978; 10(7).

114. Starks JL. Skill in field hockey: the nature of the cognitive advantage. *J Sport Psychol.* 1987;9:146.

115. Millslagle DG. Coincidence anticipation and dynamic visual acuity in young adolescents. *Percept Mot Skills.* 2004; 99(3 Pt 2):1147–1156.

116. Seiderman A, Schneider S. *The Athletic Eye: Improved Sports Performance through Visual Training.* New York: Hearst Books; 1983.

117. Reichow AW, Stern NS. Athlete and optometrist: performance oriented. *OEP Curriculum II.* 1986;59:35.

118. Teig D. Three sports vision skills every patient needs. *Contact Lens Spectr.* 1993;28(19).

119. Ginsburg AP. *Visual Information Processing Based on Spatial Filters Constrained by Biological Data.* Springfield, VA: National Technical Information Service; 1978:97–98.

120. Ginsburg AP. Specifying relevant spatial information for image evaluation and display design: an explanation of how we see certain objects. *Proc SID.* 1980;21:219.

121. Ginsburg AP. Contrast sensitivity: relating visual capability to performance. *USAF Medical Serv Dig.* 1983;34: 15–19.

122. Hoffman LG, Polan G, Powell J. The relationship of contrast sensitivity functions to sports vision. *J Am Optom Assoc.* 1984;55:747.

123. Kluka DA, Love PA, Allen S. Contrast sensitivity functions of selected collegiate female athletes. *Sport Vis.* 1989;5:18.

124. Kluka D, Love P. Contrast sensitivity in international special Olympics, women's invitational volleyball championships, and recreational volleyball players. *Palaestra.* 1992;8:11.

125. Schneider HG, Kluka DA, Love PA. Contrast sensitivity in selected professional and collegiate football players. *J Optom Vis Dev.* 1992;23(4):23.

126. Schellart NA. Contrast sensitivity of air-breathing nonprofessional scuba divers at a depth of 40 meters. *Percept Mot Skills.* 1992;75:275.

127. Love PA, Kluka DA. Contrast sensitivity function in elite women and men softball players. *Int J Sport Vis.* 1993;1:25.

128. Kluka DA, Love PA, Sanet R, et al. Contrast sensitivity function profiling: by sport and sport ability level. *Int J Sport Vis.* 1995;2:5.

129. Kluka DA, Love PA, Covington K, et al. Performance profiles of the intercollegiate softball player and what they mean for the coach. *Sport Vis.* 2000;16:22.

130. Jendrusch G, Wittmann J, Herber F, et al. Strain-induced changes in visual efficiency as exemplified by contrast sensitivity, abstract. *Int J Sports Med.* 1998;19(suppl):46.

131. Grey CP. Changes in contrast sensitivity when wearing low, medium and high water content soft lenses. *J Br Contact Lens Assoc.* 1986;9:21.

132. Nowozyckyj A, Carney LG, Efron N. Effect of hydrogel lens wear on contrast sensitivity. *Am J Optom Physiol Opt.* 1988;65:263.

133. Oxenberg LD, Carney LG. Visual performance with aspheric rigid contact lenses. *Optom Vis Sci.* 1989;66:818.

134. Kluka DA, Love PA. The effects of daily-wear contact lenses on contrast sensitivity in selected professional and collegiate female tennis players. *J Am Optom Assoc.* 1993;64:182.

135. Allen PM, Ravensbergen RHJC, Latham K, et al. Contrast sensitivity is a significant predictor of performance in rifle shooting for athletes with vision impairment. *Front Psychol.* 2018;9:950.

136. Ginsburg AP, Evans DW, Cannon MW, et al. Large sample norms for contrast sensitivity. *Am J Optom Physiol Opt.* 1984;61:80.

137. Corwin TR, Richman JE. Three clinical tests of the spatial contrast sensitivity function: a comparison. *Am J Optom Physiol Opt.* 1986;63:413.

138. Kennedy RS, Dunlap WP. Assessment of the Vistech contrast sensitivity test for repeated-measures applications. *Optom Vis Sci.* 1990;67:248.

139. Brown B, Yap MKH. Variability in repeated contrast sensitivity measures: implications for the individual patient. *Clin Exp Optom.* 1991;74:151.

140. Reeves BC, Wood JM, Hill AR. Vistech VCTS 6500 charts—within- and between-session reliability. *Optom Vis Sci.* 1991;68:728.

141. Elliott DB, Bullimore MA. Assessing the reliability, discriminative ability, and validity of disability glare tests. *Investig Opthalmol Vis Sci.* 1993;34:108–119.

142. Dougherty BE, Flom RE, Bullimore MA. An evaluation of the Mars letter contrast sensitivity test. *Optom Vis Sci.* 2005;82:970–975.

143. Zimmerman AB, Lust KL, Bullimore MA. Visual acuity and contrast sensitivity testing for sports vision. *Eye Contact Lens.* 2011;37:153–159.

144. Tomlinson A, Mann G. An analysis of visual performance with soft contact lens and spectacle correction. *Ophthalmic Physiol Optic.* 1985;5:53.

145. Mohammadi SF, Amiri MA, Naderifar H, et al. Vision examination protocol for archery athletes along with an introduction to sports vision. *Asian J Sports Med.* 2016; 7:e26591.

146. Murphy HL. Sports and vision. *Optom Mon.* 1981;72:20.

147. Griffiths G. Eye dominance in sport: a comparative study. *Optom Today.* 2003;15:34.

148. Laby DM, Kirschen DG. The refractive error of professional baseball players. *Optom Vis Sci.* 2017;94: 564−573.

149. Kirschen DG, Laby DM, Kirschen MP, et al. Optical aberrations in professional baseball players. *J Cataract Refract Surg.* 2010;36:396−401.

150. Porta GB. *De Refractione.* 1593.

151. Classe JG, Daum KM, Semes LP, et al. Association between eye and hand dominance and hitting, fielding and pitching skill among players of the Southern Baseball League. *J Am Optom Assoc.* 1996;67:81.

152. Coons JC, Mathias RJ. Eye and hand preference tendencies. *J Genet Psychol.* 1928;35:629.

153. Miles WR. Ocular dominance demonstrated by unconscious sighting. *J Exp Psychol.* 1929;12:113.

154. Miles WR. Ocular dominance in human adults. *J Gen Psychol.* 1930;3:412.

155. Cuff NB. A study of eyedness and handedness. *J Exp Psychol.* 1930;14:164.

156. Eyre MB, Schmeeckle MM. A study of handedness, eyedness, and footedness. *Child Dev.* 1933;4:73.

157. Washburn MF, Faison C, Scott R. A comparison between the miles A-B-C method and retinal rivalry as tests of eye dominance. *Am J Psychol.* 1934;46:633.

158. Buxton CE, Crosland HR. The concept of "eye preference". *Am J Psychol.* 1937;49:458.

159. Jasper HH, Raney ET. The phi test of lateral dominance. *Am J Psychol.* 1937;49:450.

160. Williams LL. A test to determine the dominant eye. *Optom Wkly.* 1942;33:33.

161. Crider B. A battery of tests for the dominant eye. *J Gen Psychol.* 1944;31:179.

162. Walls GL. A theory of ocular dominance. *AMA Arch Ophthalmol.* 1951;45:387.

163. Crovitz HF, Zener K. A group-test for assessing hand- and eye-dominance. *Am J Psychol.* 1962;75:271.

164. Gronwall DMA, Sampson H. Ocular dominance: a test of two hypotheses. *Br J Psychol.* 1971;62:175.

165. Coren S, Kaplan CP. Patterns of ocular dominance. *Am J Optom Arch Am Acad Optom.* 1973;50:283.

166. Porac C, Coren S. The dominant eye. *Psychol Bull.* 1976; 83:880.

167. Metalis SA, Niemiec AJ. Assessment of eye dominance through response time. *Percept Mot Skills.* 1984;59:539.

168. Coren S, Porac C. Monocular asymmetries in visual latency as a function of sighting dominance. *Am J Optom Physiol Opt.* 1982;59:987.

169. Brown ER, Taylor P. Handedness, footedness, and eyedness. *Percept Mot Skills.* 1988;66:183.

170. Laby DM, Rosenbaum AL, Kirschen D. Ocular dominance, central, etc. and baseball. *Binocul Vis Strabismus Q.* 1988;13:165.

171. Purves D, White LE. Monocular preference in binocular viewing. *Proc Natl Acad Sci USA.* 1994;91:8339−8342.

172. Guillon M, Dalton K, Naroo SA, Maissa CA. Ocular dominance in golf. *Optom Vis Sci.* 2011;88. E-abstract 115053.

173. Laby DM, Kirschen DG. Thought on ocular dominance − is it actually a preference? *Eye Contact Lens.* 2011;37: 140−144.

174. Dalton K, Guillon M, Naroo SA. Ocular dominance and handedness in golf putting. *Optom Vis Sci.* 2015;92: 968−975.

175. Woo TL, Pearson K. Dextrality and sinistrality of hand and eye. *Biometrika.* 1927;19:165.

176. Duke-Elder WS. *Textbook of Ophthalmology.* Vol. 1. St Louis: CV Mosby; 1938:1056−1058.

177. Berner GE, Berner DE. Relation of ocular dominance, handedness, and the controlling eye in binocular vision. *AMA Arch Ophthalmol.* 1953;50:603.

178. Porac C, Coren S. Is eye dominance a part of generalized laterality? *Percept Mot Skills.* 1975;40:763.

179. Rymar K, Kameyama T, Niwa S-I, et al. Hand and eye preference patterns in elementary and junior high school students. *Cortex.* 1984;20:441.

180. Robison S, Jacobsen S, Heintz B. Crossed hand-eye dominance: prevalence in normal and athletic populations. *J Optom Vis Dev.* 1997;28:235.

181. Thomas NG, Harden LM, Rogers GG. Visual evoked potentials, reaction time and eye dominance in cricketers. *J Sports Med Phys Fit.* 2005;45:428−433.

182. Portal JM, Romano PE. Patterns of eye-hand dominance in baseball players. *N Engl J Med.* 1988;319:655.

183. Laby DM, Kirschen DG, Rosenbaum AL, et al. The effect of ocular dominance on the performance of professional baseball players. *Ophthalmology.* 1998;105:864.

184. Portal JM, Romano PE. Ocular sighting dominance: a review and a study of athletic proficiency and eye-hand dominance in a collegiate baseball team. *Binocul Vis Strabismus Q.* 1998;13:125.

185. Stull RB. Study of hand and eye dominance and coordination of basketball players. *J Am Optom Assoc.* 1960; 31:203.

186. Shapiro IL, Kropp L. Hand and eye dominancy in target shooting—part 1. *J Am Optom Assoc.* 1964;35:761.

187. Shapiro IL, Kropp L. Hand and eye dominancy in target shooting—part 2. *J Am Optom Assoc.* 1964;35:863.

188. Adams GL. Effect of eye dominance in baseball batting. *Res Q Am Assoc Health Phys Educ.* 1965;36:3.

189. Gregg JR. Your eyes for shooting. *Optom Wkly.* 1967;58: 37.

190. Falkowitz C, Mendel H. The role of visual skills in batting averages. *Optom Wkly.* 1977;68:33.

191. Gregg JR. How to prescribe for hunters and marksmen. *J Am Optom Assoc.* 1980;51:675.

192. Tieg D. *Major League Baseball Research Project*. Ridgefield, CT: Institute for Sports Vision; 1980:1–9.
193. Gregg JR. Target the sharpshooters in your practice. *Optom Manag*. 1986;22:65.
194. Gregg JR. *Vision and Sports: An Introduction*. Stoneham, MA: Butterworth Publishers; 1987:148–154.
195. Dunham P. Coincidence-anticipation performance of adolescent baseball players and nonplayers. *Percept Mot Skills*. 1989;68:1151.
196. Noll JE. Vision considerations in shooting sports. *N Engl J Optom*. 1990;42:6.
197. Steinberg GM, Frehlich SG, Tennant LK. Dextrality and eye position in putting performance. *Percept Mot Skills*. 1995;80:635.
198. Jones LF, Classe JG, Hester M, et al. Association between eye dominance and training for rifle marksmanship: a pilot study. *J Am Optom Assoc*. 1996;67:73.
199. Milne C, Buckolz E, Cardenas M. Relationship of eye dominance and batting performance in baseball players. *Int J Sport Vis*. 1995;2:17.
200. Goss DA. The relationship of eye dominance and baseball batting: a critical literature review. *J Behav Optom*. 1998;9:87.
201. Shick J. Relationship between depth perception and hand-eye dominance and free-throw shooting in college women. *Percept Mot Skills*. 1971;33:539.
202. Sugiyama Y, Lee MS. Relation of eye dominance with performance and subjective ratings in golf putting. *Percept Mot Skills*. 2005;100:761–766.
203. Laborde S, Desseville FE, Leconte P, Margas N. Interaction of hand preference with eye dominance on accuracy in archery. *Percept Mot Skills*. 2009;108:558–564.
204. Rombouts SA, Barkhof F, Sprenger M, et al. The functional basis of ocular dominance: functional MRI findings. *Neurosci Lett*. 1996;221(1).
205. Schor CM, Flom MC. The relative value of stereopsis as a function of viewing distance. *Am J Optom Arch Am Acad Optom*. 1969;46:805.
206. Ebenholtz SM, Wolfson DM. Perceptual aftereffects of sustained convergence. *Percept Psychophys*. 1975;17:485.
207. Paap KR, Ebenholtz SM. Perceptual consequences of potentiation in the extraocular muscles: an alternative explanation for adaptation to wedge prisms. *J Exp Psychol Hum Percept Perform*. 1976;27.
208. Paap KR, Ebenholtz SM. Concomitant direction and distance aftereffects of sustained convergence: a muscle potentiation explanation for eye-specific adaptation. *Percept Psychophys*. 1977;21:307.
209. Ebenholtz SM, Fisher SK. Distance adaptation depends upon the plasticity in the oculomotor control system. *Percept Psychophys*. 1982;31:551.
210. Shebilske WL, Karmiohl CM, Profit DR. Induced esophoric shifts in eye convergence and illusory distance in reduced and structured viewing conditions. *J Exp Psychol Hum Percept Perform*. 1983;9:270.
211. Graybiel A, Jokl E, Trapp C. Russian studies of vision in relation to physical activity and sports. *Res Q Am Assoc Health Phys Educ*. 1955;26:480.
212. Pickwell D. Binocular vision in sport. *Optom Today*. 1986;26:240.
213. Schor CM, Ciuffreda KJ. *Vergence Eye Movements*. London: Butterworth; 1983.
214. Sheedy JE. Actual measurement of fixation disparity and its use in diagnosis and treatment. *J Am Optom Assoc*. 1980;51:1079.
215. Stuart JA, Burian HM. Changes in horizontal heterophoria with elevation and depression of gaze. *Am J Ophthalmol*. 1962;53:274.
216. McKee MC, Young DA, Kohl P, et al. Effect of head and eye positions on fixation disparities, phorias, and ductions at near. *Am J Optom Physiol Opt*. 1987;64:909.
217. Coffey B, Reichow AW, Colburn PB, et al. Influence of ocular gaze and head position on 4 m heterophoria and fixation disparity. *Optom Vis Sci*. 1991;68:893.
218. Coffey B, Mathison T, Viker M, et al. Visual alignment considerations in golf putting consistency. In: Cochran AJ, ed. *Science and Golf: Proceedings of the First World Scientific Congress of Golf*. London: E&FN Spon; 1990:76–80.
219. Wheatstone C. Contributions to the physiology of vision. Part the first. On some remarkable and hitherto unobserved, phenomena of binocular vision. *Phil Trans Roy Soc Lond*. 1838;128:371.
220. Hubel DH, Wiesel TN. Receptive fields of single neurones in the cat's striate cortex. *J Physiol*. 1959;148:574.
221. Nikara T, Bishop PO, Pettigrew JD. Analysis of retinal correspondence by studying receptive fields of binocular single units in cat striate cortex. *Exp Brain Res*. 1968;6:353.
222. Bishop PO, Henry GH, Smith CJ. Binocular interaction fields of single units in the cat striate cortex. *J Physiol*. 1971;216:39.
223. Regan D, Beverly KI. Electrophysiological evidence for existence of neurones sensitive to direction of depth movement. *Nature*. 1973;246:504.
224. Richards W, Regan D. A stereo field map with implications for disparity processing. *Invest Ophthalmol Vis Sci*. 1973;12:904.
225. Pettigrew JD. Binocular neurones which signal change of disparity in area 18 of cat visual cortex. *Nat New Biol*. 1973;241:123.
226. Zeki SM. Cells responding to changing image size and disparity in the cortex of the rhesus monkey. *J Physiol*. 1974;242:827.
227. Beverly KI, Regan D. The relation between discrimination and sensitivity in the perception of motion in depth. *J Physiol*. 1975;249:387.
228. Cynader M, Regan D. Neurones in cat parastriate cortex sensitive to the direction of motion in three-dimensional space. *J Physiol*. 1978;274:549.
229. Regan D, Beverley KI. Binocular and monocular stimuli for motion in depth: changing-disparity and changing-size feed the same motion-in-depth stage. *Vis Res*. 1979;19:1331.
230. Regan D, Beverley K, Cynader M. The visual perception of motion in depth. *Sci Am*. 1979;241:136.

231. Cynader M, Regan D. Neurons in cat visual cortex tuned to the direction of motion in depth: effects of positional disparity. *Vis Res.* 1982;22:967.

232. Toyama K, Kozasa T. Responses of Clare-Bishop neurones to three dimensional movement of light stimulus. *Vis Res.* 1982;22:571.

233. Schor CM, Wood IC, Ogawa J. Spatial tuning of static and dynamic local stereopsis. *Vis Res.* 1984;24:573.

234. Regan D, Erkelens CJ, Collewijn H. Necessary conditions for the perception of motion in depth. *Invest Ophthalmol Vis Sci.* 1986;27:584.

235. Regan D. Visual processing of four kinds of relative motion. *Vis Res.* 1986;26:127.

236. Regan D, Regan MP. Objective evidence for phase-independent spatial frequency analysis in the human visual pathway. *Vis Res.* 1988;28:187.

237. Hong X, Regan D. Visual field defects for unidirectional and oscillatory motion in depth. *Vis Res.* 1989;29:809.

238. Rouse MW, Tittle JS, Braunstein ML. Stereoscopic depth perception by static stereo-deficient observers in dynamic displays with constant and changing disparity. *Optom Vis Sci.* 1989;66:355.

239. Regan D. The Charles F. Prentice award lecture 1990: specific tests and specific blindnesses: keys, locks and parallel processing. *Optom Vis Sci.* 1991;68:489.

240. Nemire K. Automated system for ball launching, visual occlusion, and data acquisition in a ball hitting task. *Behav Res Methods.* 1991;23:36.

241. Regan D. Visual judgments and misjudgments in cricket, and the art of flight. *Perception.* 1992;21:91.

242. Savelsbergh GJP, Whiting HTA. The acquisition of catching under monocular and binocular conditions. *J Mot Behav.* 1992;24:320.

243. von Hofsten C, Rosengren K, Pick HL, et al. The role of binocular information in ball catching. *J Mot Behav.* 1992;24:329.

244. Graydon J, Bawden M, Holder T, et al. The effects of binocular and monocular vision on a table tennis striking task under conditions of spatial-temporal uncertainty. *Int J Sport Vis.* 1996;3:35.

245. Sheedy JE, Bailey IL, Buri M, et al. Binocular vs. monocular task performance. *Am J Optom Physiol Opt.* 1986;63:839.

246. Poffenberger AT. Reaction time to retinal stimulation with special reference to the time lost in conduction through nerve centers. *Arch Psychol N Y.* 1912;23(1).

247. Ueno T. Reaction time as a measure of temporal summation at suprathreshold levels. *Vis Res.* 1977;17:227.

248. Blake R, Martens W, DiGianfilippo A. Reaction time as a measure of binocular interaction in human vision. *Invest Ophthalmol Vis Sci.* 1980;19:930.

249. Harwerth RS, Smith EL, Levi DM. Suprathreshold binocular interactions for grating patterns. *Percept Psychophys.* 1980;27:43.

250. Jones RK, Lee DN. Why two eyes are better than one: the two views of binocular vision. *J Exp Psychol.* 1981;7:30.

251. Woodman W, Young M, Kelly K, et al. Effects of monocular occlusion on neural and motor response times of two dimensional stimuli. *Optom Vis Sci.* 1990;67:169.

252. Molia LM, Rubin SE, Kohn N. Assessment of stereopsis in college baseball pitchers and batters. *J AAPOS.* 1998;2(2):86–90.

253. Jenerou A, Bauer A, Reich K. Stereopsis' play on baseball. *Optom Vis Perf.* 2017;5:14–19.

254. Boden LM, Rosengren KJ, Martin DF, Boden SD. A comparison of static near stereo acuity in youth baseball/softball players and non-ball players. *Optometry.* 2009;80:121–125.

255. Hunfalvay M, Orr R, Murray N, Roberts C-M. Evaluation of stereo acuity in professional baseball and LPGA athletes compared to non-athletes. *Vis Dev Rehabil.* 2017;3:33–41.

256. Weissman S. Sex differences in dynamic stereoacuity, *Proceedings of the 80th Annual Convention. Am Psychol Assoc.* 1972;7:81.

257. Weissman S, Slonim P. Effects of knowledge of results on dynamic stereo acuity in males and females. *Percept Mot Skills.* 1973;36:964.

258. Slonim PS, Weissman S, Galzer E, et al. Effects of training on dynamic stereo acuity performance by males and females. *Percept Mot Skills.* 1975;40:359.

259. Solomon H, Zinn W. An introduction to dynamic sports vision. *Optom Mon.* 1983;74:569.

260. Zinn WJ, Solomon H. A comparison of static and dynamic stereoacuity. *J Am Optom Assoc.* 1985;56:712.

261. Soloman H, Zinn HJ, Vacroux R. Dynamic stereoacuity: a test for hitting a baseball? *J Am Optom Assoc.* 1988;59:522.

262. Hofeldt AJ, Hoefle FB. Stereophotometric testing for Pulfrich's phenomenon in professional baseball players. *Percept Mot Skills.* 1993;77:407.

263. Laby DM, Kirschen DG. Dynamic stereoacuity: preliminary results and normative data for a test for the quantitative measurement of motion in depth. *Bi Vis Eye Muscle Surg Q.* 1995;10:191.

264. Hofeldt AJ, Hoefle FB, Bonafede B. Baseball hitting, binocular vision, and the Pulfrich phenomenon. *Arch Ophthalmol.* 1996;114:1490.

265. Clark B, Warren N. Depth perception and interpupillary distance as factors in proficiency in ball games. *Am J Psychol.* 1935;47:485.

266. Dickinson J. *The Relationship of Depth Perception to Goal Shooting in Basketball* [dissertation]. Iowa State University; 1953.

267. Montebello RA. *The Role of Stereoscopic Vision in Some Aspects of Baseball Playing Ability.* Ohio State University College of Optometry; 1953 [thesis].

268. Olsen EA. Relationship between psychological capacities and success in college athletics. *Res Q Am Assoc Health Phys Educ.* 1956;27:79.

269. Deshaies P, Pargman D. Selected visual abilities of college football players. *Percept Mot Skills.* 1976;43:904.

270. Ridini LM. Relationship between psychological functions tests and selected sport skills of boys in junior high. *Res Q Am Assoc Health Phys Educ.* 1968;39:674.

271. Chang S-T, Liu Y-H, Lee J-S, See L-C. Comparing sports vision among three groups of soft tennis adolescent athletes: normal vision, refractive errors with and without correction. *Indian J Ophthalmol.* 2015;63:716−721.

272. Erickson G, Citek K, Yoo H, Reichow A. A Comparison of stereoacuity at 6 m of collegiate baseball players in primary gaze and batting stance [Abstract]. *J Vis.* 2010; 10(7):374. https://doi.org/10.1167/10.7.374.

273. Yoo H, Reichow A, Erickson G. Stereoacuity of athletes in primary and non-primary gazes [abstract]. *J Vis.* 2011; 11(11):331. https://doi.org/10.1167/11.11.331.

274. Garzia RP, Nicholson S. A study of binocular accommodative and vergence facility and predictive analysis of global stereopsis. *J Behav Optom.* 1991;2(3).

275. Jafarzadehpur E, Aazami N, Bolouri B. Comparison of saccadic eye movements and facility of ocular accommodation in female volleyball players and non-players. *Scand J Med Sci Sports.* 2007;17:186−190.

276. Di Russo F, Pitzalis S, Spinelli D. Fixation stability and saccadic latency in elite shooters. *Vis Res.* 2003;43: 1837−1845.

277. Griffin JR, Borsting EJ. *Binocular Anomalies: Theory, Testing and Therapy.* 5th ed. Santa Ana, CA: Optometric Extension Program Foundation; 2010:21−33.

278. Scheiman M, Wick B. *Clinical Management of Binocular Vision: Heterophoric, Accommodative, and Eye Movement Disorders.* Philadelphia: Wolters Kluwer Health; 2020:24−31.

279. Maples WC. Oculomotor dysfunctions: classification of saccadic and pursuit deficiencies. In: Press LJ, ed. *Applied Concepts in Vision Therapy.* St Louis: Mosby; 1997:120−136.

280. Feldon SE, Burde RA. The oculomotor system. In: Moses RA, Hart WM, eds. *Adler's Physiology of the Eye: Clinical Application.* St Louis: C.V. Mosby; 1987:142.

281. Bahill AT, LaRitz T. Why can't batters keep their eyes on the ball? *Am Sci.* 1984;72:249.

282. Brown S, Couper T. Visual and ocular motility performance of one hundred cricketers. *Aust Orthoptic J.* 1990; 70:175.

283. Land MF, McLeod P. From eye movements to actions: how batsmen hit the ball. *Nat Neurosci.* 2000;3: 1340−1345.

284. Lenoir M, Crevits L, Goethals M, et al. Are better eye movements an advantage in ball games? A study of pro-saccadic and antisaccadic eye movements. *Percept Mot Skills.* 2000;91:546−552.

285. Babu RJ, Lillakas L, Irving EL. Dynamics of saccadic adaptation: differences between athletes and nonathletes. *Optom Vis Sci.* 2005;82:1060.

286. Ceyte H, Lion A, Caudron S, et al. Visuo-oculomotor skills related to the visual demands of sporting environments. *Exp Brain Res.* 2017;235:269−277.

287. Whittaker SG, Eaholtz G. Learning patterns of eye motion for foveal pursuit. *Invest Ophthalmol Vis Sci.* 1982; 23:393.

288. McHugh DE, Bahill AT. Learning to track predictable target waveforms without a time delay. *Invest Ophthalmol Vis Sci.* 1985;26:932.

289. Carnahan H, Hall C, Lee TD. Delayed visual feedback while learning to track a moving target. *Res Q Exerc Sport.* 1996;67:416.

290. Adolphe RM, Vickers JN, Laplante G. The effects of training visual attention on gaze behavior and accuracy: a pilot project. *Int J Sport Vis.* 1997;4:29.

291. Elmurr P, Cornell E, Heard R. Saccadic eye movements (part 2): the effects of practice on saccadic reaction time. *Int J Sport Vis.* 1997;4:13.

292. Morrillo M, Di Russo F, Pitzalis S, Spinelli D. Latency of prosaccades and antisaccades in professional shooters. *Med Sci Sports Exerc.* 2006;38:388−394.

293. Mann DL, Spratford W, Abernethy B. The head tracks and gaze predicts: how the world's best batters hit a ball. *PLoS One.* 2013;8(3):e58289.

294. Fogt NF, Zimmerman AB. A method to monitor eye and head tracking movements in college baseball players. *Optom Vis Sci.* 2014;91:200−211.

295. Fogt N, Persson TW. A pilot study of horizontal head and eye rotations in baseball batting. *Optom Vis Sci.* 2017;94: 789−796.

296. Higuchi T, Nagami T, Nakata H, Kanosue K. Head-eye movement of collegiate baseball batters during fastball hitting. *PLoS One.* 2018:e0200443.

297. Kishita Y, Ueda H, Kashino M. Eye and head movements of elite players in real batting. *Front Sports Act Living.* 2020;2:3.

298. Kubitz K, Roberts C-M, Hunfalvey M, Murray N. A comparison of cardinal gaze speed between major league baseball players, amateur prospects, and non-athletes. *J Sport Perform Vis.* 2020;2(1):e17−28.

299. Mahadas K, Mohammand F, Samim H, et al. Timing differences in eye-hand coordination between experienced and inexperienced tennis players. *Optom Vis Perf.* 2015; 3(2):149−158.

300. Von Lassberg C, Beykirch K, Campos JL, Krug J. Smooth pursuit eye movement adaptation in high level gymnasts. *Mot Contr.* 2012;16:176−194.

301. Liu S, Edmunds FR, Burris K, Appelbaum LG. Visual and oculomotor abilities predict professional baseball batting performance. *bioRxiv.* 2020;1(21):913152.

302. Trachtman JN. The relationship between ocular motilities and batting average in little leaguers. *Am J Optom Arch Am Acad Optom.* 1973;50:914.

303. Maples WC. *Oculomotor Test Manual.* Santa Ana, CA: Optometric Extension Program Foundation; 1995.

304. Garzia RP, Richman JE, Nicholson SB, et al. A new visual-verbal saccade test: the Developmental Eye Movement test (DEM). *J Am Optom Assoc.* 1990;61:124.

305. Abernethy B. Enhancing sports performance through clinical and experimental optometry. *Clin Exp Optom.* 1986;69:189.

306. Nagano T, Kato T, Fukuta T. Visual search strategies of soccer players in one-on-one defensive situations on the field. *Percept Mot Skills.* 2004;99:968.

307. Land MF. Vision, eye movements, and natural behavior. *Vis Neurosci.* 2009;26:51−62.

308. Piras A, Lobietti R, Squatrito S. A study of saccadic eye movement dynamics in volleyball: comparison between athletes and non-athletes. *J Sports Med Phys Fit.* 2010;50:99−108.

309. Piras A, Vickers JN. The effect of fixation transitions on quiet eye duration and performance in the soccer penalty kick: instep versus inside kicks. *Cogn Process.* 2011;12:245−255.

310. Timmis MA, Turner K, van Paridon KN. Visual search strategies of soccer players executing a power vs. placement penalty kick. *PLoS One.* 2014;9(12), e115179.

311. Wilson M, Causer J, Vickers J. Aiming for excellence: the quiet eye as a characteristic of expertise. In: Baker J, Farrow D, eds. *Handbook of Sport Expertise.* London: Routledge/Taylor and Francis; 2015:22−37.

312. Vickers JN. Visual control when aiming at a far target. *J Exp Psychol Hum Percept Perform.* 1996;2:324.

313. Vickers JN. Origins and current issues in Quiet Eye research. *Curr Issues Sport Sci.* 2016;1:1−11.

314. Ruch TC. Binocular vision and central visual pathways. In: Fulton JA, ed. *A Textbook of Physiology.* Philadelphia: Saunders; 1949:471.

315. Hobson R, Henderson MT. A preliminary study of the visual field in athletics. *Proc Iowa Acad Sci.* 1941;48:331.

316. Johnson WG. *Peripheral Perception of Athletes and Non-athletes, and the Effect of Practice.* University of Illinois; 1952 [thesis].

317. Buchellew WF. *Peripheral Perception and Reaction Time of Athletes and Non-athletes.* University of Illinois; 1954 [thesis].

318. Stroup F. Relationship between measurements of field of motion perception and basketball ability in college men. *Res Q Am Assoc Health Phys Educ.* 1957;28:72.

319. Williams JM, Thirer J. Vertical and horizontal peripheral vision in male and female athletes and non-athletes. *Res Q Am Assoc Health Phys Educ.* 1976;46:200.

320. Berg WP, Killian SM. Size of the visual field in collegiate fast-pitch softball players and nonathletes. *Percept Mot Skills.* 1995;81:1307.

321. Blundell NL. The contribution of vision to the learning and performance of sports skills. Part 2: the effects of exercise, altitude and visual training. *Aust J Sci Med Sport.* 1985;17(3).

322. Fleury M, Bard C. Fatigue metabolique et performancede taches visuelles. *Can J Sport Sci.* 1990;15:43.

323. Koskela PU. The effect of jogging on visual field indices. *Acta Ophthalmol.* 1990;68:91.

324. Wood JM, Woods RL, Jack MP. Exercise does not increase visual field sensitivity. *Optom Vis Sci.* 1994;71:682.

325. Grall V, Lessing T, Jendrusch G, et al. Synchronoptical ability of differentiation—exemplified by the foot fault in tennis. *Int J Sports Med.* 1998;19:S45.

326. Grall V, Pfennig H, Jendrusch G, et al. Trainability of synchronoptical identification ability. *Int J Sports Med.* 1998;19:S45.

327. Ryu D, Abernethy B, Mann DL, et al. The role of central and peripheral vision in expert decision making. *Perception.* 2013;42:591−607.

328. Opdenacker K, Jendrusch G, Heck H. Effect of physical activity on the performance of perceptual tasks in central and peripheral vision. In: Mester J, King G, Struder H, et al., eds. Perspectives and Profiles, *Sixth Annual Congress of the European College of Sports Science, 15th Congress of the German Society of Sport Science, Cologne, July 2001.* 2001:827.

329. Beckerman SA, Zost MG. Effect of lighting levels on performance on the Wayne computerized saccadic fixator and Wayne Peripheral Awareness trainer. *J Behav Optom.* 1994;5:155.

330. Zwierko T. Differences in peripheral perception between athletes and nonathletes. *J Hum Kinet.* 2007;19:53−62.

331. Zwierko T, Głowacki T, Osinski W. The effect of specific anaerobic exercises on peripheral perception in handball players. *Kinesiol Slov.* 2008;14:68−76.

332. Zwierko T, Osinski W, Lubinski W, et al. Speed of visual sensorimotor processes and conductivity of visual pathway in volleyball players. *J Hum Kinet.* 2010;23:21−27.

333. Jiménez-Pavón D, Romeo J, Cervantes-Borunda M, et al. Effects of a running bout in the heat on cognitive performance. *J Exerc Sci Fit.* 2011;9:58−64.

334. Mankowska M, Poliszczuk T, Poliszczuk D, Johne M. Visual perception and its effect on reaction time and time-movement anticipation in elite female basketball players. *Pol J Sport Tour Sci.* 2015;22:3−8.

335. Schumacher N, Schmidt M, Reer R, Braumann K-M. Peripheral vision tests in sports: training effects and reliability of peripheral perception test. *Int J Environ Res Publ Health.* 2019;16:500.

336. Martin WF. *An Insight to Sports: Featuring Trapshooting and Golf.* Seattle: SportsVision; 1984.

337. Vickers D, Nettlebeck T, Willson RJ. Perceptual indices of performance: the measurement of "inspection time" and "noise" in the visual system. *Perception.* 1972;1:263.

338. Vickers D, Smith PL. The rationale for the inspection time index. *Pers Indiv Differ.* 1986;7:609.

339. Dumler MJ. A study of factors related to gains in the reading rate of college students trained with the tachistoscope and accelerator. *J Educ Res.* 1958;52:27.

340. Brand CR, Dreary IJ. Intelligence and "inspection time." In: Eysenck HJ, ed. *A Model for Intelligence.* New York: Springer; 1982:133−148.

341. Nettlebeck T. Inspection time and intelligence. In: *Vernon PA, Editor: Speed of Information Processing and Intelligence.* Norwood, NJ: Ablex; 1987:295−346.

342. Zhang Y, Caryl PG, Deary IJ. Evoked potential correlates of inspection time. *Pers Indiv Differ.* 1989;10:379.

343. Dreary IJ, Mitchell H. Inspection time and high-speed ball games. *Perception.* 1989;18:789.

344. Abernethy B, Russell DG. Advance cue utilization by skilled cricket batsmen. *Aust J Sci Med Sport.* 1984;16:2−10.

345. Isaacs LD, Finch AE. Anticipatory timing of beginning and intermediate tennis players. *Percept Mot Skills.* 1983;57:451.

346. Nettleton B. Flexibility of attention and elite athletes' performance in "fast ball games. *Percept Mot Skills*. 1986;63: 991.

347. Goulet C, Bard M, Fleury M. Expertise differences in preparing to returns a tennis serve: a visual information processing approach. *J Sport Psychol*. 1989;11:382.

348. Wright DL, Pleasants F, Gomez-Meza M. Use of advanced visual cue sources in volleyball. *J Sport Exerc Psychol*. 1990; 12:406.

349. Muller S, Abernethy B, Farrow D. How do world-class cricket batsmen anticipate a bowler's intention? *Q J Exp Psychol*. 2006;59:2162–2186.

350. Reichow AW, Garchow KE, Baird RY. Do scores on a tachistoscope test correlate with baseball batting average? *Eye Contact Lens*. 2011;37:123–126.

351. McLeod P. Visual reaction time and high-speed ball games. *Perception*. 1987;16:49.

352. Laby DM, Kirschen DG, Govindarajulu U, DeLand P. The effect of visual function on the batting performance of professional baseball players. *Sci Rep*. 2019; 9:16847.

353. Pylyshyn ZW, Storm RW. Tracking multiple independent targets: evidence for a parallel tracking mechanism. *Spatial Vis*. 1988;3:179–197.

354. Cavanagh P, Alvarez GA. Tracking multiple targets with multifocal attention. *Trends Cognit Sci*. 2005;9: 349–354.

355. Memmert D. Pay attention! A review of visual attentional expertise in sport. *Int Rev Sport Exerc Psychol*. 2009;2: 119–138.

356. Memmert D, Simons DJ, Grimme T. The relationship between visual attention and expertise in sports. *Psychol Sport Exerc*. 2009;10:146–151.

357. Zhang X, Yan M, Yangang L. Differential performance of Chinese volleyball athletes and nonathletes on a multiple-object tracking task. *Percept Mot Skills*. 2009; 109:747–756.

358. Faubert J, Sidebottom L. Perceptual-cognitive training of athletes. *J Clin Sport Psychol*. 2012;6:85–102.

359. Faubert J. Professional athletes have extraordinary skills for rapidly learning complex and neutral dynamic visual scenes. *Sci Rep*. 2013;3:1154.

360. Mangine GT, Hoffman JR, Wells AJ, et al. Visual tracking speed is related to basketball-specific measures of performance in NBA players. *J Strength Condit Res*. 2014;28: 2406–2414.

361. Romeas T, Faubert J. Soccer athletes are superior to nonathletes at perceiving soccer-specific and non-sport specific human biological motion. *Front Psychol*. 2015;6: 1343.

362. Alvarez GA, Franconeri SL. How many objects can you track? Evidence for a resource-limited attentive tracking mechanism. *J Vis*. 2007;7(13):14.

363. Qiu F, Pi Y, Liu K, et al. Influence of sports expertise level on attention in multiple object tracking. *Peer J*. 2018;6: e5732.

364. Finke RA. Mental imagery and the visual system. *Sci Am*. 1986;254:88.

365. Roland PE, Larsen B, Lassen NA, et al. Supplementary motor area and other cortical areas in organization of voluntary movement in man. *J Neurophysiol*. 1980;43:118.

366. Roland PE, Friberg L. Localization of cortical areas activated by thinking. *J Neurophysiol*. 1985;53:1219.

367. Deutsch G, Bourbon WT, Papanicolaou AC, et al. Visuospatial tasks compared via activation of regional cerebral blood flow. *Neuropsychologia*. 1988;26:445.

368. Naito E. Controllability of motor imagery and transformation of visual imagery. *Percept Mot Skills*. 1994;78:479.

369. Mahoney M, Avener J. Psychology of the elite athlete: an exploratory study. *Cognit Ther Res*. 1977;1:135.

370. Meyers AW, Cooke CJ, Cullen J, et al. Psychological aspects of athletic competitors: a replication across sports. *Cognit Ther Res*. 1979;3:361.

371. Greenspan MJ, Feltz DL. Psychological interventions with athletes in competitive situations: a review. *Sport Psychol*. 1989;3:219.

372. Davis H. Cognitive style and nonsport imagery in elite ice hockey performance. *Percept Mot Skills*. 1990;71:795.

373. White A, Hardy L. An in-depth analysis of the uses of imagery by high-level slalom canoeists and artistic gymnasts. *Sport Psychol*. 1998;12:387–403.

374. Callow N, Hardy L. Types of imagery associated with sport confidence in netball players of varying skill levels. *J Appl Sport Psychol*. 2001;13:1–7.

375. Cumming J, Hall C. Athletes' use of imagery in the offseason. *Sport Psychol*. 2002;16:160–172.

376. Weinberg R, Butt J, Knight B, et al. The relationship between the use and effectiveness of imagery: an exploratory investigation. *J Appl Sport Psychol*. 2003;15:26–40.

377. Arvinen-Barrow M, Weigand DA, Thomas S, et al. Elite and novice athletes' imagery use in open and closed sports. *J Appl Sport Psychol*. 2007;19:93–104.

378. MacKay DG. The problem of rehearsal or mental practice. *J Mot Behav*. 1981;13:274.

379. Hale BD. The effects of internal and external imagery on muscular and ocular concomitants. *J Sport Psychol*. 1982; 4:374.

380. Feltz DL, Landers DM. The effects of mental practice on motor skill learning and performance: a meta-analysis. *J Sport Psychol*. 1983;5:25.

381. Kohl RM, Roenker DL. Mechanism involvement during skill imagery. *J Mot Behav*. 1983;15:179.

382. Feltz DL, Landers DM, Becker BJ. *A Revised Meta-Analysis of the Mental Practice Literature on Motor Skill Learning*. Washington, DC: National Academy Press; 1988.

383. Requin J. Neural basis of movement representations. In: Requin J, Stelmach GE, eds. *Tutorials in Motor Neurosciences*. Dordrecht, The Netherlands: Kluwer; 1991:333–345.

384. Jeannerod M. The representing brain: neural correlates of motor intention and imagery. *Brain Behav Sci*. 1994;17: 187.

385. Schuster C, Hilfiker R, Amft O, et al. Best practice for motor imagery: a systematic literature review on motor imagery training elements in five different disciplines. *BMC Med*. 2011;9:75.

386. Decety J, Ingvar DH. Brain structures participating in mental stimulation of motor behavior: a neuropsychological interpretation. *Acta Psychol.* 1990;73:13.

387. Decety J, Kawashima R, Gulyas B, et al. Preparation for reaching: a PET study of the participating structures in the human brain. *Neuroreport.* 1992;3:761.

388. Decety J. Do imagined and executed actions share the same neural substrate? *Cognit Brain Res.* 1996;3:87.

389. Jacobson E. Electrophysiology of mental activities. *Am J Psychol.* 1932;44:676.

390. Ulich E. Some experiments on the function of mental training in the acquisition of motor skills. *Ergonomics.* 1967;10:411.

391. McGuigan FJ. Covert oral behavior during the silent performance of language tasks. *Psychol Bull.* 1970;74:309.

392. Harris DV, Robinson WJ. The effects of skill level on EMG activity during internal and external imagery. *J Sport Psychol.* 1986;8:105.

393. Decety J, Michel F. Comparative analysis of actual and mental movements times in two graphic tasks. *Brain Cognit.* 1989;11:87.

394. de'Sperati C, Deubel H. Mental extrapolation of motion modulates responsiveness to visual stimuli. *Vis Res.* 2006;16:2593.

395. Decety J, Jeannerod M, Preblanc C. The timing of mentally represented actions. *Behav Brain Res.* 1989;34:35.

396. Decety J. Motor information may be important for updating the cognitive processes involved in mental imagery of movement. *Eur Bull Cognit Psychol.* 1991;4:415.

397. Decety J, Jeannerod M. Fitts' law in mentally simulated movements. *Behav Brain Res.* 1996;72:127.

398. Reed CL. Chronometric comparisons of imagery to action: visualizing versus physically performing springboard dives. *Mem Cognit.* 2002;30:1169.

399. Yu QH, Fu ASN, Kho A, et al. Imagery perspective among young athletes: differentiation between external and internal visual imagery. *J Sport Health Sci.* 2016;5:211–218.

400. Montuori S, Curcio G, Sorrentino P, et al. Functional role of internal and external visual imagery: preliminary evidences from pilates. *Neural Plast.* 2018, 7235872.

401. Suin R. Removing emotional obstacles to learning and performance by visuo-motor behavior rehearsal. *Behav Ther.* 1972;3:308.

402. Suin R. Behavior rehearsal training for ski racers. *Behav Ther.* 1972;3:519.

403. Suin R. Visual motor behavior rehearsal: the basic technique. *Scand J Behav Ther.* 1984;13:131.

404. Suin R. Imagery rehearsal applications to performance enhancement. *Behav Ther.* 1985;8:155.

405. Suin R. *Seven Steps to Peak Performance: The Mental Training Manual for Athletes.* Toronto: Huber; 1986.

406. Sherman A. Overview of research information regarding vision and sports. *J Am Optom Assoc.* 1980;51:661.

407. Hall C, Buckoltz E, Fishburne G. Imagery and acquisition of motor skills. *Mem Cognit.* 1992;7:19.

408. Driskell JE, Copper C, Moran A. Does mental practice enhance performance? *J Appl Psychol.* 1992;79:481.

409. Salmon J, Hall C, Haslam I. The use of imagery by soccer players. *J Appl Sport Psychol.* 1994;6:116.

410. Zervas Y, Kakkos V. Visuomotor behavior rehearsal in archery shooting performance. *Percept Mot Skills.* 1991; 73:1183.

411. Corbin CB. Mental practice. In: Morgan WP, ed. *Ergonomic Aids and Muscular Performance.* New York: Academic Press; 1972:93–118.

412. Richardson A. *Mental Imagery.* New York: Springer; 1969.

413. Hall E, Erffmeyer SE. The effect of visuo-motor behavior rehearsal with videotaped modeling on free throw accuracy of intercollegiate female basketball players. *J Sport Psychol.* 1983;5:343.

414. Gray SW, Fernandez S. Effects of visuo-motor behavior rehearsal with videotaped modeling on basketball performance. *Psychol J Hum Behav.* 1989;26:41.

415. Guillot A, Nadrowska E, Collet C. Using motor imagery to learn tactical movements in basketball. *J Sport Behav.* 2009;32:189–206.

416. Noel RC. The effect of visuo-motor behavior rehearsal on tennis performance. *J Sport Psychol.* 1980;2:221.

417. Weinberg RS, Gould D, Jackson A, et al. Influence on cognitive strategies on tennis serves of high and low ability. *Percept Mot Skills.* 1980;50:663.

418. Dana A, Gozalzadeh E. Internal and external imagery effects on tennis skills among novices. *Percept Mot Skills.* 2017;124:1022–1043.

419. Weinberg RS, Seabourne TG, Jackson A. Effects of visuomotor behavior rehearsal, relaxation, and imagery on karate performance. *J Sport Psychol.* 1981;3:228.

420. Weinberg RS, Seabourne TG, Jackson A. Effects of visuomotor behavior rehearsal on state-trait anxiety and performance: is practice important? *J Sport Behav.* 1982;5: 209.

421. Seabourne TG, Weinberg R, Jackson A, et al. Effect of individualized practice and training of visuo-motor behavior rehearsal in enhancing karate performance. *J Sport Behav.* 1984;7:58.

422. Seabourne TG, Weinberg R, Jackson A. Effect of individualized, nonindividualized and package intervention strategies on karate performance. *J Sport Psychol.* 1985; 7:40.

423. Yamamoto K, Inomata K. Effects of mental rehearsal with past and whole demonstration models on acquisition of backstroke swimming skills. *Percept Mot Skills.* 1982;54: 1067.

424. Lee AB, Hewitt J. Using visual imagery in a floatation tank to improve gymnastic performance and reduce physical symptoms. *Int J Sport Psychol.* 1987;18:223.

425. Gray SW. Effect of visuomotor rehearsal with videotaped modeling on racquetball performance of beginning players. *Percept Mot Skills.* 1990;70:379.

426. Meacci WG, Price EE. Acquisition and retention of golf putting skill through the relaxation, visualization and body rehearsal intervention. *Res Q Exerc Sport.* 1985;56:176.

427. Meacci WG, Pastore DL. Golf: making short putts. *Strategies.* 1992;5:13.

428. Meacci WG, Pastore DL. Effects of occluded vision and imagery on putting golf balls. *Percept Mot Skills.* 1995; 80:179.

429. Kim T, Frank C, Schack T. A systematic investigation of the effect of action observation training and motor imagery training on the development of mental representation structure and skill performance. *Front Hum Neurosci.* 2017;11:499.

430. Olsson CJ, Jonsson B, Nyberg L. Internal imagery training in active high jumpers. *Scand J Psychol.* 2008;49:133–140.

431. Schack T. Knowledge and performance in action. *J Knowl Manag.* 2004;8:38–53.

432. Williams SE, Cumming J. Measuring athlete imagery ability: the sport imagery ability questionnaire. *J Sport Exerc Psychol.* 2011;33:416–440.

433. Ando S, Kida N, Oda S. Central and peripheral visual reaction time of soccer players and nonathletes. *Percept Mot Skills.* 2001;92:786–794.

434. Fullerton HS. Eye, ear, brain and muscle tests on 'Babe' Ruth. *W Optom World.* 1925;13:160.

435. Slater-Hammel AT, Stumpner RL. Batting reaction-time. *Res Q Am Assoc Health Phys Educ.* 1950;21:353.

436. Sanderson FH, Holton JN. Relationships between perceptual motor abilities and cricket batting. *Percept Mot Skills.* 1980;51:138.

437. Classe JG, Semes LP, Daum KM, et al. Association between visual reaction time and batting, fielding, and earned run averages among players of the Southern Baseball League. *J Am Optom Assoc.* 1997;68:43.

438. Montes-Mico R, Bueno I, Candel J, et al. Eye-hand and eye-foot visual reaction times of young soccer players. *Optometry.* 2000;71:775.

439. Knapp BN. Simple reaction times of selected top-class sportsmen and research students. *Res Q.* 1961;32:409.

440. Blundell NL. Critical visual-perceptual attributes of championship level tennis players. In: Howell ML, Wilson BD, eds. Kinesiological Sciences. *Proceedings of the VII Commonwealth and International Conference on Sport, Physical Education, Recreation and Dance.* Brisbane: University of Queensland; 1984:51–59.

441. Kioumourtzoglou E, Kourtessis T, Michalopoulou M, et al. Differences in several perceptual abilities between experts and novices in basketball, volleyball, and waterpolo. *Percept Mot Skills.* 1998;86:899.

442. Harbin G, Durst L, Harbin D. Evaluation of oculomotor response in relationship to sports performance. *Med Sci Sports Exerc.* 1989;21:258.

443. Nakamoto H, Mori S. Sport-specific decision-making in a Go/NoGo reaction task: difference among nonathletes and baseball and basketball players. *Percept Mot Skills.* 2008;106:163–170.

444. Dogan B. Multiple-choice reaction and visual perception in female and male elite athletes. *J Sports Med Phys Fit.* 2009;49:91–96.

445. Ak E, Kocak S. Coincidence-anticipation timing and reaction time in youth tennis and table tennis players. *Percept Mot Skills.* 2010;110(3 Pt 1):879–887.

446. Taimela S. Factors affecting reaction-time testing and the interpretation of results. *Percept Mot Skills.* 1991;73:1195.

447. Currier DP, Nelson RM. Changes in motor conduction velocity induced by exercise and diathermy. *Phys Ther.* 1969;49:146.

448. Hancock S, McNaughton L. Effects of fatigue on ability to process visual information by experienced orienteers. *Percept Mot Skills.* 1986;62:491.

449. Hascelik Z, Basgore O, Turner K. The effects of physical training on physical fitness tests and auditory and visual reaction times of volleyball players. *J Sports Med Phys Fit.* 1989;29:234.

450. Baer AD, Gersten JW, Robertson BM, et al. Effects of various exercise programs on isometric tension, endurance and reaction time in the human. *Arch Phys Med Rehabil.* 1955;36:495.

451. Gallaway M, Aimino J, Scheiman M. The effect of protective sports eyewear on peripheral visual field and a peripheral visual performance task. *J Am Optom Assoc.* 1986;57:304.

452. Dawson ML, Zabik RM. Effect of protective eyewear on reaction time in the horizontal field of vision. *Percept Mot Skills.* 1988;67:155.

453. Lange B, Hunfalvay M, Murray N, et al. Reliability of computerized eye-tracking reaction time tests in nonathletes, athletes, and individuals with traumatic brain injury. *Optom Vis Perform.* 2018;6:119–129.

454. Wells AJ, Hoffman JR, Beyer KS, et al. Reliability of the Dynavision D2 for assessing reaction time performance. *J Sports Sci Med.* 2014;13:145–150.

455. Henry M. Stimulus complexity, movement, age, and sex in relation to reaction latency and speed in limb movements. *Res Q Sports Med.* 1961;32:353.

456. Keele S. Motor control. In: Boff K, Kaufman L, Thomas J, eds. *Handbook of Perception and Human Performance.* New York: John Wiley & Sons; 1986:30–60.

457. Sherman A. A method for evaluating eye-hand coordination and visual reaction time in athletes. *J Am Optom Assoc.* 1983;54:801.

458. Mitchell JA, Nicholson DW, Maples WC. Standardization of the Wayne saccadic fixator. *J Behav Optom.* 1990;1:199.

459. Vogel GL, Hale RE. Initial norms using the Wayne Saccadic Fixator for eye-hand coordination and visual reaction times. *J Behav Optom.* 1990;1:206.

460. Kida N, Oda S, Matsumura M. Intensive baseball practice improves Go/NoGo reaction time, but not the simple reaction time. *Brain Res Cogn Brain Res.* 2005;22:257–264.

461. Nakamoto H, Mori S. Effects of stimulus-response compatibility in mediating expert performance in baseball players. *Brain Res.* 2008;1189:179–188.

462. Laby DM, Kirschen DG, Govindarajulu U, DeLand P. The hand-eye coordination of professional baseball players: the relationship to batting. *Optom Vis Sci.* 2018;95: 557–567.

463. Vogel GL, Hale RE. Does participation in organized athletics increase a child's scoring ability on the Wayne Saccadic Fixator? *J Behav Optom.* 1992;3:66.

464. Appler DV, Quimby CA. The effect of ambient room illumination upon Wayne Saccadic Fixator performance. *J Am Optom Assoc.* 1984;55:818.

465. Beckerman S, Fornes AM. Effects of changes in lighting level on performance with the AcuVision 1000. *J Am Optom Assoc.* 1997;68:243.

466. Bayly MF, Clark KJ, Perrin DH. The effects of perceived fatigue on visual reaction time. *Int J Sport Vis.* 1996;3:18.

467. Mollenberg O, Jendrusch G, Heck H. Table tennis specific eye-hand (bat) coordination and visual depth perception. In: Mester J, King G, Struder H, et al., eds. Perspectives and Profiles, *Sixth Annual Congress of the European College of Sports Science, 15th Congress of the German Society of Sport Science, Cologne, July 2001.* 2001:1249.

468. Klavora P, Esposito JG. Sex differences in performance on three novel continuous response tasks. *Percept Mot Skills.* 2002;95:49.

469. Willms A, Dalton KN. Establishment of standard methods for the measurement of eye-hand visual-motor reaction time. *Optom Vis Perf.* 2017;5(2):49–56.

470. Galpin AJ, Li Y, Lohnes CA, Schilling BK. A 4-week choice foot speed and choice reaction training program improves agility in previously non-agility trained, but active men and women. *J Strength Condit Res.* 2008;22:1901–1907.

471. Paquette MR, Schilling BK, Bravo JD, et al. Computerized agility training improves change-of-direction and balance performance independently of footwear in young adults. *Res Q Exerc Sport.* 2017;88:44–51.

472. Sharp RH, Whiting HTA. Information processing and eye-movement behavior in a ball catching skill. *J Hum Mov Stud.* 1975;1:124.

473. Franks IM, Weicker D, Robertson DGE. The kinematics, movement phasing and timing of a skilled action in response to varying conditions of uncertainty. *Hum Mov Sci.* 1985;4:91.

474. Bootsma RJ, van Wieringen PCW. Visual control of an attacking forehand drive. In: Meijer OG, Roth K, eds. *Complex Movement Behavior: The Motor-Action Controversy.* Amsterdam: North-Holland; 1988:189–199.

475. Bootsma RJ. *The Timing of Rapid Interceptive Actions: Perception-Action Coupling in the Control and Acquisition of Skill.* Amsterdam: Free University Press; 1988.

476. Jendrusch G, Tidow G, de Marees H. Precise determination of the contact point in tennis. *Int J Sports Med.* 1988;5:365.

477. Bootsma RJ. Accuracy of perceptual processes subserving different perception-action systems. *Q J Exp Psychol.* 1989; 41A:489.

478. Bootsma RJ, van Wieringen PCW. Timing an attacking forehand drive in table tennis. *J Exp Psychol Hum Percept Perform.* 1990;16:21.

479. Bootsma RJ. Predictive information and the control of action. *Int J Sport Psychol.* 1991;22:271.

480. Savelsbergh GJP, Whiting HTA, Bootsma RJ. "Grasping" tau. *J Exp Psychol Hum Percept Perform.* 1991;17:315.

481. Bootsma RJ, Peper CE. Predictive visual information sources for the regulation of action with special emphasis on catching and hitting. In: Proteau L, Elliott D, eds. *Vision and Motor Control.* Amsterdam: North-Holland; 1992:285–314.

482. Bootsma RJ, Oudejans RRD. Visual information about time-to-collision between two objects. *J Exp Psychol Hum Percept Perform.* 1993;19:1041.

483. Siegel D. Response velocity, range of movement, and timing accuracy. *Percept Mot Skills.* 1994;79:216.

484. Gray R, Regan DM. Unconfounding the direction of motion in depth, time to passage and rotation rate on an approaching object. *Vis Res.* 2006;46:2388.

485. Shea CH, Krampitz JB, Northam CC. Information processing in coincidence timing tasks: a developmental perspective. *J Hum Mov Stud.* 1982;8:73.

486. Lee DN, Young DS, Reddish PE, et al. Visual timing in hitting an accelerating ball. *Q J Exp Psychol.* 1983;35A:333.

487. Petrakis E. Sex differences and specificity of anticipation of coincidence. *Percept Mot Skills.* 1985;61:1135.

488. Payne VG. The effects of stimulus runway length on coincidence-anticipation timing performance. *J Hum Mov Stud.* 1986;12:289.

489. Magill RA. *Motor Learning: Concepts and Applications.* 4th ed. Madison, WI: Brown & Benchmark; 1993.

490. Molstad SM, Kluka DA, Love PA, et al. Timing of coincidence anticipation by NCAA Division I softball athletes. *Percept Mot Skills.* 1994;79:1491.

491. Hart MA, Reeve TG. A preliminary comparison of stimulus presentation methods with the Bassin anticipation timing task. *Percept Mot Skills.* 1997;85:344.

492. Millslagle DG. Dynamic visual acuity and coincidence-anticipation timing by experienced and inexperienced women players of fast pitch softball. *Percept Mot Skills.* 2000;90:498–504.

493. Ripoll H, Latiri I. Effect of expertise on coincident-timing accuracy in a fast ball game. *J Sports Sci.* 1997;15:573–580.

494. Williams LR. Coincidence timing of a soccer pass: effects of stimulus velocity and movement distance. *Percept Mot Skills.* 2000;91:39–52.

495. Millslagle DG. Effects of increasing and decreasing intra-trial stimulus speed on coincidence-anticipation timing. *Percept Mot Skills.* 2008;107:373–382.

496. Fogt N, Lemos E. Binocular and monocular coincidence-anticipation timing responses. *Vis Dev Rehabil.* 2018;4:186–199.

497. Duncan MJ, Stanley M, Smith M, et al. Coincidence anticipation timing performance during an acute bout of brisk walking in older adults: effect of stimulus speed. *Neural Plast.* 2015, 210213.

498. Duncan MJ, Smith M, Bryant E, et al. Effects of increasing and decreasing physiological arousal on anticipation timing performance during competition and practice. *Eur J Sport Sci.* 2016;16:27–35.

499. Akpinar S, Devrilmez E, Kirazci S. Coincidence-anticipation timing requirements are different in racket sports. *Percept Mot Skills.* 2012;115:581–593.

500. Sanders G. Sex differences in coincidence-anticipation timing (CAT): a review. *Percept Mot Skills*. 2011;112: 61–90.

501. Robertson S, Collins J, Elliott D, et al. The influence of skill and intermittent vision on dynamic balance. *J Mot Behav*. 1994;26:333.

502. Robertson S, Elliott D. The influence of skill in gymnastics and vision on dynamic balance. *Int J Sport Psychol*. 1996;27:361.

503. Robertson S, Elliott D. Specificity of learning and dynamic balance. *Res Q Exerc Sport*. 1996;67:69.

504. Croix G, Chollet D, Thouvarecq R. Effect of expertise level on the perceptual characteristics of gymnasts. *J Strength Condit Res*. 2010;24:1458–1463.

505. Witkin HA, Dyk RB, Paterson HF, et al. *Psychological Differentiation*. New York: Wiley; 1962.

506. Witkin HA, Lewis HB, Hertzman M, et al. *Personality through Perception*. Westport, CT: Greenwood; 1972.

507. Knapp B. *Skill in Sport*. London: Routledge & Kegan Paul; 1964.

508. Jones MG. Perceptual studies: perceptual characteristics and athletic performance. In: Whiting HTA, ed. *Sports Psychology*. London: Kimpton; 1972:96–115.

509. Kane JE. Personality, body concept and performance. In: Kane JE, ed. *Psychological Aspects of Physical Education and Sport*. London: Western Printing Services; 1972:91–127.

510. Hodgson CI, Christian E, McMorris T. Performance on the portable rod and frame test predicts variation in learning the kayak roll. *Percept Mot Skills*. 2010;110: 479–487.

511. Counil L. Field dependence and orientation of upside-down posture in water. *Percept Mot Skills*. 2015;120: 15–24.

512. Young HH. A test of Witkin's field-independence hypothesis. *J Abnorm Soc Psychol*. 1959;59:188.

513. Elliott R, McMichael RE. Effects of specific training on frame dependence. *Percept Mot Skills*. 1963;17:363.

514. Gallahue DL. The relationship between perceptual and motor abilities. *Res Q*. 1968;39:948.

515. Gruenfeld L, Arbuthnot H. Field independence as conceptual framework for prediction of variability in ratings of others. *Percept Mot Skills*. 1969;28:31.

516. Meek F, Skubie V. Spatial perception of highly skilled and poorly skilled females. *Percept Mot Skills*. 1971;33:1309.

517. Svinicki JG, Bundgaard CJ, Schwensohn CH, et al. Physical activity and visual field-dependency. *Percept Mot Skills*. 1974;39:1237.

518. Pargman D, Bender P, Deshaies P. Correlation between visual disembedding and basketball shooting by male and female varsity college athletes. *Percept Mot Skills*. 1975;41:539.

519. Rotella RJ, Bunker LK. Field dependence and reaction time in senior tennis players (65 and over). *Percept Mot Skills*. 1978;46:585.

520. Docherty D, Boyd DG. Relationship of disembedding ability to performance in volleyball, tennis, and badminton. *Percept Mot Skills*. 1982;54:1219.

521. Raviv S, Nabel N. Field dependence-independence and concentration as psychological characteristics of basketball players. *Percept Mot Skills*. 1988;66:831.

522. Raviv S, Nabel N. Relationship between two different measurements of field-dependence and athletic performance of adolescents. *Percept Mot Skills*. 1990;70:75.

523. Terelak J. Field dependence/independence and eye-hands-legs coordination. *Percept Mot Skills*. 1990;71: 947.

524. Liu WH. Review of recent Chinese research on field dependence-independence in high-level athletes. *Percept Mot Skills*. 1996;83:1187.

525. Pargman D. Visual disembedding and injury in college football players. *Percept Mot Skills*. 1976;42:762.

526. Gill NT, Herdtner TJ, Lough L. Perceptual and socioeconomic variables, instruction in body-orientation, and predicted academic success in young children. *Percept Mot Skills*. 1968;26:1175.

527. Leithwood KA, Fowler W. Complex motor learning in four-year-olds. *Child Dev*. 1971;42:781.

528. Wang L, Krasich K, Bel-Bahar T. Mapping the structure of perceptual and visual-motor abilities in healthy young adults. *Acta Psychol*. 2015;157:74–84.

529. Haynes HM. The distance rock test: a preliminary report. *J Am Optom Assoc*. 1979;50:707.

530. Haynes HM, McWilliams LG. Effects of training on near-far response time as measured by the distance rock test. *J Am Optom Assoc*. 1979;50:715.

531. Kavner RS. *Total Vision*. New York: A&V Publishers; 1978.

532. Kubistant T. The uses of visualization in sports medicine. *Sportsmed Dig*. 1982;4(5).

533. Silva JM, Weinberg RS. *Psychological Foundation of Sport*. Champaign, IL: Human Kinetics; 1984.

534. Clarke ND, Duncan MJ. Effect of carbohydrate and caffeine ingestion on badminton performance. *Int J Sports Physiol Perform*. 2016;11:108–115.

CHAPTER 5

Sports Vision Screening and Report Strategies

Sports vision practitioners have many opportunities to be involved with vision services for a sports team. A high percentage of professional and division I college and university sports teams in North America provide a vision screening program, and many also have an optometrist or ophthalmologist as a vision consultant.[1] Many sports programs at all levels of competition use vision screening for their athletes, but many more do not have access to this service. A survey of professional, college, and university athletic programs and optometrists concluded that a significant unmet need exists for vision care services for athletes.[1]

Many reports of vision screening results from athletes have been published.[2-18] No single standardized sports vision screening has been used in any of the studies, and journal articles that discuss vision screening for athletes rarely specify a set of evaluation procedures with detailed protocols and normative data.[3,11,19-27] The procedures chosen for sports vision screening of a team or athletic program typically result from considerations of time, location, vision task demands, and the value of the information acquired from the procedures. The result should be an efficient, high-yield battery of tests that identify vision problems that can interfere with peak sports performance and also allow comparison of athletes based on a profile of the vision skills assessed.

The results from a sports vision screening should be reported to the appropriate team personnel and the individual athletes. For those in the United States, the practitioner should ensure compliance with Health Insurance Portability and Accountability Act regulations. Many possible methods can be used to deliver this information, and the ability to communicate the findings and management recommendations effectively distinguishes the provider as an "expert." Communication skills are at a premium if the objective is compliance with recommendations.

DEVELOPING A SPORTS VISION SCREENING

Most vision screenings are conducted at a location outside a sports vision practitioner's office. A full sports vision evaluation on each athlete is usually not possible to conduct because of the limitations of time and location. The location of the screening may limit the use of some evaluation instruments because of the space available, control of lighting, availability of electricity, and portability of equipment. The amount of time available for the screening dictates the extent of testing feasible based on the number of athletes to be screened. The practitioner must also consider the available personnel to conduct the screening and determine how the athletes will proceed through the screening procedures for maximal efficiency.

Before the factors of time and location can be deliberated, the practitioner must identify the visual factors that potentially contribute to peak human performance so that these specific functions can be isolated and measured in the screening, if possible. The visual demands critical to success in sports can vary tremendously between different sports or positions. Chapter 2 provides an approach to the task analysis process essential for providing appropriate vision care to athletes. The evaluation procedures that are judged to yield the most relevant assessment of critical visual skills should be identified and contemplated for inclusion in the screening. The list of desirable procedures should then be reduced to the number of procedures that are feasible within the limitations of time and location. When determining which procedures should be selected, procedures that are the most suitable for sampling the vision skill areas identified as critical to performance are most commonly chosen.

In addition to the evaluation procedures chosen for the sports vision screening, the athlete's history must be ascertained. The limitation of time is a factor with this

Sports Vision. https://doi.org/10.1016/B978-0-323-75543-6.00006-1

75

part of the screening as well, and a questionnaire is commonly used to improve efficiency. The questionnaire should include some of the basic elements of a history for a comprehensive vision examination, including questions regarding main concerns, secondary vision concerns, and personal eye and medical history. The use of vision correction and eye protection is a crucial element to investigate in the athlete history questionnaire. Supplementary questions are listed in Chapter 4 that yield information concerning the athlete's visual performance during the sport; these can be listed in the questionnaire. The ability to relate symptoms elicited on the questionnaire to the vision skills assessed in the screening is advantageous. The athlete history questionnaire should be verbally reviewed with the athlete, and thorough follow-up information should be obtained if time permits.

The decision of whether to include procedures for the evaluation of ocular health status is difficult. The range of procedures necessary to assess internal and external health is challenging to perform within the limitations of time and location. With the advent of new ocular health imaging technologies, documentation of elements of the athlete's ocular health may be possible; however, these new technologies should be combined with a thorough ocular health assessment and not be used in isolation. Because an incomplete assessment of the elements of ocular health can be intolerably misleading, it is not recommended as part of a sports vision screening. A legal disclaimer stating the limitations of the screening and recommendation of routine comprehensive vision care should be included in the report materials provided to the team (see sample vision screening form in Appendix B).

As the practitioner gains experience with a variety of teams and sports, sport-specific screenings can be developed for use in subsequent screenings. The assessment areas and procedures used can be modified as needed on the basis of the results of further research and the practitioner's own experience.

CONDUCTING THE SPORTS VISION SCREENING

Many aspects of a successful sports vision screening must be addressed before conducting the screening. Recording forms for the athlete data, a list of equipment and supplies to bring to the screening site, assessment protocols for each procedure, training of any ancillary staff who will be assisting in data collection, and development of the flow of athletes through the screening are all required elements.

Recording Forms

The recording forms for the screening should be developed in a manner that enhances the efficiency of the screening. Each assessment procedure should have a recording method that minimizes the amount of time needed to record each athlete's results. Because a comparison of vision skills among athletes on the team is often performed, the screening form should also facilitate easy transfer to the comparison instrument that will be used. Ideally, athlete data would be directly entered on a computer spreadsheet for assessment at the conclusion of the screening, eliminating the need for paper forms. If a copy of the sports vision screening form will be provided to the team personnel and/or athlete, it will need to be designed in a manner that clearly communicates the results and recommendations as well as have a professional appearance.

Equipment and Supply List

For an off-site screening, the instrumentation selected for the screening should be portable and prepared for transportation. Some equipment will need to be adapted for use at the screening site. For example, the Senaptec Sensory Station (www.senaptec.com) has developed several visual performance assessments that can be conducted on a tablet computer in order to facilitate ease of screening outside a typical clinic location (Fig. 5.1). Lighting can be a factor that should be prepared for. Any supplies and spare parts that may be needed for any instrument should be included in the list of items to bring, such as extra light bulbs, batteries, electric adaptors, extension cords, and power strips. Administrative supplies are usually needed, including clipboards, pens, staplers, masking tape, measuring tape, and name tags. The functioning of all equipment should be checked, and any batteries should be charged before departing for the screening.

Screening Protocols and Staff Training

Stringent assessment protocols should be established for each procedure used in a screening. If the goal is to compare vision skill performance among the team members, all team members must receive the same instructions and performance feedback. The instructions to the athletes before evaluation with each procedure should be standardized as much as possible to minimize the influence of variable instructions on performance. Modification of the instructions or screening protocols during the screening may be tempting; however, any modifications diminish the ability to compare athlete performance. The best way to avoid modifying assessment protocols is to master the procedures and

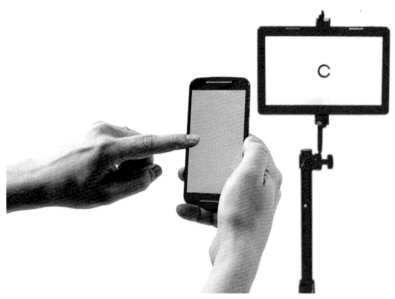

FIG. 5.1 Senaptec Sensory Station's tablet-based assessments.

fine-tune the instructions before conducting the screening. A trial run through the screening with a volunteer "athlete" is a good way to find any issues that need adjusting, and it should also provide an estimation of the time needed for each athlete to complete the screening.

The screening staff should all be thoroughly trained to administer the procedures with the established protocols. If the staff masters the procedure administration, the screening will be much more efficient. For some assessment procedures, a few practice trials are useful to familiarize the athlete with the performance demands prior to measurement. The number of practice trials should also be standardized for all athletes. The protocols should also include methods to motivate the athletes to demonstrate peak performance and ignite their competitive nature. On a procedure such as eye-hand coordination, the highest score achieved (so far) on that procedure by members of the team could be posted next to the apparatus to motivate each athlete to try to post the highest score for the team. Other than the use of the highest score on a particular procedure, each athlete should get minimal feedback on performance during the screening. For each procedure, the athlete should be told he or she is doing well and the results of the screening will be communicated at a later time. Under no circumstances should the athlete be told that he or she has failed any portion of the screening or that visual performance is below normal. The communication of visual performance results is highly sensitive and should be conducted in a manner that facilitates effective management. Therefore communication of screening results is typically reserved for the final report to the team personnel and the athlete.

The instructions to each athlete for each procedure should educate them about the nature of the vision skill being evaluated. The relevance of the vision skill to specific task demands of the sport should be explained to the athlete to help encourage proper motivation during the screening. The better the athlete is motivated to perform on each procedure, the more accurate the measurement of ability becomes. The staff conducting the screening should also be trained to elicit any additional case history information as the athlete proceeds through the screening.

The Flow of the Screening

How the athletes will flow through the screening should be determined in advance. One common setup is to have a number of stations that the athlete moves through where specific assessment procedures are conducted. Ideally, each station should take the athlete the same amount of time to complete so that backup does not occur at certain stations. This ideal situation is not always possible when one procedure takes significantly more time to administer than other procedures in the screening.

Consideration should be given to the importance of the sequence of the screening because altering the sequence of the screening may be tempting for some athletes if a considerable backup is present at particular stations. However, in general, every athlete should go through the screening sequence identically to facilitate comparison of athlete performance. For example, if one athlete performed a visual motor speed assessment at the beginning of the screening and another performed it at the end of the screening, the results may be tainted by the difference in screening sequence. Although this is an important consideration, it is also recognized that assessment sequence may not significantly alter performance results.

The station-to-station approach can be efficient because the staff have mastered the administration of the procedures at their particular station (Figs. 5.2 and 5.3). However, if a group of sports vision practitioners is conducting the screening, each practitioner may take individual athletes through every station of the screening. By having a single practitioner conduct all the procedures, the practitioner may develop more insight into the performance and issues with each individual athlete. The additional insight gained by the practitioner conducting all the screening procedures may be translated into more effective recommendations for that athlete.

No matter which method of screening athletes is chosen, each athlete should proceed through the screening expeditiously. For the team personnel, the time available as a team is extremely valuable. The impression that the team's time is being wasted sitting or standing around during a screening should be avoided. A meeting with the team personnel before the screening is highly recommended to discuss potential scheduling schemes for the team. A reasonable flow of athletes through the screening can be scheduled in coordination with other team training activities. Demonstrating an understanding of the needs of the team and creativity in finding mutually beneficial solutions are greatly appreciated by team personnel.

A meeting time in advance of the screening also affords an excellent opportunity to preview the screening area that will be used. This preview should provide valuable information for designing the floor plan for the screening stations and developing the most effective flow for the screening. Team personnel should also complete the sports vision screening because this will impart useful firsthand experience with the visual skills assessed. The consultation with the team personnel to discuss the screening results is more effective if the team personnel have firsthand knowledge of the vision skills being discussed.

An additional consideration when developing a sports vision screening is the need for supplementary testing. A vision problem may be detected in an athlete during the screening that requires further testing. For example, a cover test may be performed when an athlete has significantly reduced stereopsis in order to

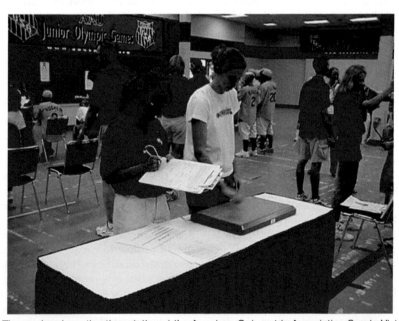

FIG. 5.2 The eye-hand reaction time station at the American Optometric Association Sports Vision Section screening for the Amateur Athletic Union Junior Olympic Games.

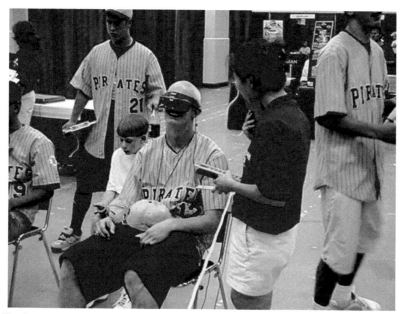

FIG. 5.3 The far stereopsis station at the American Optometric Association Sports Vision Section screening for the Amateur Athletic Union Junior Olympic Games.

determine a possible cause of the reduced stereopsis. The practitioner will need to decide what additional testing may be needed on-site and bring the necessary equipment to conduct that testing. Conversely, the practitioner may choose to simply refer any athletes for follow-up care when vision problems are identified during the course of a screening.

GENERATING REPORTS FOR SPORTS VISION SCREENINGS AND SPORTS VISION EVALUATIONS

Reporting the results of a sports vision screening or sports vision evaluation is absolutely critical for the success of any sports vision program. The report should be communicated to the team personnel and/or individual athletes in a timely manner, such as within 2 weeks of the screening or evaluation. Ideally, a report would be generated immediately at the conclusion of the evaluation. Keep in mind that the interested parties need to know the following five *W*'s[28]:

- *What* needs to be done?
- *When* does it need to be done?
- *Who* should carry out the recommendations?
- *Where* does it need to be done?
- *Why* does it need to be done?

Many methods can be used to construct a report letter for a vision evaluation and no single method is

superior.[28] When reporting the results of a sports vision assessment, the inclusion of a vision skill performance profile is recommended to communicate the relative strengths and potential disadvantages demonstrated by the athlete. I prefer to describe subpar performance as an "opportunity to improve" rather than a weakness. The development of a performance profile is easier when conducting a team assessment because the peer group data are available for direct comparison. When an individual assessment has been performed on an athlete, the practitioner must use available normative data or compare performance to other athletes previously evaluated. See Appendix C for a sample sports vision evaluation summary letter for an individual athlete.

Many computer spreadsheet software programs are available that provide a simple method for comparing vision skill performance by athletes on a team. The data from each athlete can be entered on a spreadsheet when numeric results are present, allowing calculation of performance averages and standard deviations for each procedure. Most data spreadsheet programs have functions for making many statistical calculations. The practitioner must appraise each performance average and standard deviation to determine if the values are appropriate for comparison and recommendations. For example, if a team has demonstrated an unusually high level of visual acuity and 20/20 (6/6) is more than 1 standard deviation below average performance, what recommendations will be made for an athlete who achieved "only" 20/20 visual acuity? Team data can also be compared with available normative data to help determine the validity of the results.

Many possible methods can be used to present visual performance profile information to the team personnel and athletes. The presentation should be easy to interpret by the intended audience. A simple bar graph can be effective for showing relative strengths and weaknesses. The average performance on each skill should be apparent from each athlete's profile, and a benchmark scale illustrating relative performance should also be readily apparent. When appropriate, a scale of 1−5 for the vertical axis of a bar graph can be used, with 3 always representing the performance average for the team on each procedure (see Appendix D). The standard deviation for performance on each procedure is represented by each whole number step on the graph. Specifically, the average is represented by number 3 on the y-axis, and 1 standard deviation above and below the average is represented by numbers 4 and 2, respectively.

To perform a statistical analysis of the visual skill performance of an individual athlete compared with team data or normative data in the context of the scale from 1 to 5, two simple calculations can be performed. If a higher numeric value indicates better performance, such as a score on a Go/No Go assessment, the following calculation is applied:

$$[(\text{Athlete score} - \text{Average score}) / \text{Standard deviation}] + 3$$

Therefore if an athlete scored 85 on the eye-hand co-ordination test and the performance average for his or her team was 79, he or she would have a performance profile rating of 4.20 when the standard deviation is 5, as follows:

$$[(85 - 79) / 5] + 3 = 4.20$$

A lower number indicates better performance on many visual skill procedures, such as stereoacuity. The calculation for this statistical analysis is performed in the same manner, with the exception that the athlete score is subtracted from the average, as follows:

$$[(\text{Average score} - \text{Athlete score}) / \text{Standard deviation}] + 3$$

Therefore if an athlete achieved 25 arc sec on the assessment of stereopsis, and the performance average for his or her team was 15 arc sec, he or she would have a performance profile rating of 1.57 when the standard deviation is 7, as follows:

$$[(15 - 25) / 7] + 3 = 1.57$$

Most computer spreadsheet programs will produce a graphic presentation of data selected from a spreadsheet. The performance profile rating for each visual skill is selected for inclusion in the bar graph and the x-axis coordinates are labeled to match a description key for the visual skill areas. The description key is a short summary of each skill assessed and its relevance to sports performance. The description key is vital for successful communication of the relevance of each factor in the performance profile, and the language used in the description key should be routinely fine-tuned to enhance the efficacy of this important tool (see Appendix D).

The result of the statistical analysis is a graphic presentation of the performance profile for each individual athlete, with an explanation of the sports performance value of each visual skill assessed. Additional graphs can be generated for the team personnel that compare performance on any individual assessment procedure for all members of the team. For example, the coach may want to see a relative ranking of performance on visual-motor reaction times for the team. To protect athlete identity, numbers are assigned to each athlete for this type of graph. A key denoting which individual athlete corresponds to which athlete number is provided to the appropriate team personnel with an explanation of the issues regarding healthcare confidentiality. To be compliant with the Health Insurance Portability and Accountability Act regulations in the United States, each athlete should sign a release of healthcare information before the release of any information to team personnel.

A short narrative should be provided for each athlete's performance on a sports vision screening. This narrative can be in paragraph form or presented as a bulleted list. The narrative should summarize any issues revealed during the athlete history as well as the relative strengths and "opportunities to improve" based on the athlete's performance in the screening. Recommendations for further vision care should be clearly stated with an explanation of the potential benefits of that care. The disclaimer regarding health assessment is included in the athlete narrative. See Appendix D for a sample athlete profile and narrative.

Computer-Based Assessment Systems

Computer-based instruments that measure various aspects of vision allow individual athlete performance to be compared to a database of other athletes. As described in Chapter 4, computerized assessment and training devices such as the Senaptec Sensory Station (http://senaptec. com), Sports Vision Performance from M&S (http://

www.mstech-eyes.com/products/category/sports-vision-p erformance), RightEye (https://www.righteye.com/tests-therapies/vision-performance), and Vizual Edge Performance Trainer (http://vizualedge.com), and the sports vision software available from Centro de Optometria Internacional have been developed to measure a broad set of visual, cognitive, and sensorimotor skills. The comparative analysis offered with these systems provides information about performance across the visual performance measures in order to identify areas of strength and potential disadvantages. This type of analysis can provide valuable information to athletes about what interventions and training procedures may benefit them the most, and the information is generated quickly and easily with these systems. A sample athlete profile from the Senaptec Sensory Station is shown in Fig. 5.4.

Meeting with the team personnel to review the reports is tremendously valuable. Many issues and questions can be properly addressed at this time. If possible, a short consultation with each athlete in the presence of the appropriate team personnel or other interested parties represents the best opportunity for effective communication of the results and recommendations. A fundamental aspect of these consultations is discussing how to use the acquired information to improve the sports performance of the athletes and the team. As previously mentioned, the word "fail" should not be used when describing the visual performance of an athlete. More positive word selection, such as "opportunities to improve," minimizes any negative impact on athlete confidence. It is also quite helpful to describe how aspects of visual performance may limit the potential for peak sports performance.[15] The time with the team personnel is also an appropriate occasion to review issues of contact lens replacement, eye protection, and eye injury management.

Sports vision screenings are a common aspect of sports vision care. A practitioner's ability to maximize the potential inherent in this opportunity often determines success. Proper preparation for a team screening

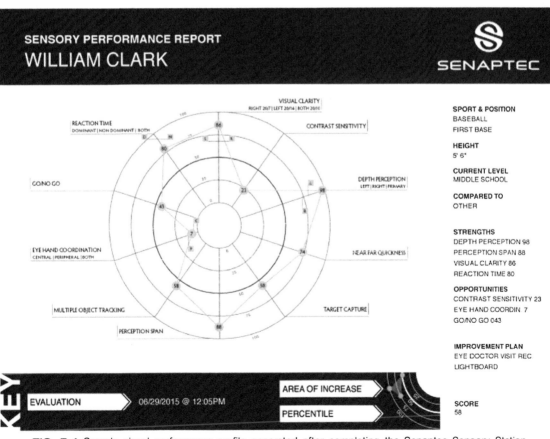

FIG. 5.4 Sample visual performance profile generated after completing the Senaptec Sensory Station assessments.

and timely and effective communication of the screening results can provide the foundation for a successful relationship with a team or organization. Success often is determined by the length of relationships with teams or organizations rather than by how many solitary opportunities were obtained.

REFERENCES

1. Zieman BG, Reichow AW, Coffey B, et al. Optometric trends in sports vision: knowledge, utilization, and practitioner role expansion potential. *J Am Optom Assoc.* 1993; 64:490.
2. Martin WF. A research study on athletes' vision. *Contacto.* 1963;7(5).
3. Bauscher WA. Vision and the athlete. *Optom Wkly.* 1968; 59:21.
4. Garner AI. What a practitioner should know about an athlete's vision. *Contacto.* 1976;20:24.
5. Garner AI. An overlooked problem: athletes' visual needs. *Phys Sportsmed.* 1977;5:75.
6. Erenstone R, Miller NP, Silagy ZS. Optometry at the 1980 Winter Olympics. *J Am Optom Assoc.* 1981;52:647.
7. Harris PA, Blum DS. AOA sports vision section screening of basketball officials. *J Am Optom Assoc.* 1984;55:130.
8. Sports vision gets gold at the Barcelona Olympics. *Calif Optom.* 1992;18:6.
9. Milne DC, Lewis RV. Sports vision screening of varsity athletes. *Sports Vision.* 1993;1(8).
10. Goldsmid MA. Visual fitness and performance in tennis athletes. *Eye Quest Mag.* 1994;38.
11. Berman AM. Sports performance vision testing. *Optom Today.* 1996;4:28.
12. Laby DM, Rosenbaum AL, Kirschen DG, et al. The visual function of professional baseball players. *Am J Ophthalmol.* 1996;122:476.
13. Beckerman S, Hitzeman SA. The ocular and visual characteristics of an athletic population. *Optometry.* 2001;72:498.
14. Beckerman S, Hitzeman SA. Sports vision testing of selected athletic participants in the 1997 and 1998 AAU Junior Olympic Games. *Optometry.* 2003;74:502.
15. Laby DM, Kirschen DG, Pantall P. The visual function of Olympic-level athletes — an initial report. *Eye Contact Lens.* 2011;37:116.
16. Beatty RM, Bakkum BW, Hitzman SA, et al. Sports vision screening of amateur athletic union junior Olympic athletes: a ten-year follow-up. *Optom Vis Performance.* 2016; 4:97.
17. Sanghera NK, Baas EA, Bakkum BW, et al. Sports vision evaluation findings in an elite athlete population. *Optom Vis Performance.* 2016;4:107.
18. Jorge J, Fernandes P. Static and dynamic visual acuity and refractive errors in elite football players. *Clin Exp Optom.* 2019;102:51.
19. Wilson TA, Falkel J. *Sports Vision Training for Better Performance.* Champaign, IL: Human Kinetics; 2004:1−13.
20. Reichow AW, Stern NS. Guidelines for screening and testing the athlete's visual system—part I. *OEP Curriculum II.* 1987;59:243.
21. Jones DE, Gillilan RW. Optometric services for the athletic department. *J Am Optom Assoc.* 1973;44:1060.
22. Screening athletes: how important is sports vision care? *Rev Optom.* 1977;114:14.
23. Farnsworth CL. How to serve sports vision patients. *Rev Optom.* 1984;121:64.
24. Berman AM. Starting a sports vision practice. *Optom Manag.* 1990;25:30.
25. Schwartz CA. Sports screening for success. *Optom Econ.* 1994;4:12.
26. Wilson TA. Sports vision: getting into the game. *Optom Manag.* 1997;32:20s.
27. Hubbs L. Take it from the pros part I: 10 steps for attracting sports-minded patients. *Optom Manag.* 2000;35:116.
28. Ettinger ER. *Professional Communications in Eye Care.* Boston: Butterworth-Heinemann; 1994.

CHAPTER 6

Prescribing for the Athlete

The eye care practitioner is in a unique position to provide expert consultative services to athletes regarding vision correction and the potential uses and benefits of ophthalmic products. The practitioner should consider the nature of the athletic activity (contact vs. noncontact sports) as well as the weather and atmospheric conditions that may be encountered by the athlete. These aspects oblige the practitioner to consider and analyze the following environmental factors:

- the presence of ocular hazards;
- the need for protection from impact for the eye, face, and head;
- the need for protection from solar radiation;
- issues of visibility and mechanical forces with protection;
- issues with sunlight conditions (variability and glare);
- issues with artificial lighting (color perception and glare);
- temperature issues that may affect ophthalmic products;
- humidity conditions, especially low humidity with contact lens (CL) wear;
- altitude factors that may affect oxygen transmission in CL wear;
- dust and foreign body potential;
- sweat, fogging, and precipitation effects with ophthalmic products;
- the need for product flexibility because of environmental variability.

These environmental factors will be addressed in the following sections to assist the practitioner in determining the advantages and disadvantages of the available options. Each athlete has individual variables that affect ophthalmic recommendations. The gender, age, level of participation, combination of sports activities, and previous history of product use influence the choice of available options. Some athletes seek a single product to meet all visual performance needs, whereas others seek the optimal products for a variety of highly specific uses. Effective patient counseling begins with a thorough history to determine the specific needs and profile for the individual. Many patients would like to make informed decisions about the use of ophthalmic products; therefore a thorough case history coupled with comprehensive education and recommendations establish the practitioner as a valuable resource for the athlete.

REFRACTIVE COMPENSATION

Studies conducted on populations of teenaged and professional adult athletes have found similar incidence of refractive error and visual symptoms as in the general population (approximately 20%–40%), dispelling the impression that athletes have a lower incidence of refractive error and vision problems.[1-5] Athletes who currently use vision correction require an evaluation to determine if the prescription is providing optimal visual performance for the specific sport demands. A task analysis of the sport will assist in determining the specific visual demands, and a careful refractive analysis can establish the best refractive compensation for use in that sport. For example, a myopic baseball player may benefit from an additional 0.25 D of minus to improve contrast judgment or when playing in twilight conditions. This prescription becomes the sport-specific prescription and is not intended for general use. Other sports, such as billiards, have specific viewing distances that should be considered, especially for the presbyopic athlete.

The eye care practitioner should advise athletic patients about the advantages and disadvantages of spectacles, protective eyewear, CLs, and refractive surgery for specific sports. The athlete should be able to make an informed decision about the best option for his or her individual needs. If spectacles are an option, the athlete should be counseled on the best lens characteristics, frame designs, tint characteristics, and protection factors. CLs offer a method to minimize many of the disadvantages found with most spectacle corrections, specifically poor optics, distortion, lack of safety, and lack of comfort.[6-8] Refractive surgery offers the potential advantage of eliminating the need for optical devices; however, surgical procedures have safety and suboptimal vision performance outcome concerns. Orthokeratology offers an alternative to refractive surgery for some athletes.

Sports Vision. https://doi.org/10.1016/B978-0-323-75543-6.00012-7

For the approximately 80% of athletes who do not use vision correction, some may benefit from a sport-specific refractive prescription. To determine the possible benefits of a refractive prescription, the eye care provider should consider the athlete's entering unaided visual acuities, the visual demands of the sport, and the effort exerted by the athlete to achieve clarity. For example, a golfer with unaided visual acuities of 20/25 (6/7.5) may appreciate the improved ability to judge the terrain of the course and find the ball when wearing a −0.25 DS prescription. This amount of myopia is typically insignificant, but the lack of compensation may have an impact on golf performance. Similarly, an uncorrected hyperope may find relief from eye strain with a prescription when playing tennis.

Guidelines have been published to assist the practitioner in determining when refractive compensation should be considered (Table 6.1).[9] Any patient with myopia of −0.25 D or more should be counseled on the possible benefits of refractive compensation. Astigmatism has a similar effect on visual resolution as myopia, especially against-the-rule and oblique astigmatism. Refractive compensation should be considered with −0.50 D or more astigmatism, although with-the-rule astigmatism compensation may not yield as much improvement on clinical measures. Low amounts of hyperopia are often well tolerated without correction; however, hyperopia of +1.00 D or greater may require a significant amount of effort from the athlete to achieve and maintain clarity. Low amounts of anisometropia are not always compensated for, especially when the refractive errors are low. Anisometropia of 0.50 D or more can have a detrimental effect on depth perception, and some athletes may be sensitive to that effect. Additionally, the effects of meridional anisometropia should be considered in athletes with asymmetric astigmatism.

These guidelines are useful for the practitioner to trigger the discussion of the potential benefits of a refractive prescription; the athlete ultimately makes the decision whether to experiment with the prescription.

When an athlete decides to experiment with a refractive prescription and he or she has not previously worn a correction, the timing of the experimentation should be discussed. The best time to experiment is during the off-season. The athlete is typically not competing at that time, so adaptation to the prescription will not directly affect critical performance. Athletes generally use the off-season to rest, work on biomechanical skills, and prepare their physical conditioning for the next season. This presents a perfect opportunity to experiment with refractive compensation. If a new prescription is introduced during the competitive season, the athlete may find that performance is negatively affected during the adaptation to the magnification effects induced by spectacle lens wear. For example, a basketball player who wears a myopic prescription for the first time will need to adjust to the change in spatial perception induced by the lenses (e.g., the basket can appear closer).

Presbyopia potentially presents a prescribing challenge in some sports activities. In many sports, a near addition is unnecessary because near visual acuity has a minimal impact on performance. In tennis, for example, clarity of near vision provides no advantage to performance. In golf, near visual acuity does not affect performance; however, clear near vision is desirable for seeing the score card and identifying the ball during play. A spectacle prescription with near addition lenses can interfere with the golfer's view when addressing the ball and adjusting swing mechanics. A small, low-set segment set in one lens in the opposite viewing direction from the putting view angle has been recommended as a solution to this problem. For example, offset the segment in right gaze (lower temporal corner of the right lens) for a right-handed golfer.[10] A better option may be CLs for playing the game and a near spectacle addition to use when scoring. Alternatively, a progressive addition lens (PAL) may be prescribed with a short corridor and narrow near zone set low to minimize peripheral distortion effects. For example, the Definity Fairway Transitions SOLFX and Oakley True Digital Golf PALs are designed for use in golf. Pilots and boat operators may require a double segment design, with positioning of the near additions to allow them to read instruments in downgaze and upgaze positions. Placing a small segment at the top of the lens and a traditional segment at the bottom of the lens typically provides a solution to the near-vision

TABLE 6.1 Guidelines for Refractive Compensation in Athletes.	
Refractive Status	**Consider Prescribing at**
Myopia	−0.25 D or more
Hyperopia	+1.00 D or more
Astigmatism	0.50 D or more[a]
Anisometropia	0.50 D or more[b]

[a] Against-the-rule astigmatism and oblique astigmatism are more detrimental than with-the-rule astigmatism.
[b] Consider meridional effects with asymmetric astigmatism.

challenge (although this lens design is not currently available with polycarbonate lenses). Billiards players often use a single-vision intermediate-distance prescription during play, and the optical centers may need to be carefully measured in the billiards viewing position with strong prescriptions to minimize induced prism effects. Scuba divers may need a multifocal CL or spectacle prescription bonded to the face mask or attached as an insert within the mask to allow the diver to see the equipment, instruments, and underwater environment clearly. In these cases, a spectacle prescription must be adjusted for the significant increase in vertex distance created by the mask. For dynamic reactive sports, spectacle lenses produced better reaction times at near distances in presbyopes than CLs.[11] Several companies offer PALs in high base (wrap) designs for use in sports.

The toughest challenge with presbyopia is created by shooters. Shotgun shooters are not significantly affected by the loss of accommodation because the task does not require critical alignment of sights on the target.[12] Rifle shooting requires that the shooter clearly focus the target at a far distance while carefully aligning the front and rear sights of the rifle with the target. For the presbyope, the rifle's front sight (intermediate distance) and rear sight (just beyond the spectacle plane) cannot be viewed with the same clarity as they were before the onset of presbyopia, and bifocal, trifocal, and multifocal lens designs do not offer an effective solution. Some shooters are happy with the distance correction slightly overplussed, creating a tolerable amount of blur for both the target and sights.[13] Telescopic sights also have been recommended for this situation to allow clarity and accurate alignment without the need for near accommodation.[12] Aiming scopes are available for archery as well; however, the increased magnification offered by these converging lenses does not improve visual acuity of the target because of the presence of significant dioptric blur.[14] If spectacles are worn by the shooter, the lens material should protect the athlete and the eye relief distance should be sufficient to protect against rifle recoil.[12,13] As described with billiards, the optical centers may need to be carefully marked with the athlete in the shooting position(s) with a strong refractive prescription to minimize the induced prism effects.

Pistol shooters are particularly affected by presbyopia because the front and rear sights must be aligned with exacting precision as a result of the shorter length of the weapon. Again, the front sight is positioned at an intermediate distance from the eyes, and the difference in accommodative demand between the sights and the far target creates significant blur for one distance when focusing at the other. Presbyopic pistol shooters are particularly disturbed by the loss of image clarity and often want a solution that provides image clarity at both distances. A pinhole aperture can be created by punching a tiny hole in black electric tape and carefully aligning the tape on the spectacle lens of the aiming eye to allow adequate acuity at both distances for the early presbyope.[12] As the pistol shooter approaches absolute presbyopia, the pinhole will no longer provide adequate relief and a bifocal spectacle will need to be carefully measured to allow clarity of the distant target through the upper lens and clarity of the pistol sights through the near addition lens. This movement between the distance correction and near correction should occur with 1 mm of head movement up or down when in the shooting position, and the practitioner should meticulously measure this position (with clear tape to simulate the add position) for a special-purpose shooting prescription.[12] An executive or FT40 segment design will not induce a vertical image jump when moving into the near segment. A flip-down lens design that would allow clarity at two distances also has been recommended,[12,13] but the effect on alignment created by flipping the lenses may be unacceptable.

NONPROTECTIVE SPORTS EYEWEAR

A nonprotective spectacle correction is only recommended for use in some noncontact sports. In sports with a low incidence of contact (e.g., volleyball), other risks for eye injury exist, such as injury from the ball. In most sports the use of CLs or appropriate protective eyewear is preferred over the use of dress eyewear. Dress eyewear does not offer the impact resistance necessary to protect the wearer from the possible hazards encountered in many sports. There may be a need for education among non–eye care sports professionals regarding the advantages of CLs for use in sports.[15]

The American National Standards Institute (ANSI) has established industry standards for the impact resistance of ophthalmic lenses. Dress eyewear performance standards are detailed in the ANSI Z80.1 standard,[16] and the industrial strength (safety) eyewear standards are detailed in the ANSI Z87.1 standard.[17] Outside the United States, there are regional (European Committee for Standardization) and global (International Organization for Standardization [ISO]) governing bodies that work cooperatively to develop eye protection standards. The use of polycarbonate, Trivex (PPG Industries, Pittsburgh, Pennsylvania), or NXT (Intercast Europe,

Parma, Italy) lens materials can provide significantly improved impact attenuation properties over conventional glass and CR-39 lens materials.[11,18–22] Trivex and NXT materials deliver impact resistance similar to polycarbonate while also providing better optical clarity (higher Abbe value), lighter weight materials (lowest density), and improved scratch and crack/chip resistance. However, the frame construction of dress eyewear does not withstand the forces encountered in many sports. The ANSI Z80.3 standard for nonprescription sunglasses and dress eyewear and standards for sports protective eyewear are discussed later in this chapter.

Spectacle prescriptions are not commonly recommended for use in sports. The main concerns besides the lack of adequate eye protection provided by dress eyewear is the potential impact of optical aberrations of the lenses and visual field restriction created by the frames. Four of the seven monochromatic, or Seidel, lens aberrations can degrade the optical image transmitted through the off-center portions of the lens; radial or oblique astigmatism, power error caused by the curvature of the lens, lateral chromatic aberration, and distortion can each decrease the useful field of view through a lens.[20,23] The reduction in the useful field of view can have a detrimental impact on performance in sports. For example, a right-handed golfer viewing the hole during a putt looks through the left field portions of his or her spectacle lenses, and the image can be significantly altered in large refractive errors because of these aberrations. Stronger refractive prescriptions also produce larger amounts of prismatic effects when viewing away from the optical centers of the lenses, and the effect is increased with larger angles of view as approximated by Prentice's rule.[20,24] Therefore lens design and optical center measurements are critical features of crafting the optimal spectacle correction for an athlete. Wrap lens designs potentially can eliminate or reduce some of the aberration and visual field problems found in nonwrap lenses; however, these designs are more commonly found in performance sun eyewear rather than dress eyewear. Wrap design frames and lenses may create problems with induced prismatic effects; therefore careful measurement of the optical centers is necessary with stronger prescriptions.

Spectacle lenses may be a good prescribing option for some noncontact sports and recreational athletes who do not require high-performance optics. Many who participate in golf, tennis, running, cycling, fishing, archery, and shooting sports perform satisfactorily with spectacle corrections. These athletes should be prescribed a suitable impact-resistant lens material and counseled regarding the risks of eye injury with dress eyewear. These athletes also may appreciate the visual performance benefits of CLs, such as elimination of the four field-of-view aberrations and expanded visual fields. Many shooters and archers prefer spectacles over CLs because of the stability of clear vision obtained with spectacle lenses. Because peripheral vision is not a significant factor in most aiming sports, the enhanced visual field does not offer a significant benefit. The shooter or archer is not typically bothered by lens aberrations off the optical center; however, the lenses may need to be fit with the optical centers set for eye position used when aiming with strong prescriptions. The athlete should bring the weapon, carefully unloaded, to the office for this measurement. The practitioner can also arrange to meet the athlete at his or her training facility to make the measurement to generate interest in sports vision services. Additionally, CL movement on the eye can produce undesirable visual fluctuations during prolonged gaze behavior (without blinking) that many shooters and archers develop.

Lens Treatment Options

Ophthalmic lenses are available with a variety of lens treatment options. Most athletes will be bothered by reflections from the lens surface, and reflections off the back surface of the lens are particularly distracting. For example, the tennis player who sees a reflection of the leaves on a tree behind him or her fluttering in a breeze may be bothered by this distraction during the serve or service return. Antireflective coatings are a particularly valuable lens treatment option, and the improvements in technology that allow multilayer antireflective coating have improved the performance of this lens option.[20] The athlete should be warned that antireflective coatings are easy to scratch if the spectacles are not cleaned properly or not kept in a protective case when not in use and that the coating will make dirt and smudges more visible. If polycarbonate lenses are prescribed, an abrasion-resistant coating is provided by the manufacturer because polycarbonate is an inherently soft material and is easily scratched.

Lens fogging and precipitation are two other factors that should be considered in spectacle wearers who compete in predisposing environmental conditions. Condensation appears on spectacle lenses when the temperature of the lenses is lower than the dew point of the surrounding air.[20] Rain, fog, and other moisture in the environment also will produce water drops on the lens surface that can dramatically degrade the athlete's vision through the lenses. Antifog coatings are available to make the lens surface more wettable so that the moisture forms a thin film on the lens rather than droplets.[20] These coatings also help slough water off the lens surface quicker in wet environments. An antifog coating does, however, interfere with the efficacy of an antireflective coating.

Lens coatings reduce the impact resistance properties of the lens because of the change in surface tension created by the coatings. However, polycarbonate and Trivex lens materials with antireflection coatings have reduced penetration resistance to sharp objects, especially in lenses with reduced center thickness.[22,25]

PROTECTIVE EYEWEAR

In many sports, participation exposes the athlete to significant risk for eye injury. Sports involving a ball or fast-moving object, a racquet, a stick, a bat, or body contact have a significant potential for eye injuries (see Table 6.2 for sport risk categories).[26] In 2019, Prevent Blindness America estimated that more than 30,000 eye injuries occur each year from sports participation in the United States.[27] This estimate is recognized as only a fraction of the true incidence of sport-related eye injuries because these injuries represent only those reported from a core of hospital emergency departments in the United States and its territories.[27] There are other methods for determining the true incidence.[28] The Coalition to Prevent Sports Eye Injuries estimates that more than 600,000 eye injuries related to sports and recreation occur each year. Many of the eye injuries sustained during sports participation are preventable with the use of appropriate eye protection. Primary eye care providers must educate all patients about the risks for eye injury during vocational and avocational pursuits, provide information regarding the options for prevention of eye injuries, and direct the patient to ophthalmic services for ocular protection during sports and recreational activities.[29]

As previously discussed, dress eyewear or occupational safety eyewear does not offer the impact resistance necessary to protect the wearer from the possible hazards encountered in many sports. Polycarbonate, Trivex, or NXT lens materials provide significantly improved impact attenuation.[18–22] However, the frame construction of dress eyewear cannot withstand the forces encountered in many sports. Specifically, the materials used for dress eyewear and potentially vulnerable construction of the temple and bridge create endangerments. Similarly, CLs do not offer eye protection for athletes; in fact, rigid CLs may increase the damage to the cornea if they break from a

blunt trauma.[30] Many manufacturers have designed eyewear and equipment to protect the athlete during sports participation, and performance standards have been developed to ensure adequate protection for specific sport purposes.[31,32]

The American Society for Testing of Materials (ASTM) is a nongovernmental group that has developed performance standards (F803) for eye and head protection in many sports, including basketball, baseball, racquet sports, field hockey, and women's lacrosse. ASTM performance standards are established for each sport individually, and the forces potentially encountered in a sport are used to determine appropriate testing parameters. Typically, the protective eyewear is placed on a standard head form and the ball, puck, stick, finger, or elbow is directed at the eyewear from a variety of angles at the predetermined velocity. For example, the eyewear designed for racquet sports must protect the eye and orbit from a squash or racquetball projected at 90 mph from several angles. More details regarding the development of standards and evaluation methods can be found at the ASTM web site (www. astm.org). Additional ASTM standards are available for sports in which traditional eyewear designs are inadequate, including protection attached to a helmet for youth baseball batters and base runners (F910), ice hockey (F513), paintball (F1776), airsoft sports (F2879), and skiing goggles and shields (F659). All protective eyewear are also tested for standard D1003, which covers the evaluation of specific light-transmitting and wide-angle, light-scattering properties of transparent materials. The ISO also has sports eye protection standards for skiing goggles (ISO 18527-1) and racquet sports (ISO 18527-2).

Several groups certify equipment to ensure compliance with the ASTM standards for various sports. The Canadian Standards Association (CSA) certifies products that meet Canadian standards for racquet sports (similar to the ASTM standards). The Protective Eyewear Certification Council (PECC) certifies protectors that meet ASTM F803 standards. The Hockey Equipment Certification Council certifies helmets and face shields for use in hockey. For baseball and football helmets and face protectors for football and men's lacrosse, the National Operating Committee on Standards for Athletic Equipment offers certification. Athletes should use equipment that displays the logo of these certifying bodies to ensure safety (Fig. 6.1). The ASTM standards have proven to be extremely effective in preventing sports eye injuries; no severe eye injuries have been reported for an athlete wearing appropriate eye protection.

TABLE 6.2
Recommended Eye Protectors for Selected Sports[a].

Sport	Minimal Eye Protector	Comment
Baseball/softball (youth batter and base runner)	ASTM F910	Face guard attached to helmet
Baseball/softball (fielder)	ASTM F803 for baseball	ASTM specifies age ranges
Basketball	ASTM F803 for basketball	ASTM specifies age ranges
Bicycling	Helmet plus streetwear/fashion eyewear	
Boxing	None available; not permitted in sport	Contraindicated for functionally one-eyed athletes
Fencing	Protector with neck bib	
Field hockey (men and women)	ASTM F803 for women's lacrosse Goalie full-face mask	Protectors that pass for women's lacrosse also pass for field hockey
Football	Polycarbonate eye shield attached to helmet-mounted wire face mask	
Full-contact martial arts	None available; not permitted in sport	Contraindicated for functionally one-eyed athletes
Ice hockey	ASTM F513 face mask on helmet Goaltenders ASTM F1587	HECC- or CSA-certified full-face shield
Lacrosse (men)	Face mask attached to lacrosse helmet	
Lacrosse (women)	ASTM F803 for women's lacrosse	Optional helmet
Paintball	ASTM F1776 for paintball	
Racquet sports (badminton, tennis, paddle tennis, handball, squash, and racquetball)	ASTM F803 for selected sport	
Soccer	ASTM F803 for selected sport	
Street hockey	ASTM 513 face mask on helmet	Must be HECC or CSA certified
Track and field	Streetwear with polycarbonate lenses/fashion eyewear[b]	
Water polo, swimming	Swim goggles with polycarbonate lenses	
Wrestling	No standard available	Optional custom-protective eyewear

ASTM, American Society for Testing of Materials; *CSA*, Canadian Standards Association; *HECC*, Hockey Equipment Certification Council.
[a] Joint policy statement of the American Academy of Pediatrics Board of Directors, February 1996, and the American Academy of Ophthalmology Board of Trustees, February 1995. Revised and approved by the American Academy of Pediatrics Board of Directors, June 2011, and the American Academy of Ophthalmology Board of Trustees, 2013.
[b] Eyewear that passes ASTM F803 is safer than streetwear eyewear for all sports activities with impact potential.

To assist athletes in selecting appropriate sports eye protection, the American Academy of Ophthalmology issued a joint policy statement with the American Academy of Pediatrics containing recommended eye protectors for selected sports (Table 6.2).[33] Many publications have provided recommendations for eye protection in sports.[26,34–51] Two basic types of protective eyewear designs are available: a goggle style worn similarly to dress eyewear (Fig. 6.2) and shield-style protection attached to a helmet (Fig. 6.3). Protective sports eyewear must be correctly fit to ensure adequate protection for the athlete. If a young athlete has facial features that are too small to fit any available protective sports eyewear correctly, polycarbonate lenses of 3 mm

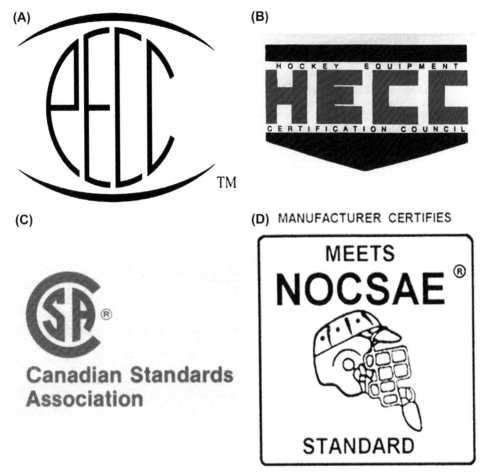

FIG. 6.1 Certifying logos from the **(A)** Protective Eyewear Certification Council, **(B)** Hockey Equipment Certification Council, **(C)** Canadian Standards Association, and **(D)** National Operating Committee on Standards for Athletic Equipment. (Courtesy of Paul Vinger, MD, Concord, Massachusetts.)

center thickness should be placed in a children's frame that meets ANSI Z87.1 standards. This design offers the best chance of eye protection in this situation, although it may not completely protect the athlete from the forces encountered in many sports.[26]

Eye protection can prevent ocular damage in many sports. This chapter focuses on the more common sports in which eye protection is used.

Racquet Sports

As discussed in Chapter 7, a significant portion of sport-related eye injuries are caused by racquet sports.[31,52–57] Racquet sports include badminton, handball, racquetball, squash, and tennis; the CSA and ASTM F803 standard and ISO 18527-2 standard are designed to provide protection for any racquet sport. The ball or shuttlecock is hit with tremendous force and can travel at dramatic speeds (Table 6.3). As previously mentioned, the eyewear must protect the eye and orbit from a squash or racquetball projected at 90 mph from several angles, including the side. The hinges are also tested to ensure protection from the forces directed at this potentially weak area. Hingeless frames with straps are recommended when feasible.

Even though the balls used in some racquet sports are larger than the average orbital opening, the compression forces can push the ball deep inside the orbit.[31] The first protective eyewear was designed for use in handball and consisted of a lensless rubber-covered wire frame to reduce the orbital opening (Fig. 6.4). These open eye guards were subsequently

(A)

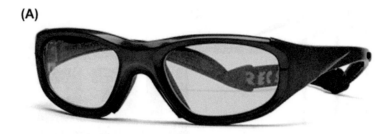

Bright Blue / Black

(B)

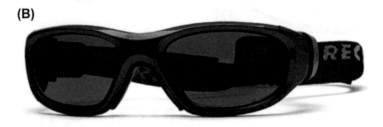

Crimson / Black

FIG. 6.2 Goggle-style sports eye protectors: **(A)** Liberty MAXX frame with temples and **(B)** Liberty MAXX frame with straps. (Courtesy of Liberty Sport, Fairfield, New Jersey.)

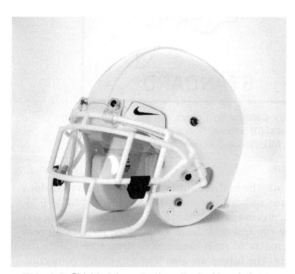

FIG. 6.3 Shield-style protection attached to a helmet.

TABLE 6.3
Estimated Ball or Shuttlecock Speed Records in Competition.

Sport	Shot Type/Record	Speed in kph (mph)
Badminton	Smash	426 (264.7)
Racquetball	Serve	307 (191)
Squash	Serve	281.6 (176)
Table tennis	Smash record	116 (72)
Tennis	Men's serve record	253 (157)
	Women's serve record	210.8 (131)

See Guinness Book of World Records.

used for protection in squash and racquetball. Studies demonstrated that the lack of a protective lens allowed penetration of the ball, potentially resulting in significant eye trauma.[58–63] The ability of the lensless eye guard to compress the ball actually may increase the risk to the ocular tissues by essentially funneling the ball into the orbit.[61,63] Additionally, lensless eye guards

offer only limited protection from a racquet injury and are never recommended for use.

Performance requirements for prescription and nonprescription sports protective eyewear for racquet sports (racquetball, squash, and tennis) will have a new ASTM international standard, F3164. The new standard will expand on F803 to address specific requirements for racquet sports and to update the standards to match the advances in these sports.

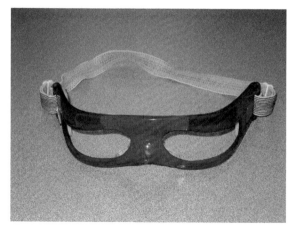

FIG. 6.4 Lensless eye guard previously used for racquet sports.

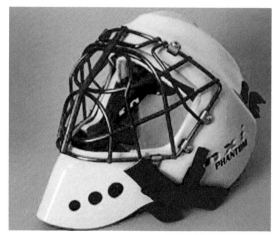

FIG. 6.5 Hockey goaltender face and eye protection. (Courtesy of NxI Defense Systems, Lake Orion, Michigan.)

Many have advocated for protective eyewear use in squash and racquetball and for promoting education regarding the ineffective protection provided by dress eyewear.[57–74] Dress eyewear with glass or CR39 lenses may increase the risk of severe ocular trauma in racquet sports if the lens shatters on impact.[53,59,64,67,75,76] Most racquet sport organizations for handball, racquetball, and squash mandate the use of appropriate protective eyewear during competition, and many athletic clubs have instituted eye protection requirements for club play. Similar consideration should be given for mandating appropriate protective eyewear for badminton, especially considering the speed of the shuttlecock in competition.[77]

Ice and Field Hockey
In ice hockey the most common cause of eye injury is from the stick, followed by the puck or opponent.[31,52,78–85] With the mandate for face protection in all levels of hockey, except the National Hockey League (NHL), the incidence of eye injuries has significantly declined.[86–90] No eye injuries have been reported with a full-face shield in use; however, significant trauma has been incurred with a half-face shield.[90] It was unfortunate that for many years the NHL resisted issuing a mandate for face protection, with each season producing examples of the ocular effects of this decision. Beginning with the 2013–14 season, the NHL mandated that all players who have fewer than 25 games of NHL experience must wear a visor properly affixed to their helmet. Furthermore, visors are to be affixed to the helmets in such a fashion as to ensure adequate eye protection. A retrospective study of 10 NHL seasons found significantly increased risk

of eye injuries in players who did not wear a visor, and those players were found to be involved in more fights, hits, and penalty minutes.[91] At this time, more than 90% of NHL players use a visor. There are many styles of face protection approved for hockey by ASTM (F513 and F1587) and CSA (CAN3-Z262.2-M78) standards: full-face masks for goaltenders and full-face masks or half visors for other positions (Fig. 6.5). Because of the improved eye safety profile, full-face shields are recommended.

The ASTM F803 standard is recommended for eye protection in field hockey. Similar to the update to the F803 standard described for tennis, field hockey now has a new standard (F2713) specific to the requirements of the sport. A study found significantly higher rates of eye injuries and concussions in states with no protective eyewear mandate for field hockey compared with those that had mandates.[92,93] In the states with no mandate, players were more than five times likely to sustain a hockey-related eye injury than those in a state with a mandate. The eye injuries were more serious in states without a mandate and were virtually eliminated in those with a mandate. In addition, the concussion rates were similar between the states, indicating that the use of protection did not result in more aggressive or physical play in the states with a mandate.

Lacrosse
Lacrosse has risks for eye injury that are similar to hockey in that the stick and ball present significant hazards. Men's lacrosse mandates head and face protectors, thereby minimizing the risk for ocular injury. Women's lacrosse did not mandate face protection until recently, and the incidence and severity of eye injuries that

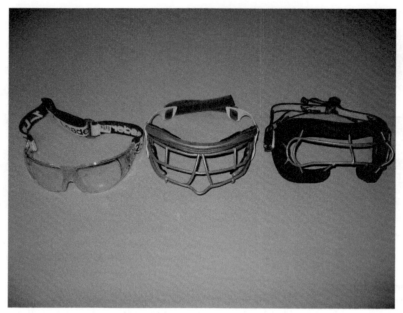

FIG. 6.6 Wire mesh eye protector for women's lacrosse.

caused many to advocate for compulsory eye protection appear justified by a significant reduction in the number of eye injuries in the year following the mandate.[31,94–100] The ASTM F803 standard is recommended for protection in women's lacrosse, and wire mesh protectors are favored by the athletes (Fig. 6.6). The women's lacrosse ball is shot at 45 mph at the eyewear during ASTM testing to determine effective attenuation of the forces encountered in the sport. Similar to the update to the F803 standard described for tennis and field hockey, lacrosse now has a new standard (F3077) specific to the requirements of the sport.

Baseball
Baseballs have a high incidence of reported eye injuries in the United States, and the sport of baseball has been reported as the leading cause of sport-related eye injuries in children in the United States.[31,57,101–104] Risks include being hit with a pitch or a batted or thrown baseball. Spectators are also at risk of injury from batted balls or errant throws. The hardness of the ball has been related to the potential risk for head injury but does not have a significant effect on ocular injuries; the harder the ball, the greater the risk for head and brain injury.[105] The ASTM F910 standard is designed to provide protection for batters and base runners in youth baseball. Approved face guards have provided excellent protection and have good acceptability by athletes and parents.[106] A significant portion of youth baseball players

reported vision obstruction (40%) and discomfort (23%) and that they played worse with the face guard (12%); however, 81% believed playing with the face guard was acceptable.[106]

Paintball and Airsoft Sports
War games with paintball guns present a tremendous risk for ocular injury when proper protection is not used.[107–115] The paint pellet is shot with sufficient energy to cause severe eye trauma; the ASTM F1776 standard therefore establishes specifications for eye protection (Fig. 6.7). Eye injuries have not been reported with the use of ASTM F1776 approved eyewear, although eye injury can occur from a shot that displaces loosely fitting eyewear.[111] Airsoft sports are covered by the F2879 standards; however, other shooting sports are not specifically covered by ASTM standards. The ASTM F803 standard is generally recommended for use as "combat goggles,"[47] and polycarbonate lenses with side shields have been recommended to protect against shotgun spray.[116]

Alpine Skiing
The risk of ocular trauma is relatively low for cross-country and downhill skiers. Tree branches can cause problems and ski pole tips can result in significant damage.[117] The ASTM F659 standard is designed to protect against lens breakage from a ski pole impact. Because the amount of ultraviolet (UV) radiation markedly

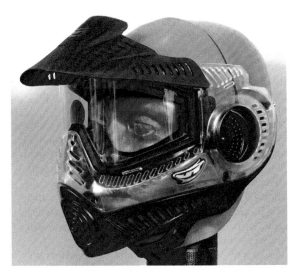

FIG. 6.7 Eye and face protection for paintball.

increases at higher elevations, and snow reflects 85% of the UV radiation, additional risk of photokeratitis exists when appropriate UV filters are not used.[118] Many goggle designs are available with prescription inserts for those who do not wear CLs, although CLs are typically the preferred method for refractive compensation.

Swimming and Water Sports

Swimming and water sports also do not present a significant risk of eye trauma. A study of ocular pathology prevalence in swimmers using goggles for at least 5 years compared with nonswimmers found no significant differences.[119] The elastic band tension, however, can cause swim goggles to snap back and cause severe ocular injuries.[31] Many swim goggles are commercially available, and many designs are available with prescription lenses.[120,121] Most swimmers and divers use a goggle or face mask so that no adjustment is necessary to the habitual prescription to compensate for the difference in the index of refraction of the water medium.[47] Some goggle designs have ventilation holes to reduce lens fogging in highly active water sports such as water skiing, surfing, windsurfing, and endurance swimming.[121] A variety of dive masks are also available with prescription inserts or corrective lenses affixed to the faceplate. The air space of the dive mask eliminates the need to change the habitual prescription; however, the increased vertex distance may necessitate an adjustment to the prescription. Water polo presents a risk of blunt trauma from fingers, elbows, or the ball to the improperly protected eye. Swim goggles for water

polo should contain polycarbonate lenses to prevent lens breakage, particularly for goalkeepers, who are at a higher risk for facial injury from the ball.

Soccer

The soccer ball is responsible for most ocular traumas in soccer, although the incidence of eye injuries is relatively low.[55,57,122–127] Although the soccer ball is significantly larger than the orbital opening, a portion of the ball will deform and enter the orbit during contact with the high velocities at which the ball is kicked.[126,127] A work item for eye protection in soccer (WK1237) was initiated under an ASTM committee for F803, but there were no recommendations produced. Most practitioners recommend the use of ASTM F803 standard eyewear for racquet sports with a secure strap for protection in soccer.

Other Sports

Eye protection may be desirable in many other sports and recreational activities, but no standards exist for those activities. Protective eyewear that meets the ASTM standard for squash often offers the best available protection for athletes unless custom-fabricated protective eyewear can be acquired.

Issues With Protective Eyewear

Some of the common issues causing athletes to be resistant to using protective eyewear are eyewear discomfort, adjustment to wearing eyewear, lens fogging, poor vision (especially visual field constriction), cosmetic appearance, and the perception that it is unnecessary. Athletes who do not habitually wear a spectacle prescription have more difficulty adjusting to wearing eyewear. Adjustment can occur quickly if the eyewear is worn for an extended period (e.g., several hours continuously), and this should be done outside the sport situation to minimize athlete stress during adaptation. This eyewear adaptation training should also help the athlete adjust to the change in peripheral visual field size that may be induced by the frame.

Early studies found that sports protective eyewear constricted the peripheral visual field.[128–130] The constricted visual field was perceived by 12.5% of subjects using racquetball protectors[128] and was reported to affect visual reaction time (especially with flat lens design eyewear).[130] A study of several types of protective eyewear found that all restricted peripheral vision to some degree but that the restriction did not affect a peripheral reaction task.[129] Some recent studies did not find that sports eye protectors constricted visual fields,[131,132] whereas a comparison of hockey visor and sports goggles did find field restrictions but no effect on visual acuity, contrast sensitivity, color vision, or foveal threshold.[133] The decision to wear eye protection becomes a balance between the cost to peripheral vision versus the risk of vision loss.

In highly active sports, and humid or cold environmental conditions, problems with eyewear fogging can occur. All approved protective eyewear has an antifog coating on the lenses and additional antifog solutions are available for supplemental use. Athletes should remove the eyewear when not actively participating in the sport to prevent the rising body heat from condensing on the lenses.[64]

Many athletes are concerned about cosmetic appearance and protective eyewear is not typically appealing to the athlete. Fortunately, protective eyewear has evolved into more fashionable designs with vibrant colors and more options to select from, which will hopefully help earn greater acceptability in some sports. Athletes and sports in which a prevailing attitude of machismo impedes the use of appropriate eye protection will always exist.

Squash is a sport with a significant risk for eye injury and has received the attention of several studies to determine the issues related to the low rates of protective eyewear use in the sport. Many players believe that prescription dress eyewear offers adequate protection,[69−72] and lensless eye guards may continue to be sold as protection.[66] Among those who do not wear any eyewear during squash, most believed that protective eyewear was unnecessary because of inadequate knowledge of the risks.[71,72,134] The misperception that experience and expertise reduce the risk for eye injury in squash also exists[134]; in fact, the amount of time playing squash and the increased speeds encountered at higher levels of play actually increase the risk for injury.[67,135] Some squash players were concerned with poor vision and comfort[34]; however, studies suggest that education regarding injury risk and prevention is an effective motivator to increase eye protection use (especially because a previous eye injury increases use).[66,69,71−73,133,134,136−138]

Functionally Monocular Athletes

Some athletes would like to compete in sports but have some level of loss of function in one eye. Best corrected visual acuity less than 20/40 (6/12) is often used to determine loss of visual function because this level of impairment begins to affect academic and occupational performance as well as driving privileges. A study of children with an enucleated eye found good compliance with protective eyewear use in sports and that

subsequent eye injury to the remaining eye had been successfully averted.[41] In the functionally monocular athlete, the main risk is severe injury to the better eye. Children with amblyopia have a risk of blindness that is more than 15 times higher than those with normal vision (1.75/1000 compared with 0.11/1000), and trauma (including sports trauma) accounts for more than 50% of the resulting blindness.[139]

Functionally monocular athletes should use protective eyewear that meets relevant standards for participation in all sports activities.[39] These same athletes should wear well-built dress eyewear frames containing polycarbonate or Trivex lenses for nonsport activities. Functionally monocular athletes should be discouraged from participating in sports with a risk for serious eye injury in which an effective method of eye protection does not exist, such as boxing, wrestling, and martial arts.[39,140]

Athletes who have had eye trauma or eye surgery that has resulted in a weakening of the ocular tissues should be counseled about the risk of eye trauma in sports. Recommendations for eye protection in sports and recreational activities are made similar to those for the functionally monocular athlete.[26] Specifically, athletes who have undergone radial keratotomy (RK) should be adequately counseled because the procedure significantly weakens the corneal integrity.[31] Modern ablation methods of laser refractive surgery have a lower risk profile compared with RK; however, there is an increased risk of flap dislocation in post-laser in situ keratomileusis (LASIK) eyes for athletes in some sports.[141,142]

Clinicolegal Issues for Protective Eyewear

Eye care providers are in a position that requires appropriate patient counseling regarding eye injury risks and suitable prevention measures. All prescribed or recommended ophthalmic materials are potential sources of legal liability. Legal liability claims can be based on either practitioner negligence or product-based liability resulting from problems with the lenses or frames.[143−146] Plano eyewear and plano sun eyewear can also be a source of potential liability for the practitioner if proper counseling is not provided. Patients who use CLs or who have undergone laser refractive surgery also need appropriate counseling regarding supplemental eye protection during sports and recreational activities.[147]

Good patient counseling begins with a thorough patient history to determine the specific needs and risk profile for the individual. A lack of knowledge regarding a patient's sports participation does not protect a practitioner in a liability case if an attempt to elicit that information was not made. Any eyewear recommendations must be made with a thorough knowledge of how that eyewear will be used.

A claim of professional negligence is particularly troubling for a practitioner. Negligence claims involving sports and recreational eyewear typically stem from failure to prescribe the appropriate lens material, failure to warn of potential for breakage (especially with non-impact-resistant materials), or failure to inspect and verify the eyewear before dispensing.[143,145] Industry standards play an important role in determining legal liability, and practitioners are expected to understand and comply with those standards. As previously mentioned, polycarbonate or Trivex lenses offer increased impact resistance compared with glass or CR-39; therefore these materials clearly are the recommended choice.[18–22] The lens material preference should be clearly stated on the prescription provided to the patient; if the patient refuses the recommended lens material, that fact should be adequately documented in the patient record and the patient should be warned of the diminished impact resistance of the alternate material. The impact resistance of a lens material should be discussed without using the words shatterproof or unbreakable because even polycarbonate material will shatter if hit with sufficient force.[143] If a practitioner offers ophthalmic dispensing services, the ancillary personnel responsible for verification and dispensing should be properly educated regarding the industry standards. The lenses should be inspected to ensure that the impact resistance is not compromised by surface treatments[22] or improper edging.[143]

Eye care practitioners are also obligated to counsel the patient on suitable frames for sports and recreational activities. The frames should meet any prevailing ASTM, CSA or ISO performance standards, and the practitioner and dispensing personnel must understand the proper uses for the eyewear and any liability issues. For example, claims have resulted from the recommendation of lensless eye guards for racquetball.[144,148] If a patient selects a frame that is not suitable for protection, that fact should be adequately documented in the patient record and the patient should be warned of the diminished impact resistance of both the frame and the lenses (because the frame may not adequately prevent the lenses from displacing back into the eye on impact).

PRESCRIBING FILTERS AND PERFORMANCE SUN EYEWEAR

Athletes who participate in outdoor sports and recreational activities require protection from solar radiation. On a bright sunny day, illuminance ranges from 1000 to 10,000 footlamberts, saturating the retina and reducing finer levels of contrast sensitivity.[149] Dark sunglasses aid in recovery of contrast sensitivity and dark adaptation after photoreceptor saturation.[150] The commonly accepted benefits of sun eyewear include protection from sun exposure and ocular trauma, and the reduction of eye fatigue, squinting, and glare disability. The ability of properly selected filters to reduce glare and improve contrast may also produce an enhancement in the ability to discern crucial details and judge depth.

The ocular effects of UV radiation depend on the duration of exposure and the wavelength of the radiation.[151] Prolonged exposure to the middle UV-B waveband has been associated with a variety of ocular problems, including pterygium, pinguecula, cataract, and keratopathy.[152–154] UV protection provides patients with decreased risks of cataracts, photokeratitis, corneal burns, anterior uveitis, and retinal lesions.[152,153] The American Optometric Association recommends 99% −100% protection from near- and middle-UV (UV-A, UV-B) radiation for sun eyewear.[155]

Research on the hazards of high-intensity blue light, defined by European sunglass standards as 380−500 nm, has shown that short-wavelength visible light may create deleterious retinal changes, specifically retinal lesions.[156,157] The most harmful wavelength in the visible spectrum for the production of retinal injury appears to be radiation near 440 nm.[154]

The visible light portion of the electromagnetic spectrum is between approximately 380 and 760 nm (Fig. 6.8). The human eye is capable of discerning the entire spectrum of color because of the different wavelengths of light that comprise the chromatic spectrum. Part of the eye's ability to see artificial (or enhanced) depth is because of the natural chromatic aberration that occurs when monochromatic light is focused on the retina. Because of the differences of wavelength, different colors will refract through the ocular media with different focal points. The difference in focal power between the shorter wavelengths (blue spectrum) and the longer wavelengths (red spectrum) is approximately 2.3 D of focal length.[158] This chromatic aberration results in image blur. Chromatic aberration is cited as the most significant aberration in the well-corrected human eye,[158,159] and filters that diminish transmission of the short-wavelength (blue) portion of the visible light spectrum improve retinal image quality by reducing the amount of chromatic aberration.[160]

Visible light is responsible for glare that can cause significant interference with an athlete's ability to see the visual details critical for successful performance. For example, direct glare from the sun is evident in a blue sky because it affects the visibility of a lofted ball. Reflected glare is exceptionally troubling for athletes when the sun is reflected off surfaces such as water, snow, pavement, and sand. These surfaces reflect horizontally polarized light that can produce substantial glare, particularly water surfaces that are constantly moving. Vertically polarized filters are effective by virtually eliminating horizontally polarized light in the environment.

For an athlete who must compete during the twilight transition hours, the exposure to bright sunlight impedes the initial phase of dark adaptation.[151,161–163] The final level of dark adaptation is elevated, and daily prolonged sun exposure can produce decrements in visual acuity and contrast sensitivity.[161,162,164] Excessive exposure to bright visible light can result in erythropsia, which is often reported as "red vision" when the individual returns indoors after many hours in the sun.[165] The judicious use of sun eyewear can minimize the impact of bright sunlight on the dark adaptation process and thereby assist the athlete during the transition to artificial lighting conditions. Additionally, the transmission levels of sun eyewear lenses may need to be periodically adjusted in changing sun conditions (e.g., variable cloud cover). An athlete may benefit from a variety of sun eyewear products or a single product with interchangeable lenses or photochromic lenses. Skeet and trap shooters are particularly sensitive to the effects of changing light levels and typically possess eyewear incorporating several filter hues with several tint densities (Fig. 6.9).

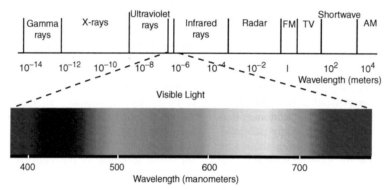

FIG. 6.8 Electromagnetic spectrum.

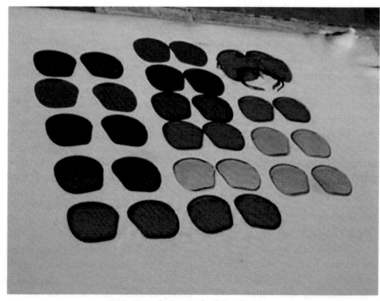

FIG. 6.9 A shooter's tint selection.

Sun eyewear is a tremendous market, and growth in the sports sun eyewear segment has been impressive. Significant innovations in frame design have been made to suit sports demands better, and a trend toward sport-specific lens tinting has been growing. Many manufacturers have invested heavily in research and design to develop light transmission characteristics that purportedly offer performance enhancement features for specific sport demands. Continued innovation in this area can be expected as frame and lens technologies continue to push the envelope of individualized and sport-specific performance. Separating the hype from solid evidence of performance benefits is often difficult, and tint preference is still broadly influenced by individual variations. The transmittance characteristics for each filter are based on the tint colors used, the amount of tint used, and the lens material used.[150,157,166] The resulting spectral transmission curve is often proprietary for the manufacturer and protected by patent law. The general filter recommendations in this chapter are presented as a guide.

Neutral Gray Tints

Neutral gray tints absorb all wavelengths of the visible light spectrum approximately equally; therefore the natural appearance of colors is preserved. Gray filters often have the lowest transmission properties, so that they perform best in very bright conditions. These filters are preferred by athletes who are sensitive to color information in their sport and who do not appreciate even subtle alteration of the natural environment. Neutral gray tints are often favored by those participating in golf, skiing, and mountaineering activities. Athletes must make critical performance decisions based on subtle terrain details in these sports and distortion of natural contour cues can lead to poor decisions.

Yellow-Brown Range Tints

The process of filtering some of the visible spectrum through the attenuation of the transmittance of the shorter wavelength colors (blue) decreases the chromatic aberration between the longer red wavelengths and the transmitted midrange greens. The reduction in chromatic aberration leads to improved image clarity, and the selective transmission of yellow wavelength light concentrates the visible information at the most sensitive portion of the visible light spectrum. Therefore yellow-range tints filter the glare produced by the short-wavelength light while transmitting peak visible light information with reduced chromatic aberration. Studies have not always been successful in quantifying the improvement in visual acuity and contrast sensitivity

reported with yellow tints.[150] Yellow filters have been shown to improve depth perception, contour recognition, and reaction times.[167–179] Of note, many of these studies were conducted under indoor artificial lighting conditions that are far below the intensity (in candelas per square meter) of natural sunlight and this factor may obfuscate the enhancement effects.

Many athletes appreciate the improvement in contrast with yellow-range tints, especially in low-light conditions such as twilight (dawn and dusk), fog, and heavy cloud cover. Early studies found that objects were more visible in fog with a yellow tint in front of a light.[180,181] Of note, outdoor low-light conditions are still substantially more intense than indoor artificial lighting. The common response is that these filters brighten and sharpen the details while enhancing subtle contrast features; however, the effect may be uncomfortable for photosensitive athletes. The improved contrast judgment is most likely caused by the reduction in chromatic aberration induced by the filter. Yellow and brown tints are popular with shooting and snow sport athletes and perform well in fog and low-light conditions.[182] Mountaineers use yellow tints in whiteout conditions to enhance the contrast of environmental features.[183] Thick fog and whiteout conditions produce a Ganzfeld effect, and the reduced chromatic aberration serves to enhance the visibility of low-contrast images. Yellow tints have been used for driving, boating, or flying in low-light conditions; however, the filters distort color perception and can cause problems with traffic signal recognition. A yellow-range tint may be helpful in sports in which an object must be located or tracked against the background of a blue or overcast sky, such as tennis, baseball, and soccer. Studies have demonstrated improved perception of low-contrast contours and faster reaction time for low-contrast targets with yellow tints.[167,168]

Green-Range Tints

Information in the green portion of the visible light spectrum is selectively transmitted by green-range tints. This allows green information to be enhanced and other colors to be relatively muted. Green tints may be preferred in golf, tennis, and woodland shooting. For golf, the green tint enhances the contour information of the grass, and the tint will accentuate the contrast of a brown animal against the green foliage for hunters. Green-range tints have been advocated in tennis to enhance the contrast of the yellow tennis ball against the blue sky; however, the tint can effectively mask the ball against a green background—a common paint color for the court surface and windscreen around the court.[184]

Red-Range Tints

Red-range tints are designed to transmit information selectively at the far end of the visible light spectrum. These filters are widely used in trap and skeet shooting because the reddish orange sporting clay is enhanced against the background of brown dirt, grass, green foliage, or blue sky. Red-range filters also absorb short-wavelength light that contributes to the poor image quality effects of chromatic aberration. These tints are popular in sports in which sharp image clarity is crucial, especially in heavy overcast or foggy conditions. Skiers favor red-range tints for "flat" light conditions and often report enhancement of contrast judgment and depth information with red-range goggles.

Blue-Range Tints

Blue-range tints do not offer a substantive benefit for most sports. The selective transmission of short-wavelength visible light does not serve to diminish glare or enhance contrast. In fact, most athletes report that contrast sensitivity is degraded when blue tints are worn outdoors. Some performance sun eyewear appears to have blue-tinted lenses; however, this impression is created by the metallic or iridescent coatings applied to the lens surface.

Polarized Filters

As previously mentioned, polarized filters are excellent for reducing the effects of reflected glare off horizontal surfaces, especially water, snow, pavement, and sand. Polarized lenses are available in gray, brown, and photochromic lens options. The athlete can choose the lens option best suited for his or her sport demands. Many sports performance sun eyewear products are available with polarized filters and are potentially beneficial for fishing, water sports, driving, and cycling (especially useful for wet surfaces). Despite the widespread acceptance of polarized filters, they may remove important details in some sports. Although the amount of reflected glare from the snow surface is considerable in downhill skiing, crucial details regarding surface conditions (e.g., ice) and contours can be masked by the filters. Several companies offer a variety of golf sun eyewear with polarized lenses; however, one study found that polarized filters did not offer any statistically significant advantage or disadvantage on putting performance over nonpolarized filters.[185] It may be that polarized lenses remove some of the reflectance information from the blades of grass when judging the contours of the green. Another disadvantage of polarized filters is that many liquid crystal displays utilize a polarizer that is set at 45 degrees to aid visibility, which can significantly reduce visibility when viewed through vertically oriented polarized filters. Polarized lenses may interfere with the ability to see instrument displays used in some sport activities, such as cycling, motor sports, or flying.

Photochromic Filters

Photochromic lenses change transmission characteristics in response to changes in light or UV radiation.[186] Photochromic lenses were initially only available in glass lenses, making them unsuitable for many sports activities. Photochromic lenses are now available in CR-39, polycarbonate, and Trivex lens materials, which significantly improve their suitability for some sports. Most photochromic lenses have a gray or brown tint that darkens with exposure to intense sunlight; a photochromic lens that darkens with a polarized filter is also now available. A study comparing activated photochromic lenses with clear lenses found significant improvements in glare disability, glare discomfort, heterochromatic contrast thresholds, and photostress recovery time.[187] Photochromic lenses can be an excellent option for recreational athletes who participate in noncontact sports and who wish to have sun eyewear that is flexible with changing environmental conditions. Many persons who participate in golf, tennis, running, cycling, and fishing perform satisfactorily with spectacle corrections containing photochromic tints. For the competitive athlete, the optical performance of this option may not provide the high performance sought in performance sun eyewear.

Lens Coatings

Premium sun lenses typically have coatings to help achieve a higher level of optical performance. Most manufacturers use high-vacuum technology to apply several thin layers of coatings. These vacuum deposition coatings are designed to reduce reflections, attenuate transmission of UV and infrared radiation, selectively transmit portions of the visible spectrum (in particular, reduce transmission of short-wavelength light), minimize lens fogging, and improve scratch resistance.[188] The exact nature of the lens coatings, the sequence of the coatings, and the number of layers applied remain proprietary information protected by the manufacturer.

Metallic coatings are used to create a mirrored surface on the front of the lens that effectively reflects incident light. There are two basic types of mirror coatings: metallized and dielectrically coated. The main difference is that metallized coatings not only reflect light, like dielectrically coated mirrors, but also absorb some of the light to reduce overall transmission.

Dielectrically coated mirrors can be made in almost any color, and is distinguished from "flash" coatings that have more transparency and less reflection. The use of mirror coatings significantly decreases the amount of light reaching the eye; these coatings are exceptionally effective in sports in which sun intensity can be high, such as snow sports, water sports, beach volleyball, running, and cycling. As some mirror coatings reflect infrared radiation, which produces extra heat, these coatings are useful in sports where the ocular tissues can become overheated, such as endurance sports including running and cycling.

The use of sun eyewear results in a reduction of overall mean luminance. A natural scene in sports contains fine spatial detail that is often of low contrast, which requires a lot of light stimulating the retina in order to resolve some important details (judging a fly ball in baseball, softball, or cricket). The use of filters reduces mean luminance, which means that the ball must subtend a larger area on the retina in order to be seen. This explains why filters may not be useful in some sport situations because the object would need to be closer before the important details could be detected.[189] The issue of visibility and contrast sensitivity at far distances reinforces the need to balance filter color with visible light transmission properties so that the filter is not too dark to discern the target; sometimes more light transmission (e.g., a lighter tint) is optimal in sports applications.

The ANSI standard Z80.3 establishes impact and UV attenuation standards for plano (nonprescription) dress eyewear applied to sun eyewear.[190,191] Athletes should be counseled regarding the modest protection offered by premium sun eyewear with polycarbonate or Trivex lenses compared with glass or CR-39 lenses. Sun eyewear should offer protection from both UV-A and UV-B radiation, although manufacturer transmittance claims have been shown to be overestimated.[192] The transmittance curve of a lens product helps determine the level of UV protection. Any polycarbonate lens offers better UV protection than do uncoated glass or CR-39 lenses.

Prismatic effects induced by the lens design of the sun eyewear are another factor that may be noticed by athletes. Contributing factors to prismatic effects include the steep front and back lens curves, the tilt of the lens, lens thickness, and manufacturing abnormalities. Premium sports eyewear was found to have significant amounts of prism in both primary and lateral gaze.[193] Prismatic effects induced by eyewear designs may affect the athlete's ability to judge depth and location. For example, with yoked horizontal prisms the image is displaced laterally, but if the prisms are oriented in opposing horizontal directions, both the perceived size and distance of the object appear to change.[194] Changes in lateral displacement or apparent size and distance may cause critical errors in sport situations such as golf putting. Most ophthalmic professionals are concerned about the amount of optical distortion present in sun eyewear.

Face-form (wrap) design sun eyewear offers improved coverage of the ocular surface tissues and a wider field of view than traditional designs. The improved coverage increases UV protection by preventing light leakage around the frame and protects the eye from the harmful effects of wind and dust. The expanded visual field afforded by wrap-design eyewear is often offset by the induced prismatic effects of this design. Several eyewear manufacturers have used innovative optical designs to minimize the amount of induced prism, especially in the peripheral aspects of the lens. The result has been wrap-design lenses with an enhanced "sweet spot" viewing area with minimal prismatic distortion. The Nike and Oakley (Oakley.com) eyewear designs were found to have the least amount of induced prism in both primary gaze and 30 degrees of lateral gaze directions.[193] Of note, prescription eyewear with a wrap design may need to have the prescription power adjusted to compensate for the wrap.[195]

An excellent fit is required when dispensing sun eyewear for sports use. The frame needs to fit snugly to the face to prevent issues with vertex distance and visual field obstruction from the frame; however, a snug fit can reduce wind exposure while creating fogging problems. Many sports frames are designed to minimize fogging through improved ventilation around the frame and through the nosepiece (Fig. 6.10). The frame should also stay secured to the head so that movement does not dislodge the eyewear. Many manufacturers use rubber and silicone to softly grip the frame to the head at its contact points on the nose bridge and around the ears. The frames should be adjusted so that the touch points of the frame do not create discomfort and the optical centers are aligned in the primary viewing position. Some sports frames have adjustable or changeable temples and nose bridges to provide the athlete with the best possible fit. The specific needs of the female athlete have begun to be addressed by the sun eyewear industry, resulting in better-fitting frames and sport-specific designs.[196] Finally, eyewear designs obviously need to be aesthetically pleasing for any athlete to use it!

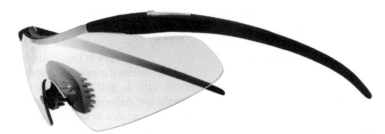

FIG. 6.10 Sun eyewear highlighting ventilation and nosepiece design to prevent fogging.

CONTACT LENSES

The value of "plastic" CLs for refractive compensation in athletes has been readily recognized since the advent of plastic lenses.[197–201] The advent of CLs provided many young athletes with significant refractive conditions the potential to compete with the rest of their peers. Testimonials were written by elite athletes regarding the marvels of CLs for sports purposes.[202,203] Many of the disadvantages of spectacle corrections are eliminated by the use of CLs, especially in contact sports in which eyewear can become a limitation to the athlete. The available options for eye care practitioners increased from the limited applications of custom-fit scleral (haptic) lenses and polymethyl methacrylate lenses to modern rigid gas permeable (RGP) and hydrogel (soft) lens choices. Indeed, CLs have become the method of choice for refractive compensation in most sports.

Considerations for Performance Contact Lenses

The field-of-view aberrations, visual field restriction, optical distortion, frame comfort, frame stability, surface reflections, lens fogging, and precipitation issues described with spectacle lenses can largely be avoided by moving the optics onto the cornea. The induced prismatic effects evident with most spectacle lenses when the athlete views off the optical centers of the lenses are eliminated by CLs. The potential visual field impediment created by eyewear frames is eliminated with CLs, as are the issues of lens reflection and fogging that compromise visual performance with eyewear. The peripheral visual field is increased by approximately 15% with CLs.[204] Athletes often report compromised comfort from eyewear frames as well, and the precision of the frame fit is often further compromised by the handling of the eyewear. CLs are an excellent option in highly dynamic sports because no frame can be dislodged and no lenses can fog up. Dynamic sports include baseball, basketball, football, gymnastics, hockey, lacrosse, racquet sports, skiing sports, skating sports,

soccer, surfing sports, and volleyball (see Box 2.3). Although CL comfort certainly is an issue to contend with, the frame issues of eyewear are removed with this option. The combination of these advantages elevates the use of CLs as the method of choice for refractive compensation for most athletes.

The main objective of CL corrections is to provide an excellent optical image that is stable in all conditions encountered during sports performance. Excellent visual acuity is typically a critical factor in sports performance, and measurement of visual acuity through CLs is a standard part of an assessment. Snellen-type visual acuity measurements may not be sensitive to the subtle visual discrimination tasks inherent in many sports because the acuity task is usually performed only under high-contrast conditions. Measurement of contrast sensitivity function has been recommended in athletes because many sports involve visual discrimination tasks in suboptimal lighting caused by environmental variability (see Chapter 4). Contrast sensitivity may also be degraded in CL wearers if the lenses are not optimal, even when visual acuity appears acceptable.[205–208] Therefore contrast sensitivity measurement is an essential part of the evaluation of athletes who wear CLs during sports participation.

Spherical refractive errors are most easily compensated for with CLs, whereas astigmatism can present a complex fitting predicament. If excellent visual acuity cannot be achieved with a spherical lens, a soft toric lens or RGP lens should be considered. The amounts of corneal and lenticular astigmatism combine to result in the manifest astigmatism, and this combination ultimately affects the lens choices for optimal compensation. Many options are available in hydrogel and RGP materials to provide the best features for the athlete.

Aiming sports typically require prolonged fixation to achieve proper alignment with the target. As previously mentioned, many shooters and archers prefer spectacles over CLs because of the stability of clear vision obtained with spectacle lenses. Lens dehydration and surface irregularities can create significant problems in athletes with insufficient blinking or tear quality.[6] CL movement on the eye can also produce undesirable visual fluctuations during prolonged gaze behavior (without blinking) that many shooters and archers develop. CL movement has been shown to degrade contrast sensitivity.[329]

Many sports involve rapid saccadic movements as the athlete quickly assesses crucial visual information. The amount of lens movement during saccadic eye movements relates to the stability of the vision achieved with CLs. A tighter fit is generally preferred for CLs used during sports to minimize the effects of lens movement on visual performance. Lens centration should also be carefully evaluated to ensure excellent optical performance. Centration is important to assess in the pertinent gaze positions for the particular sport or position, in addition to measurements in primary gaze. Because many sports require the athlete to view information in nonprimary gaze directions (see Chapter 2), visual performance of CLs in these gaze directions is a critical aspect to assess. For example, in cycling, much of the visual information is acquired in an upgaze eye position. CL performance for a cyclist should be assessed in an upgaze position, and the factors of wind and debris should be addressed for that athlete with lens materials and supplemental protection.

The length of time that the athlete participates in the sport activity may direct the CL choices. An analysis of sports determined that the majority of competitions are completed within 2 h.[7] Even considering the travel time to participate, a sport-specific CL can be prescribed to avoid potential physiologic consequences from different fit characteristics used by some practitioners.[6,121,209,210] The sport-specific CL is worn solely for use during sports participation and a habitual prescription is used the remainder of the time. Some endurance sports necessitate a lens modality for extended use. These lenses ideally remain on the eyes throughout the event and require minimal care. In high-altitude mountaineering, long-distance sailing, or long-distance motor racing, the athlete experiences extreme conditions over a long period. The CLs should provide excellent visual performance throughout the event while sustaining good ocular health. For example, in high-altitude mountaineering, the lens needs to provide good oxygen transmission and visual performance. Removal and insertion of lenses is not practical in an extremely cold climate and the care solutions may freeze. CLs have been successfully worn on climbs of Mount Everest, and they offer a degree of protection from low temperatures and wind-driven ice and snow without fogging or breaking in the cold.[210–214] To maximize oxygen transmission at high altitudes, a higher water content hydrogel lens must be used (e.g., 70% water content), even though higher water content lenses dehydrate faster in the cold, dry climate of high mountains. The performance of these lenses should be assessed after a period of extended wear before participation in an endurance event.

CL wearers must contend with the effects of environmental conditions on CL performance. For athletes, issues of humidity, debris, wind, and UV exposure may need to be addressed when determining the best CL option. As previously mentioned, low-water-content lenses typically perform better in low-humidity climates. Larger, thicker CLs are beneficial to prevent further dehydration. Low-humidity climates include desert environments, alpine environments, and artificial indoor environments. These same lens recommendations apply to sports in which considerable wind or airflow hits the face. Wind hastens drying of CLs, so the athlete needs additional counseling in proficient blink behavior and the benefits of supplemental eyewear or goggles. For problems with dirt and debris, soft CLs are preferred because they do not trap debris under the lenses as readily as rigid lenses. Supplemental protection may also be warranted in sports with significant exposure to UV radiation. Some soft CLs are available with a UV-absorbing tint to reduce the effects of intense UV exposure on the ocular tissues. UV-absorbing CLs only provide protection to the ocular tissues covered by the CL; therefore they provide the best protection when used in combination with quality sun eyewear. UV-absorbing CLs may also offer a degree of protection for athletes at risk for pterygium formation or those who have had surgical treatment for pterygia. Light incident at the temporal cornea is focused by the peripheral anterior eye to the nasal limbus, the usual site of pterygium formation.[215]

Many athletes are affected by dry eye syndrome. Many events precipitate or exacerbate the pathophysiologic conditions implicated in the development of dry eye disease.[216] For athletes, the cumulative effects of UV exposure and dehydrating conditions (e.g., low humidity, wind exposure, airflow) can play a significant role in the development of dry eye problems. Additionally, sympathetic responses to competitive stress and the effects of heightened attention on blink behavior further contribute to the pathogenesis of dry eye disease. Athletes who are CL wearers typically have dry eye symptoms more often than those who do not wear CLs. Many treatment options are available for specific aspects of dry eye disease,[216] and athletes should receive aggressive treatment of this condition so that it does not interfere with sports performance. Several CL materials and lens care products are designed to minimize the effects of dry eye on CL wear, and these options should be considered for the athlete with dry eye syndrome. Senofilcon A CLs, such as Acuvue Oasys (Vistakon), have demonstrated greater relief of subjective ocular discomfort associated with lens wear in adverse environmental conditions than in habitual lenses of CL wearers and also provided better comfort than with no lens wear.[217] In addition to pharmaceutical treatment, the athlete should be thoroughly educated on proper lid hygiene, good blink behavior, the potential benefits of rehydrating drops for the CLs, and the rewards of a suitable diet and fluid consumption.

Performance-Tinted Contact Lenses

Tints designed to enhance performance have been incorporated into CLs for use in certain sports. By moving the tint from the spectacle plane to the corneal plane, the numerous benefits of tinted spectacles are combined with the advantages inherent to CL wear. Former home run champion Mark McGwire reported increased peripheral vision and glare reduction as well as clearer and crisper vision while wearing amber-tinted CLs.[218]

Some practitioners tint commercially available lenses with in-office systems, and some manufacturers have developed sport-specific tints. Suntacts was originally a green-tinted CL designed for surfers,[219] although the manufacturer claimed generalization to other sports, such as baseball and golf. There is a newer tinted CL product that is also called Suntacts (https://suntacts.weebly.com/), although there is very limited information available about the specifications and uses of this lens. Prosoft was a teal-tinted CL based on Bolle's Competivision tint in sun eyewear that claimed to provide a

visual performance edge for tennis players, although availability of this lens is very limited at this time. No published studies have confirmed the efficacy of either the original Suntacts or Prosoft CLs for performance enhancement, and one study demonstrated that the Prosoft tint may actually mask the appearance of a tennis ball.[184]

SportSight CL technology began as a gray tint with a 20% visible light transmission in a gas permeable CL designed to reduce glare and brightness. Subsequent tint developments evolved from gray to yellow and finally to amber and gray-green tinted B&L Nike MAXSIGHT soft CLs (Fig. 6.11). The tints enhanced certain aspects of subjective and objective visual information and improved contrast recognition by filtering short-wavelength light in the visible spectrum and manipulating transmission of wavelengths above 500 nm.[220] The amber lens was developed for use in dynamic reactive sports to cause the ball or other moving objects to "pop" out from the background environment. The gray-green lens was engineered to enhance details of the environment, such as the grass on a golf course or the water's surface in activities such as kayaking, surfing, windsurfing, or kiteboarding. Research results indicated that the B&L Nike MAXSIGHT lenses provided improved contrast discrimination, speed of visual recovery, and subjective visual performance in natural sunlight compared with tinted spectacles or clear CLs.[220,221] A study comparing B&L Nike MAXSIGHT lenses and Eye Black grease only found improvements in low-contrast visual acuity with the tinted CLs in natural sunlight; however, this lens is no longer commercially available from B&L Nike.[222]

Recently, Johnson & Johnson and Transitions have partnered to create a photochromic CL, Acuvue Oasys with Transitions Light Intelligent Technology. These silicone hydrogel CLs contain a photochromic additive

(A)

(B)

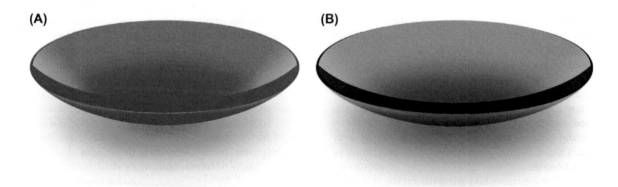

FIG. 6.11 Nike MAXSIGHT **(A)** amber and **(B)** gray-green contact lenses.

throughout the lens that enables them to actively shift between darkened and clear filtering states based on external light levels. Research results indicate that the photochromic CL provides significant improvements in glare disability and discomfort, faster photostress recovery, and enhanced chromatic contrast when compared to an untinted control CL.[223] Similarly, photochromic CLs have been shown to improve the effects of light scatter when compared to nonphotochromic CLs, even in the inactivated state under lower illuminance.[224] The study authors suggest that these improvements in visual function are likely based on simple filtering effects. The lenses have also been found to be noninferior to untinted CLs or spectacle photochromic lenses during daytime and nighttime driving conditions.[225]

Contact Lens Recommendations

The practitioner is fortunate to have a large selection of CL materials and designs to choose from. A review of all commercially available lenses is beyond the scope of this chapter; a discussion of general recommendations is presented to guide the practitioner in focusing on specific lens features. As previously discussed, the first step in choosing the best lens option is to determine the specific demands of the sport and the individual athlete.

The first major decision is to determine the best lens category for the sport. The main decision compares performance aspects of RGP versus hydrogel CLs, although scleral lenses or hybrid lens designs may also factor into the decision. RGP lenses may offer a slight advantage in terms of visual clarity, especially in athletes with significant corneal astigmatism. However, for most athletes the advantages of hydrogel lenses far outweigh this slim advantage. RGP lenses have a considerably greater risk of dislodgement in contact and water sports, are more susceptible to debris under the lenses, may produce flare symptoms in low-light conditions, and require a drastically longer adaptation period to adjust to the discomfort of lens wear. The subjective discomfort of RGP lens wear, with the requisite adaptation period, is perhaps the most discouraging feature for athletes, especially those who only need to use the lenses during sports participation. Hydrogel lenses offer a solution to most of the disadvantages of RGP designs: good optical clarity, minimal risk of dislodgement, reduced risk of foreign material under the lens, marginal reports of flare in low-light conditions, and virtually instantaneous lens comfort. Additionally, hydrogel lenses offer the potential for extended wear and disposable modalities.

Scleral lenses are similar to RGP lenses and offer the advantage of virtually no risk of dislodgement. Scleral lenses were used for athletes in contact sports early in the development of CLs; however, they must be custom made and cannot be worn for more than a few hours. This lens type was rarely prescribed for these reasons; however, there has been a resurgence in the use of scleral CLs for challenging corneal conditions.[226–228]

Combination RGP and hydrogel lens options have been produced to provide the visual clarity of an RGP lens with the comfort of a soft lens. The Saturn II and SoftPerm lenses were the original hybrid lens designs, however there were complications such as corneal neovascularization, poor tear exchange, and tearing of the lens at the junction of the soft and RGP portions. SynergEyes has introduced some of the latest hybrid CLs (see Fig. 6.12), and these provide an option for athletes who may benefit from this design, especially those with a large amount of corneal astigmatism or keratoconus. Although comfort is improved over conventional gas permeable lenses with the soft skirt, one study found that patients rated soft toric CLs higher in overall comfort as compared to the SynergEyes lens.[229] The same study also found that visual acuity was preferred with SynergEyes over the soft toric lens. Recent advances in SynergEyes lens designs include the addition of a silicone hydrogel (as opposed to the previously used HEMA hydrogel) skirt material to help eliminate concerns about oxygen transmission and the risk of corneal neovascularization. Some practitioners find that a "piggyback" setup offers better performance for the athlete than the hybrid lenses. A piggyback design is a soft lens with an RGP lens fit on top of it, "piggybacking" over the soft lens, which is chosen for its high oxygen transmission (e.g., a silicone hydrogel lens). Comfort and acuity are factors that practitioners must weigh on an individual basis to determine the best custom option for each patient.

Larger diameter RGP and soft lenses are frequently recommended for athletes to compensate for some of the environmental challenges encountered in sports.[6,7,121,209,210,230] Larger lens diameters are useful in RGP lenses to improve lid attachment, enlarge the optic zone to reduce flare symptoms, or diminish lens lag during large saccadic eye movements.[6,230] Soft lenses with larger diameters are recommended to improve lens stability during extreme body movements and forceful contact, enhance visual performance in extreme gaze positions and following saccadic eye movements, and resist dehydration from airflow and low humidity.[7] Large-diameter soft lenses are also recommended in water sports to minimize the probability

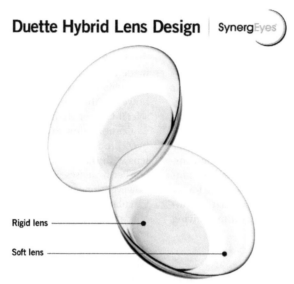

Duette Hybrid Lens Design | SynergEyes

Rigid lens

Soft lens

FIG. 6.12 The Duette hybrid contact lens design by SynergEyes. (Courtesy of SynergEyes, Carlsbad, California.)

of lens loss.[121] A hybrid lens design also typically centers well on the cornea due to the large diameter of these lenses.

Rigid Lens Recommendations

The basic fit of RGP lenses can be modified to create a more stable fit during saccadic and body movement. Typically, the modifications include a larger diameter (with an enlarged optic zone to account for pupil size), a slightly steeper lens to make the fit tighter, and steeper peripheral curves to improve adherence to the eye. A lid attachment design, also known as a Korb lens, offers good lens positioning and stability by the positioning of the lens with the superior lid.[6] Lens materials should be chosen that have negligible flexure during blinking and that wet well for use in low-humidity or high-airflow conditions. A lens that is not wetting properly may need robust cleaning or replacement. The peripheral curve can be modified with heavy blends to prevent irritation and edema from a tight-fitting lens and to enhance the tear exchange under the lens.[6] As previously mentioned the lens positioning should be assessed in relevant gaze directions for the sport.

Soft Lens Recommendations

The main considerations for hydrogel lenses are the material composition and water content, and the diameter and thickness of the lens prescribed. In general, higher water content lenses dehydrate faster than low- to medium-water-content CLs. Therefore thicker low- to medium-water-content lenses or silicone hydrogel lenses should be used to preserve lens hydration for athletes who have dehydration problems.[209] High-water-content CL materials may be needed for prolonged lens wear situations in which oxygen transmission is a crucial factor. As previously mentioned, larger diameter lenses are also recommended for better stability and hydration.[231,330,331]

The ultimate goal of the soft lens fit is stability of lens positioning and visual performance. CLs for sports use should fit tighter than traditional fitting practices dictate. The lens should have minimal movement after a blink and maintain a good centering position in extreme gaze directions. For athletes, the lens material should also handle easily so that insertion and removal can be readily performed under adverse conditions.

An alternative to engineering a specialty lens for an athlete is the use of one-day disposable lenses. The advent of disposable, single-use lenses offered an excellent alternative for many athletes who want the advantages of CLs for sports without the hassles of caring for the lenses. These CLs are wonderful for the weekend athlete or recreational scuba diver, for example, to provide the correction benefits of CLs. It is also an outstanding option for elite athletes who want immaculately clean and fresh CLs before starting a competition and uncomplicated replacement of lenses at any time during competition. The main obstacle to success with single-use CLs is the temptation to overuse them. The potential risks of overwear or overnight wear should be clearly communicated to the athlete.

Visual Performance Variables With Contact Lenses

First and foremost, the fit of the CLs and ocular health of the athlete should be meticulously evaluated. Any indications of trouble with the fit or anterior segment health should be aggressively managed. The visual acuity through the CLs as well as dynamic visual acuity for sports with dynamic vision demands should be assessed. The body positions and gravitational forces generated in some sports, such as gymnastics or aerial ski jumping, may require a ballasted toric lens designed to maintain optimal lens alignment. As previously mentioned, contrast sensitivity measurement is essential with CLs to ensure optimal performance. For athletes receiving a first refractive prescription, the effect of the lenses on ocular alignment should be measured to determine any potential impact on spatial localization. An adaptation period for any new prescription is strongly encouraged before use in competition when feasible.

Contact Lenses and Water Sports

Good vision is important for athletes who participate in water sports. With the development of CLs, the application of this form of vision correction to aqueous environments was investigated. Early literature explored the use of haptic or scleral lenses for underwater vision correction without a dive mask.[232–236] However, most eye care practitioners focus on providing vision correction with a combination of CLs and masks or goggles. While CLs are not approved for use in water, athletes who need vision correction and participate in water sports most commonly use CLs. CLs offer an advantage over prescription masks or goggles through reduced tendency for lens fogging, less restriction on peripheral vision, and clear vision without the goggle or mask on.[237–240] The main concerns regarding CL wear in water sports are lens loss and risk for infection.

Lens loss is a concern for any athlete participating in water sports. The risk for lens loss is considerably greater with RGP lenses than soft CLs. Many studies have demonstrated that hydrogel lenses adhere to the cornea when exposed to hypotonic water, such as fresh water and swimming pools.[241–248] The intensity of the lens adherence increases as the salinity of the water decreases. The adherence of the lens is theoretically caused by the osmolarity gradient between the precorneal tear film and the aqueous environment as well as by the resulting increase in overall diameter of the hydrophilic lens when immersed in water with low salinity. Lens adherence and larger overall diameter are cited as major factors in the low incidence of lens loss with soft CLs in many water sports.[248–251] A low incidence of soft CL loss has also

been reported with ocean sports despite the hypertonic environment of salt water.[238,251] The use of large-diameter lenses is credited for minimizing lens loss in this environment. The athlete should splash some water in his or her eyes before entering the water to facilitate adhesion of the soft CLs to the cornea. Removal of the CLs should be avoided for at least 30 min after water activity to allow the adhesion of the lens to the corneal epithelium to diminish.[243] Saline may also be instilled in the eyes to shorten the recovery time to normal lens movement and prevent corneal denuding.[240,243,245,246] RGP lenses do not typically adhere to the cornea in water environments,[245] so the risk of lens loss is significant unless the lids can adequately hold the lens in place. The athlete should understand the risks of lens loss in water sports and be properly counseled on precautions to minimize lens loss. Precautions include lid closure with a hard entry into the water, squinting when splashed, and the use of goggles or masks. Excessive water on the eyes should be removed by rapid blinking rather than eye rubbing.[240]

The risk for eye infection or tissue damage from CL wear is another concern that must be addressed. Despite proper sanitation practices, public swimming pools contain bacteria that pose a potential risk for infection.[252] The presence of *Acanthamoeba* species is a particular concern because of the destructive nature of a potential keratitis. Athletes should therefore remove and thoroughly clean CLs shortly after water activity or discard disposable lenses.[240,246] The risk for infection is elevated when the integrity of the corneal epithelium has been compromised.[253] RGP lenses have a greater chance of compromising the integrity of the cornea, and scuba diving may result in bubble formation under the lens that can cause corneal edema.[237,250,253] Polymethyl methacrylate lenses, and some RGP lenses, inhibit the nitrogen and carbon dioxide gas exchange during decompression. For swimmers, hydrogel CLs prevent the corneal thickness changes, stipple staining, and superficial corneal erosions noted in swimmers with no CLs,[242,246] although the use of goggles can prevent this problem.

Large-diameter lenses should be used for athletes who participate in water sports. The larger diameter CLs will reduce the risk of lens loss and improve the stability of vision through the CLs.[121,231,238,249] The water content of the hydrogel lens material may have an impact on the adherence of the lens in water,[247] although no measurable difference in corneal or conjunctival response has been noted.[246] Lens wear is contraindicated in athletes with compromised corneal integrity or a history of poor lens care compliance.

Orthokeratology (Corneal Reshaping)

Orthokeratology is a procedure used to temporarily reduce myopia and astigmatism with specially designed RGP lenses. First described by Jessen in 1962,[254] the methods for attaining predictable and effective results were revolutionized in the 1980s and 1990s with the advent of RGP materials and innovative lens designs. Current orthokeratology uses RGP lenses to flatten the central corneal curvature to reduce myopia and improve visual acuity.[255–261] Reverse geometry lens designs with uniquely constructed curves on the posterior lens surface have been responsible for allowing greater myopia reduction in shorter periods. The corneal response to orthokeratology appears to be robust in patients younger than 36 years, with a reduced response with increasing age (older than 36 years).[262] The RGP lenses are typically worn overnight during sleep and are removed shortly after awakening in the morning. Studies have demonstrated immediate corneal flattening and precorneal tear film chemistry changes after a single night of reverse geometry lens wear.[263–266] The corneal changes caused by lens wear at night remain for several hours during the day and allow clear vision without corrective lenses. The treatment effect with overnight wear of reverse geometry lenses is typically achieved in 7–40 days.[267–270] Orthokeratology has become an effective option for slowing myopia progression in children.[271]

Recently, many reverse geometry lens designs have been marketed for overnight orthokeratology; however, the fitting methods for each of these designs vary. The use of computer-assisted keratoscopes offer an effective means for controlling the procedure effects, and fitting adjustments can be made to achieve a more desirable outcome. The exact nature of the mechanisms involved in producing the corneal effects of orthokeratology is not currently well understood. Studies demonstrate thinning of the central corneal epithelium with thickening of the mid-peripheral cornea.[272–275] Some evidence shows that the posterior corneal surface is also flattened with reverse geometry lenses.[275] The procedure appears to be safe regarding maintenance of corneal integrity, and the effects are reversible with discontinuation of lens wear.[258,262,273,276,277] Some concern still exists regarding the long-term safety of the procedure for children[278] and for the increasing incidence of corneal pigmented arc formation with prolonged orthokeratology.[279] Concern also exists over the incidence of the development of microbial keratitis in patients who undertake orthokeratology, although whether the incidence is higher than that in general CL wearers is not clear.[280,281] Overall, a review found sufficient evidence to suggest that orthokeratology is a safe option[282]; however, these issues highlight the importance of appropriate patient selection and follow-up care in the success of orthokeratology.[260,283]

Orthokeratology offers a reasonable alternative to traditional refractive correction for athletes with myopia between −0.75 D and −4.00 D.[256] It is also potentially beneficial for with-the-rule astigmatism less than 1.50 D.[256] The potential disadvantage for the athlete is the increased presence of higher order aberrations and spherical aberration after orthokeratology.[284,285] The increase of higher order aberrations is speculated to cause a reduction in low-contrast visual acuity and this reduction is exacerbated with increasing pupil size.[285] However, orthokeratology remains an attractive option for athletes, especially young myopic athletes who are not yet eligible for refractive surgery.

Issues With Contact Lenses for Athletes

Special considerations apply to athletes who wear CLs during sports. The main concern is the availability of replacement CLs during sports participation, especially during competition. At least one set of spare CLs should be immediately available for the athlete and care solutions should be easily accessible to manage any issues with the lenses. Team personnel (e.g., coaches and athletic trainers) should be aware of the CL needs of the athlete and the appropriate support personnel should be facile in CL insertion, removal, and problem solving. This situation offers an excellent consultation opportunity for the eye care practitioner.

The athlete should be thoroughly counseled in the care of the CLs, including replacement schedule, cleaning regimen, troubleshooting of common problems, and follow-up care. Every effort should be made to instill the importance of excellent compliance with CL recommendations. The athlete's family and support personnel should also help the athlete maintain outstanding compliance. Most CL wearers are not 100% compliant with at least one step in the care recommendations and athletes are no exception. The most common compliance problems are failure to wash the hands before handling lenses and failure to replace CLs at the recommended interval. Describing the potential effects of noncompliance on ocular health and vision may be valuable as well as connecting those issues to the potential impact on athletic performance.

Athletes often gravitate to CLs to avoid using eyewear during sports. However, the eye care practitioner must counsel athletes who participate in sports that expose the athlete to significant risk of eye injury regarding the need for supplemental protective eyewear.

CLs offer almost no protection to the ocular tissues and adequate protective eyewear is essential for preventing serious injury.

REFRACTIVE SURGERY

For an athlete with significant refractive error, laser refractive surgery is an appealing prospect for eliminating the need for spectacles or CLs. A few high-profile athletes have reported successful outcomes with refractive surgery and even suggested that sports performance is enhanced by the results. In contrast, a study of major league baseball players found no difference in on-base percentage or batting average before laser refractive surgery compared with after surgery.[286] Similar to orthokeratology, the candidate for refractive surgery has moderate amounts of myopia or astigmatism; however, larger amounts of myopia and astigmatism can be corrected by contemporary procedures and low to moderate hyperopia and presbyopia may also be effectively managed. Also similar to orthokeratology, most refractive surgery modifies the corneal curvature to produce refraction results at or near emmetropia. The differences compared to orthokeratology are that some refractive surgery results have limited potential to be reversed and candidates must be adults (generally older than 21 years) with stable refractive error. All athletes must meet the relevant profile for success before proceeding with any refractive surgery procedure.

The main surgical methods apply incisions, corneal implants, or laser ablation to the corneal surface. Many procedure variations exist; some have widespread acceptance and application and others are rarely used. The refractive surgery options available in the United States include RK, astigmatic keratotomy (AK), limbal relaxing incisions, photorefractive keratectomy (PRK), transepithelial photorefractive keratectomy (T-PRK), LASIK, epipoloic laser in situ keratomileusis (epi-LASIK), femtosecond laser in situ keratomileusis (FS-LASIK), laser subepithelial keratomileusis (LASEK), femtosecond lenticule extraction (FLEx), small-incision lenticule extraction (SMILE), intracorneal ring segments (ICRSs), laser thermokeratoplasty, conductive keratoplasty, phakic intraocular lenses, clear lens extractions, and scleral expansion.[287]

Incisional Methods

RK is the most common procedure using corneal incisions to reduce myopic refractive error. The method involves radial incisions made in the mid-peripheral cornea to flatten a central optical zone (usually 3.0–4.5 mm in diameter). For AK, arcuate incisions

are applied in the mid-periphery, and RK and AK can be combined for compound myopia. Before the innovations afforded with laser technology, RK and AK were the popular methods of refractive surgery. The use of incisional methods has significantly declined since the advent of PRK and LASIK approaches. The main visual disadvantages of RK and AK are glare from the peripheral wounds and fluctuating vision throughout the day. For athletes in particular, the incisions may increase the potential for significant damage to the cornea in blunt eye trauma. The cornea is weakened with RK and AK, and blunt trauma forces may cause globe rupture at the site of the corneal incisions.[288–290] The positive aspect of RK compared to laser ablation procedures is that the central cornea is not directly altered, thereby preserving a central optical zone.

Laser Ablation Procedures

Forms of LASIK, including epi-LASIK and FS-LASIK, are the most common refractive surgeries performed for refractive errors between −9.00 and +3.00 D and astigmatism up to 2.50 D; PRK and LASEK are also commonly used.[287] Many surgeons are performing custom ablations using wave-front-guided LASIK to reduce both lower and higher order aberrations[291–293]; it also allows for the creation of larger corneal topographic effective optical zones compared with standard LASIK.[293] In LASIK, a microkeratome is used to create a thin flap in the corneal tissue. The flap is raised and the excimer laser ablates the exposed stromal bed, creating a specified ablation zone. The use of a femtosecond laser to create the flap in LASIK (FS-LASIK) improves the consistency of shape, placement, size, and depth of the flap.[294] FS-LASIK also creates a more stable flap postsurgically so that there is less risk of flap dislocation. Subsequent laser ablation procedures are usually required to achieve optimal results, referred to as enhancements, as some refractive regression is not uncommon.[295]

PRK was a precursor procedure to LASIK and LASEK. PRK removes a very thin layer of anterior corneal surface tissue with an excimer laser to alter the curvature of the central cornea and results in some degree of subepithelial tissue deposition responsible for haze symptoms. T-PRK removes the corneal epithelium mechanically with a motorized brush or by excimer laser ablation. LASEK and epi-LASEK entail a similar procedure where no corneal flap is created. All laser ablation procedures affect the central cornea and include a risk for corneal haze or scarring.

With the advent of femtosecond lasers for refractive surgery, a new ablation procedure was developed that did not create a flap. FLEx creates a lenticule within the cornea containing the refractive correction properties, which is then extracted through a small corneal incision. This procedure has evolved to the current SMILE, which may have biomechanical advantages over LASIK due to the absence of a flap.[296,297]

Common symptoms after laser refractive surgery include glare, halo, starbursts, and other night vision disturbances, and these are caused by higher order aberrations.[298–300] These symptoms may appear in daylight conditions if the athlete has physiologically large-diameter pupils, although wave front technology has minimized this complication.[301–306] Early forms of LASIK could also reduce contrast sensitivity compared to best corrected pre-LASIK vision; however, advances in wave-front-guided LASIK has been shown to provide some patients better post-LASIK contrast sensitivity by using ablation algorithms.[307–309] Dry eye symptoms are a common complication after LASIK surgery, although assessment for dry eye presurgically combined with advances in technique have reduced the frequency of this problem.[310–317] The cause of dry eye symptoms is most likely related to the integration of the ocular surface and lacrimal gland function. Damage to the ocular surface under dry eye conditions can produce continued alteration in tear production, creating a recurring cycle of chronic dry eye symptoms.[317,318] SMILE may offer an advantage over LASIK by retaining better corneal biomechanical strength and producing less dry eye complications.[319–321] A meta-analysis found that dry eye after both SMILE and FS-LASIK usually occurs transiently, and although SMILE does not show better outcomes compared to FS-LASIK, it may produce milder subjective symptoms.[322] The athlete should also be counseled that mid-peripheral visual field sensitivity may also be reduced after LASIK.[323] Despite anecdotal reports of improved sports performance after LASIK, an analysis of on-base percentage and batting average of major league baseball players did not reveal any statistically or practically significant differences in performance following refractive surgery.[286]

Laser ablation and lenticule extraction procedures do not impair the corneal integrity to the same degree as incisional methods. The potential for globe rupture from blunt trauma in post-LASIK eyes is equivalent to that of normal eyes. The main risk is corneal flap dislocation, which is more likely to occur within days of the procedure. The long-term susceptibility to flap-related trauma is uncertain; however, some indications exist that sport-related ocular trauma can cause flap dislocation.[141,142] Surface ablation procedures do not appear to involve a risk for weakened corneal integrity and do not entail a risk of flap dislocation.

Intracorneal Ring Segments

The implantation of intrastromal corneal rings to correct low myopia has been studied and approved in the United States.[324,325] The procedure involves the insertion of polymethyl methacrylate ring segments into the corneal stroma to alter the corneal curvature. Unlike laser ablation procedures, ICRSs do not directly disturb the central cornea and no corneal flap is generated. Implantation of ICRS is a reversible procedure and the rings can be explanted in the event that adequate success is not achieved.[326] The effects of trauma in athletes with ICRSs are relatively unknown; however, the stromal healing profile does not indicate increased fragility.[290] This refractive surgery option is not commonly used due to less predictable refractive and visual outcomes; however, it is sometimes an option for patients with keratoconus.[327]

All athletes considering refractive surgery should receive comprehensive counseling regarding the potential visual and ocular affects as well as potentially increased vulnerability in the event of ocular trauma. All athletes who have had refractive surgery should be encouraged to be conscientious in the use of appropriate protective eyewear during participation in sports. Overall, there is not a significant difference in the efficacy, safety, or visual quality outcomes with the commonly used procedures, and FS-LASIK appears to have better predictability.[328]

The eye care practitioner has a variety of resources to help the athlete attain the best vision for his or her sports pursuits. Consideration must be given to the athlete's individual profile, the task demands of the sport, and the environmental conditions encountered by the athlete. For athletes requiring vision correction, the eye care practitioner should present the advantages and disadvantages of spectacle correction, sun eyewear and filter options, protective eyewear, CLs, and refractive surgery. All athletes who participate in outdoor sports should receive counseling in sun eyewear to protect the ocular tissues, and all athletes should be encouraged to use appropriate protective eyewear if they participate in sports that expose them to a significant risk of eye injury. The eye care practitioner has a duty to correct and protect the athlete and may offer options to enhance sports performance.

REFERENCES

1. Beckerman SA, Hitzeman S. The ocular and visual characteristics of an athletic population. *Optometry*. 2001;72:498.
2. Beatty RM, Bakkum BW, Hitzman SA, Beckerman S. Sports vision screening of amateur athletic union junior olympic athletes: a ten-year follow-up. *Optom Vis Perf*. 2016;4(3):97.
3. Laby DM, Kirschen DG. The refractive error of professional baseball players. *Optom Vis Sci*. 2017;94:564–573.
4. Omar R, Kuan YM, Zuhairi NA, et al. Visual efficiency among teenaged athletes and non-athletes. *Int J Ophthalmol*. 2017;10:1460–1464.
5. Jorge J, Fernandes P. Static and dynamic visual acuity and refractive errors in elite football players. *Clin Exp Optom*. 2019;102:51–56.
6. Spinell MR. Contact lenses for athletes. *Optom Clin*. 1993;3:57.
7. Efron N. Sports vision correction with contact lenses. In: Loran DFC, MacEwen CJ, eds. *Sports Vision*. Oxford: Butterworth-Heinemann; 1995:127–147.
8. Zieman B, Reichow A, Coffey B. Optometric trends in sports vision: knowledge, utilization, and practitioner role expansion potential. *J Am Optom Assoc*. 1993;64:490.
9. Obstfeld H, Pope R. Sports vision correction with spectacles. In: Loran DFC, MacEwen CJ, eds. *Sports Vision*. Oxford: Butterworth-Heinemann; 1995.
10. Runninger J. Rx for sports. *Optom Manag*. 1979:55. June.
11. Brown B, Collins MJ, Bowman KJ. Reaction times in a complex task by presbyopic observers with spectacle and contact lens corrections. *Clin Exp Optom*. 1988;71:94.
12. Breedlove HW. Prescribing for marksmen and hunters. *Optom Clin*. 1993;3:77.
13. Gregg JR. Prescribing for the sports nut. *Optom Manag*. 1974;10:19.
14. Long WF, Haywood KM. The optical characteristics of aiming scopes in archery. *J Am Optom Assoc*. 1990;61:777.
15. Zeri F, Livi S, Maffioletti S. Attitudes towards visual correction in sport: what coaches, physical education teachers and sports physicians think. *Contact Lens Anterior Eye*. 2011;34:71–76.
16. *American National Standards Institute: Ophthalmics: Prescription Ophthalmic Lenses—Recommendations*. New York: American National Standards Institute; 2005.
17. *American National Standards Institute: Occupational and Educational Personal Eye and Face Protection Devices*. New York: American National Standards Institute; 2003.
18. Davis JK. Perspectives on impact resistance and polycarbonate lenses. In: Vinger P, ed. *Prevention of Ocular Sports Injuries*. Boston: Little, Brown; 1981:215–218.
19. Stern NS. The effects of racquetball impact on spectacles and lenses. *Optom Monthly*. 1982;73:343.
20. Stephens GL, Davis JK. Spectacle lenses. In: Duane TD, Jaeger EA, eds. *Clinical Ophthalmology*. Philadelphia: Harper and Row; 1994.
21. Vinger PF. Eye safety testing and standards. *Ophthalmol Clin N Am*. 1999;12:345.
22. Chou BR, Hovis JK. Effect of multiple antireflective coatings on impact resistance of Hoya Phoenix spectacle lenses. *Clin Exp Optom*. 2006;89:86.
23. Fry GA. *Geometrical Optics*. Philadelphia: Chilton; 1969:177.
24. Fannin TE, Grosvenor T. *Clinical Optics*. Boston: Butterworth; 1987.
25. Chou BR, Gupta A, Hovis JK. The effect of multiple antireflective coatings and center thickness on resistance of polycarbonate spectacle lenses to penetration by pointed missiles. *Optom Vis Sci*. 2005;82:964.
26. Vinger PF. A practical guide for sports eye protection. *Phys Sportsmed*. 2000;28:49.
27. *Prevent Blindness America: Sports Eye Injuries by Type/Age* (detailed), https://preventblindness.org/wp-content/uploads/2020/06/FS09_SportsInjuriesbyAge-detailed2020.pdf, Accessed July 1, 2020.
28. Leivo T, Haavisto AK, Sahraravand A. Sports-related eye injuries: the current picture. *Acta Ophthalmol*. 2015;93:224–231.
29. Ong HS, Barsam A, Morris OC, et al. A survey of ocular sports trauma and the role of eye protection. *Contact Lens Anterior Eye*. 2012;35:285–287.
30. Easterbrook M. Eye protectors for sport. In: Loran DFC, MacEwen CJ, eds. *Sports Vision*. Oxford: Butterworth-Heinemann; 1995.
31. Vinger PF. The eye and sports medicine. In: Duane TD, Jaeger EA, eds. *Clinical Ophthalmology*. Philadelphia: Harper and Row; 1994.
32. Vinger PF, Parver L, Alfaro 3d DV, et al. Shatter resistance of spectacle lenses. *J Am Med Assoc*. 1997;277:142.
33. Protective eyewear for young athletes. A joint statement of the American Academy of Pediatrics and the American Academy of Ophthalmology. *Ophthalmology*. 1996;103:1325.
34. Protective eyewear for young athletes. *Ophthalmology*. 2004;111:600.
35. Gregg JR. *Optom Manag*. 1979;15:86.
36. Kleinstein RN. Preventing eye injuries in athletes. *Optom Monthly*. 1979;70:168.
37. Vinger PF. Sports-related eye injury. A preventable problem. *Surv Ophthalmol*. 1980;25:47.
38. Vinger PF, Easterbrook M, Hirschfelder D. Sports eye injuries. A model for prevention. *J Am Med Assoc*. 1983;250:3322.
39. Vinger PF. The one-eyed athlete [editorial]. *Phys Sportsmed*. 1987;15:48.
40. Knuttgen HG. Eye injuries and eye protection in sports: a position statement from the International Federation of Sports Medicine. *Int J Sports Med*. 1988;9:474.
41. Drack A, Kutschke PJ, Stair S, et al. Compliance with safety glasses wear in monocular children. *J Pediatr Ophthalmol Strabismus*. 1993;30:249.
42. Kirman S, Kirman G, Kirman B, et al. Make your dispensary special. *Optom Manag*. 1993:37. Nov.
43. Vinger PF. Prescribing for contact sports. *Optom Clin*. 1993;3:129.

44. Jeffers JB. Concepts of eye protection. *Ophthalmol Clin N Am.* 1999;12:407.

45. Monica ML. Sports and eye safety: patient awareness prevents injuries and builds the practice. *Refract Eyecare Ophthalmol.* 1999;3.

46. Vinger PF. Injury prevention: where do we go from here? *J Am Optom Assoc.* 1999;70:87.

47. Woods TA. Protective eyewear. *Ophthalmol Clin N Am.* 1999;12:381.

48. Vinger PF, Woods TA. Prescription safety eyewear: impact studies of lens and frame failure. *Optometry.* 2000;71:91.

49. Halstead DP. Performance testing updates in head, face and eye protection. *J Athl Train.* 2001;36:322.

50. Rodriguez JO, Lavina AM, Agarwal A. Prevention and treatment of common eye injuries in sports. *Am Fam Physician.* 2003;67:1481.

51. Sinclair SA, Smith GA, Xiang H. Eyeglasses-related injuries treated in U.S. emergency departments in 2002-2003. *Ophthalmic Epidemiol.* 2006;13:23.

52. Diamond GR, Quinn GE, Pashby TJ, et al. Ophthalmologic injuries. *Prim Care.* 1984;11:161.

53. Easterbrook M. Ocular injuries in racquet sports. *Int Ophthalmol Clin.* 1988;28:232.

54. Jones NP. One year of severe eye injuries in sport. *Eye.* 1988;2:484.

55. Jones NP. Eye injury in sport. *Sports Med.* 1989;7:163.

56. Jones NP. Eye injuries in sport. In: Loran DFC, MacEwen CJ, eds. *Sports Vision.* Oxford: Butterworth-Heinemann; 1995.

57. Orlando RG, Doty JH. Ocular sports trauma: a private practice study. *J Am Optom Assoc.* 1996;67:77.

58. Bishop PJ, Kozey J, Caldwell GC. Performance of eye protectors for squash and racquetball. *Phys Sportsmed.* 1982;10:63.

59. Easterbrook M. Eye injuries in squash and racquetball: an update. *Phys Sportsmed.* 1982;10:47.

60. Pashby TJ, Bishop PJ, Easterbrook M. Eye injuries in Canadian racquet sports. *Can Fam Physician.* 1982;28:967.

61. Feigelman MJ, Sugar J, Jednock N, et al. Assessment of ocular protection for racquetball. *J Am Med Assoc.* 1983;250:3305.

62. Clemett RS, McKenzie KD, Glogau TH, et al. Eye protectors for squash players. *Aust N Z J Ophthalmol.* 1987;15:151.

63. Easterbrook M. Eye protection in racket sports: an update. *Phys Sportsmed.* 1987;15, 180-186, 192.

64. Easterbrook M. Prevention of eye injuries in racquet sports. *Ophthalmol Clin N Am.* 1999;12:367.

65. US Squash. *Protective Eyewear Policy.* www.us-squash.org/ussra/protectiveeyewear.html.

66. David DB, Shah P, Whittaker C, et al. Ocular protection in squash clubs: time for a change? *Eye.* 1995;9:575.

67. Easterbrook M. Eye injuries in squash: a preventable disease. *Can Med Assoc J.* 1978;118:298.

68. Easterbrook M. Eye protection in racquet sports. *Clin Sports Med.* 1988;7:253.

69. Eime R, McCarty C, Finch CF, et al. Unprotected eyes in squash: not seeing the risk of injury. *J Sci Med Sport.* 2005;8:92.

70. Eime R, Finch C, Owen N, et al. Do squash players accurately report use of appropriate protective eyewear? *J Sci Med Sport.* 2005;8:352.

71. Eime RM, Finch CF, Sherman CA, et al. Are squash players protecting their eyes? *Inj Prev.* 2002;8:239.

72. Finch C, Vear P. What do adult squash players think about protective eyewear? *Br J Sports Med.* 1998;32:155.

73. Genovese MT, Lenzo NP, Lim RK, et al. Eye injuries among pennant squash players and their attitudes towards protective eyewear. *Med J Aust.* 1990;153:655.

74. Leyland B. Eye protection for squash players. *Aust J Optom.* 1972;55:225.

75. Ingram DV, Lewkonia I. Ocular hazards of playing squash rackets. *Br J Ophthalmol.* 1973;57:434.

76. North IM. Ocular hazards of squash. *Med J Aust.* 1973;1:165.

77. Luong M, Dang V, Hanson C. Traumatic hyphema in badminton players: should eye protection be mandatory? *Can J Ophthalmol.* 2017;52:e143−e146.

78. Stuart MJ, Smith AM, Malo-Ortiguera SA, et al. A comparison of facial protection and the incidence of head, neck, and facial injuries in junior A hockey players. A function of individual playing time. *Am J Sports Med.* 2002;30:39.

79. Pashby TJ, Pashby RC, Chisholm LD, et al. Eye injuries on Canadian hockey. *Can Med Assoc J.* 1975;113:663.

80. Vinger PF. Ocular injuries in hockey. *Arch Ophthalmol.* 1976;94:74.

81. Pashby TJ. Eye injuries in Canadian hockey. Phase II. *Can Med Assoc J.* 1977;117:677.

82. Pashby TJ. Eye injuries in Canadian amateur hockey. *Am J Sports Med.* 1979;7:254.

83. Pashby TJ. Eye injuries in Canadian hockey. Phase III. *Can Med Assoc J.* 1979;121:643.

84. Pashby TJ. Ocular injuries in hockey. *Int Ophthalmol Clin.* 1988;28:228.

85. Benson B, Meeuwisse W. Ice hockey injuries. In: Maffulli N, Caine DJ, eds. *Epidemiology of Pediatric Sports Injuries: Team Sports.* 49. 2005:86. Med Sport Sci.

86. Antaki S, Labelle P, Dunas J. Retinal detachment following ice hockey injury. *Can Med Assoc J.* 1977;117:245.

87. Horns RC. Blinding hockey injuries. *Minn Med.* 1977;60:255.

88. Pashby TJ. Summary of eye injuries in Canadian sports. *Can J Ophthalmol.* 1990;25:284.

89. Pashby RC, Pashby TJ. Ocular injuries. In: Torg JS, Welsh P, Shephard R, eds. *Current Therapy in Sports Medicine.* St Louis: Mosby−Year Book; 1990:241.

90. Devenyi RG, Pashby RC, Pashby J. The hockey eye safety program. *Ophthalmol Clin N Am.* 1999;12:359.

91. Micieli JA, Zurakowski D, Ahmed IIK. Impact of visors on eye and orbital injuries in the National Hockey League. *Can J Ophthalmol.* 2014;49:243−248.

92. Kriz PK, Comstock RD, Zurakowski D, et al. Effectiveness of protective eyewear in reducing eye injuries among high school field hockey players. *Pediatrics*. 2012;130: 1069–1075.

93. Kriz PK, Zurakowski D, Almquist JL, et al. Eye protection and risk of eye injuries in high school field hockey. *Pediatrics*. 2015;136:521–527.

94. Lapidus CS, Nelson LB, Jeffers JB, et al. Eye injuries in lacrosse: women need their vision less than men? *J Trauma*. 1992;32:555.

95. Livingston LA, Forbes SL. Eye injuries in women's lacrosse: strict rule enforcement and mandatory eyewear required. *J Trauma*. 1996;40:144.

96. Webster DA, Bayliss GV, Spadaro JA. Head and face injuries in scholastic women's lacrosse with and without eyewear. *Med Sci Sports Exerc*. 1999;31:938.

97. O'Grady C. Safety in the women's game. *Lacrosse Magazine*. 2002:73. May.

98. Waicus KM, Smith BW. Eye injuries in women's lacrosse players. *Clin J Sport Med*. 2002;12:24.

99. Mantz SO, Nibbelink G. Injuries in intercollegiate women's lacrosse. *Am J Sports Med*. 2004;32:608.

100. Lincoln AE, Caswell SV, Almquist JL, et al. Effectiveness of the women's lacrosse protective eyewear mandate in the reduction of eye injuries. *Am J Sports Med*. 2012;40: 611–614.

101. Vinger PF. The incidence of eye injuries in sports. In: Vinger PF, ed. *Ocular Sports Injuries*. Boston: Little, Brown; 1981:21–46.

102. Strahlman E, Elman M, Daub E, et al. Causes of pediatric eye injuries: a population-based study. *Arch Ophthalmol*. 1990;108:603.

103. Napier SM, Baker RS, Sanford DG, et al. Eye injuries in athletics and recreation. *Surv Ophthalmol*. 1996;41:229.

104. Witherspoon CD, Kuhn F, Morris R, et al. Epidemiology of general and sports eye injuries. *Ophthalmol Clin N Am*. 1999;12:333.

105. Vinger PF. Baseball hardness as a risk factor for eye injuries. *Arch Ophthalmol*. 1999;117:354.

106. Danis RP, Hu K, Bell M. Acceptability of baseball face guards and reduction of oculofacial injury in receptive youth league players. *Inj Prev*. 2000;6:232.

107. Easterbrook M, Pashby TJ. Eye injuries associated with war games. *Can Med Assoc J*. 1985;133:415.

108. Randall KA. War games: a new sport that can cause eye casualties. *Sightsaving*. 1985;54(2).

109. Ryan EH, Lissner G. Eye injuries during "war games,". *Arch Ophthalmol*. 1986;104:1435.

110. Tardif D, Little J, Mercier M, et al. Ocular trauma in war games. *Phys Sportsmed*. 1986;14:90.

111. Martin PL, Magolian JJ. Eye injury during "war games" despite the use of goggles. *Arch Ophthalmol*. 1987;105: 321.

112. Easterbrook M, Pashby TJ. Ocular injuries and war games. *Int Ophthalmol Clin*. 1988;28:222.

113. Wellington DP, Johnstone MA, Hopkins RJ. Bull's-eye corneal lesion resulting from war game injury. *Arch Ophthalmol*. 1989;107:1727.

114. Hargrave S, Weakley D, Wilson C. Complications of ocular paintball injuries in children. *J Pediatr Ophthalmol Strabismus*. 2000;37:338.

115. Fineman MS. Ocular paintball injuries. *Curr Opin Ophthalmol*. 2001;12:186.

116. Varr WF, Cook RA. Shotgun eye injuries: ocular risk and eye protection efficacy. *Ophthalmology*. 1992;99:867.

117. Eichler J. Eye accidents due to ski pole injuries [in German]. *Dtsch Gesundheitswesen*. 1972;375:375.

118. Classe JG. Prescribing for noncontact sports. *Optom Clin*. 1993;3:111.

119. Dyer B, Masci D, Sakkas D, et al. Ocular protection for competitive swimmers. *Clin Exp Optom*. 1989;72(3):74.

120. Morgan E. In the swim. *Eyecare Bus*. 2000;14:82.

121. Legerton JA. Prescribing for water sports. *Optom Clin*. 1993;3:91.

122. Larrison WI, Hersh PS, Kunzweiler T, et al. Sports-related ocular trauma. *Ophthalmology*. 1990;97:1265.

123. Burke MJ, Sanitato JJ, Vinger PF, et al. Soccerball-induced eye injuries. *J Am Med Assoc*. 1983;249:2682.

124. Horn EP, McDonald HR, Johnson RN, et al. Soccer ball-related retinal injuries: a report of 13 cases. *Retina*. 2000;20:604.

125. Capao-Filipe JA, Fernandes VL, Barros H, et al. Soccer-related ocular injuries. *Arch Ophthalmol*. 2003;121:687.

126. Capao-Filipe JA. Soccer (football) ocular injuries: an important eye health problem. *Br J Ophthalmol*. 2004; 88:159.

127. Vinger PF, Capao-Filipe JA. The mechanism and prevention of soccer eye injuries. *Br J Ophthalmol*. 2004;88:167.

128. Yee CT, Drescher RJ. The effect of racquetball goggles on peripheral vision and distortion. *Optom Monthly*. 1984; 75:220.

129. Gallaway M, Aimino J, Scheiman M. The effect of sports eyewear on peripheral visual field and a peripheral visual performance task. *J Am Optom Assoc*. 1986;57:304.

130. Dawson ML, Zabik RM. Effect of protective eyewear on reaction time in the horizontal field of vision. *Percept Mot Skills*. 1988;67:115.

131. Wingert TA, Long WF, Martin WG. Hockey faceguards and visual field scotomas. *Can J Optom*. 1992;54:143.

132. Miller BA, Miller SJ. Visual fields with protective eyewear. *J Orthop Sports Phys Ther*. 1993;18:470.

133. Ing E, Ing T, Ing S. The effect of a hockey visor and sports goggles on visual function. *Can J Ophthalmol*. 2002;37: 161.

134. Eime RM, Finch CF. Have the attitudes of Australian squash players towards protective eyewear changed over the past decade? *Br J Sports Med*. 2002;36:442.

135. Eime R, Finch C, Owen N, et al. Knowledge, beliefs and attitudes of squash venue operators relating to use of protective eyewear. *Inj Contr Saf Promot*. 2004;11:47.

136. Loran D. Eye injuries in squash. *Optician*. 1992;27:18. March.

137. Eime R, Owen N, Finch C. Protective eyewear promotion: applying principles of behaviour change in the design of a squash injury prevention programme. *Sports Med*. 2004; 34:629.

138. Eime R, Finch C, Wolfe R, et al. The effectiveness of a squash eyewear promotion strategy. *Br J Sports Med.* 2005;39:681.

139. Tommila V, Tarkkanan A. Incidence of loss of vision in the healthy eye in amblyopia. *Br J Ophthalmol.* 1981;65:575.

140. Keates RH. Preventing eye injuries in sports: some questions and answers. *Phys Sportsmed.* 1988;16:122.

141. Melki SA, Talamo JH, Azar DT, et al. Late traumatic dislocation of laser in situ keratomileusis corneal flaps. *Ophthalmology.* 2000;107:2136.

142. Booth MA, Koch DD. Late laser in situ keratomileusis flap dislocation caused by a thrown football. *J Cataract Refract Surg.* 2003;29:2032.

143. Classe JG, Scholles J. Liability for ophthalmic materials. *J Am Optom Assoc.* 1986;57:470.

144. Classe JG. Legal aspects of prescribing for athletes and sportsmen. *J Am Optom Assoc.* 1987;58:674.

145. Classe JG. Legal aspects of sports vision. *Optom Clin.* 1993;3:27.

146. Classe JG. Sports related ocular trauma: a preventable epidemic. *J Am Optom Assoc.* 1996;67:66.

147. Miller PJ. Sports vision—are you legally prepared? *Contact Lens Forum.* 1990;15:11.

148. Classe JG, Gold AR, Harris MG. A review of five recent cases of significance for optometrists. *J Am Optom Assoc.* 1988;59:964.

149. Michaels D. *Visual Optics and Refraction: A Clinical Approach.* 3rd ed. St Louis: Mosby—Year Book; 12–13.

150. Clark BAJ. Color in sunglass lenses. *Am J Optom Arch Am Acad Optom.* 1969;46:825.

151. Sliney DH. Ocular injury due to light toxicity. *Int Ophthalmol Clin.* 1988;28:246.

152. West S, Duncan D, et al. Sunlight exposure and risk of lens opacities in a population based study. *J Am Med Assoc.* 1999;280:714.

153. Pitts DG. The ocular effects of ultraviolet radiation. *Am J Optom Physiol Optic.* 1978;55:19.

154. Pitts D, Kleinstein R. *Environmental Vision.* Boston: Butterworth-Heinemann; 1993, 164-177, 306.

155. *Ocular Ultraviolet Radiation Hazards and Sunlight: A Cooperative Initiative of National Society to Prevent Blindness (Prevent Blindness America).* the American Academy of Ophthalmology, and the American Optometric Association. A position statement; 1993.

156. Ham WT, Mueller HA, Sliney DH. Retinal sensitivity to damage from short wavelength light. *Nature.* 1976;260:153.

157. European Committee for Standardization. *Personal Eye Protection—Sunglasses and Sunglare Filters for General Use.* Brussels. 1997. European Standards 6 EN 1836.

158. Thibos LN, Bradley A, Zhang X. Effect of ocular chromatic aberration on monocular visual acuity. *Optom Vis Sci.* 1991;68:599.

159. Bradley A. Glen A: fry Award Lecture 1991: perceptual manifestations of imperfect optics in the human eye: attempts to correct for chromatic aberration. *Optom Vis Sci.* 1992;69:515–521.

160. Chou BR, Cullen AP. Spectral characteristics of sports and occupational tinted lenses. *Can J Optom.* 1985;47:77.

161. Clark B, Johnson ML, Dreher RE. The effect of sunlight on dark adaptation. *Am J Ophthalmol.* 1946;29:828.

162. Hecht S, Hendley CD, Ross S, et al. The effect of exposure to sunlight on night vision. *Am J Ophthalmol.* 1948;31:1573.

163. Bergmanson J, Sheldon T, Cullen A. A sting in the rays. *Optician.* 1996;212:17.

164. Kinney JAS. Night vision sensitivity during prolonged restriction from sunlight. *J Appl Psychol.* 1963:828.

165. Hart WM. Visual adaptation. In: Moses RA, Hart WM, eds. *Adler's Physiology of the Eye. Clinical Application.* St Louis: Mosby—Year Book; 1987:413.

166. Borgwardt B, Fishman GA, Meullen DV. Spectral transmission characteristics of tinted lenses. *Arch Ophthalmol.* 1981;99:293.

167. Kinney JS, Schlichting CL, Neri D, et al. *Various Measures of the Effectiveness of Yellow Goggles.* report no. 941. Groton, CT: Naval Submarine Medical Research Laboratory; 1980 (Naval Submarine Medical Research Laboratory).

168. Kinney JS, Schlichting CL, Neri DF, et al. Reaction time to spatial frequencies using yellow and luminance-matched neutral goggles. *Am J Optom Physiol Optic.* 1983;60:132.

169. Kinney JAS, Luria SM, Schlichting CL, Neri DF. The perception of depth contours with yellow goggles. *Perception.* 1983;12:363.

170. Kelly SA, Goldberg SE, Banton TA. Effect of yellow-tinted lenses on contrast sensitivity. *Am J Optom Physiol Optic.* 1984;61:657.

171. Yap M. The effect of a yellow filter on contrast sensitivity. *Ophthalmic Physiol Optic.* 1984;4:227.

172. Corth R. The perception of depth contours with yellow goggles—an alternative explanation. *Perception.* 1985;14:377.

173. Kinney JAS. The perception of depth contours with yellow goggles—comments on letter by Richard Corth. *Perception.* 1985;14:378.

174. Kelly SA. Effect of yellow-tinted lenses on brightness. *J Opt Soc Am A.* 1905;7:1990.

175. Zigman S. Vision enhancement using a short wavelength light-absorbing filter. *Optom Vis Sci.* 1990;67:100.

176. Rieger G. Improvement of contrast sensitivity with yellow filter glasses. *Can J Ophthalmol.* 1992;27:137.

177. Zigman S. Light filters to improve vision. *Optom Vis Sci.* 1992;69:325.

178. Rabin J, Wiley R. Differences in apparent contrast in yellow and white light. *Ophthalmic Physiol Optic.* 1996;16:68.

179. Lee JE, Stein JJ, Prevor MB, et al. Effect of variable tinted spectacle lenses on visual performance in controlled subjects. *CLAO J.* 2002;28:80.

180. Luckiesh M. *Color and its Applications.* New York: Van Nostrand; 1915:116—160.

181. Luckiesh M, Moss FK. *The Science of Seeing.* New York: Van Nostrand; 1937:400—453.

182. Jendrusch G, Senner V, Schaff P, et al. Vision—an essential factor for safety in skiing: visual acuity, stereoscopic depth perception, effect of colored lenses. In:

Johnson RJ, ed. *Skiing Trauma and Safety*. Vol. 12. West Conshohocken, PA: American Society for Testing and Materials; 1999:23–34.

183. Ross J. Sunglasses: skiers must emphasize substance over style. *Optom Manag*. 1991;26:52.
184. Marmor MF. Double fault! Ocular hazards of a tennis sunglass. *Arch Ophthalmol*. 2001;119:1064.
185. Reichow AW, Citek K, Erickson GE, et al. The effect of polarized lenses on golf putting performance [abstract]. *Optom Vis Sci*. 2002;79:239.
186. Stephens GL, Davis JK. Ophthalmic lens tints and coatings. In: Duane TD, Jaeger EA, eds. *Clinical Ophthalmology*. Philadelphia: Harper & Row; 1994: 11–13.
187. Renzi-Hammond LM, Hammond BR. The effects of photochromic lenses on visual performance. *Clin Exp Optom*. 2016;99:568–574.
188. Woods TA. Ophthalmic lenses for athletes and sportsmen. *Optom Clin*. 1993;3:33.
189. Sterling P, Cohen E, Smith RG, Tsukamoto Y. Retinal circuits for daylight: why ballplayers don't wear shades. In: Eekman FH, ed. *Analysis and Modeling of Neural Systems*. Kluwer Academic Publixhers; 1992:143–162.
190. American National Standards Institute. *ANSI Z80.3-2001, Ophthalmics – Non-prescription Sunglasses and Fashion Eyewear Requirements*. New York: American National Standards Institute; 1986.
191. Davis JK. The sunglass standard and its rationale. *Optom Vis Sci*. 1990;67:414.
192. Dain SJ, Hoskin AK. Ultraviolet protection in spectacle and sunglass lenses: claims vs performance. *Clin Exp Optom*. 1993;76:136.
193. Cooper SC, Smith JA, Katz M, et al. Nonprescription tinted eyewear optical accuracy study. *Optometry*. 2001; 72:510.
194. Scheiman M, Wick B. *Clinical Management of Binocular Vision: Heterophoric, Accommodative, and Eye Movement Disorders*. Philadelphia: Wolters Kluwer Health; 2020: 96–97.
195. Stephens GL. Sports eyewear takes off. *Optom Econ*. 1994; 4:10.
196. Morgan E. The women's movement. *Eyecare Bus*. 2001: 42–47. April.
197. Player HS. An investigation on the use and satisfaction of contact lenses in sports. *J Am Optom Assoc*. 1958;30: 33–36.
198. Yarwood RA. The use on contact lenses in all kinds of sports. *J Am Optom Assoc*. 1960;31:633.
199. Levey EM. The sports wearer of contact lenses—a new approach. *Am J Optom Arch Am Acad Optom*. 1965;42:21.
200. Jessen GN. Baseball and contact lenses—possible solution to the problem. *Am J Optom Arch Am Acad Optom*. 1966;43:320.
201. Firestone LE. Contact lens use for sports. *J Am Optom Assoc*. 1971;42:279.
202. Tym A. Contact lenses for tennis players. *Optom Wkly*. 1970;61:41.
203. Berry R. Contact lenses for contact sports. *Optom Manag*. 1975;11:16.
204. Benjamin WL. Visual optics of contact lenses. In: Bennett ES, Weissman BA, eds. *Clinical Contact Lens Practice*. Philadelphia: J.B. Lippincott; 1991.
205. Grey CP. Changes in contrast sensitivity when wearing low, medium and high water content soft lenses. *J Br Contact Lens Assoc*. 1986;9:21.
206. Nowozyckyj A, Carney LG, Efron N. Effect of hydrogel lens wear on contrast sensitivity. *Am J Optom Physiol Opt*. 1988;65:263.
207. Oxenberg LD, Carney LG. Visual performance with aspheric rigid contact lenses. *Optom Vis Sci*. 1989;66:818.
208. Kluka DA, Love PA. The effects of daily-wear contact lenses on contrast sensitivity in selected professional and collegiate female tennis players. *J Am Optom Assoc*. 1993;64:182.
209. Gardner JJ. Doctor's playbook: the X's and O's of fitting athletes. *Rev Optom*. 2001;138:73.
210. Bennett ES. Athletics. In: Bennett ES, Weissman BA, eds. *Clinical Contact Lens Practice*. Philadelphia: J.B. Lippincott; 1991.
211. Kolstad A, Opsahl R. Cold injury to corneal epithelium. A cause of blurred vision in cross country skiers. *Acta Ophthalmol*. 1969;47:656.
212. Clarke C. Contact lenses at high altitude: experience on Everest south-west face 1975. *Br J Ophthalmol*. 1976;60: 479.
213. Socks JF. Contact lenses in extreme cold environments: responses of rabbit corneas. *Am J Optom Physiol Optic*. 1982;59:297.
214. Socks JF. Use of contact lenses for cold weather activities. Results of a survey. *Int Contact Lens Clin*. 1983;10:82.
215. Maloof AJ, Ho A, Coroneo MT. Influence of corneal shape on limbal light focusing. *Invest Ophthalmol Vis Sci*. 1994; 35:2592.
216. Marshall LL, Roach JM. Treatment of dry eye disease. *Consult Pharm*. 2016;31:96.
217. Ousler GW, Anderson RT, Osborn KE. The effect of senofilcon A contact lenses compared to habitual contact lenses on ocular discomfort during exposure to a controlled adverse environment. *Curr Med Res Opin*. February 2008;24:335–341.
218. Kopp JD. Eye on the ball: an interview with Dr. C. Stephen Johnson and Mark McGwire. *J Am Optom Assoc*. 1999;70:79.
219. Petersen WL. Contact lenses and surfing: the need to ensure safety in the sport has prompted some interesting studies. *Contact Lens Spectr*. 1989;159:59.
220. Citek K, Reichow AW. Visual performance comparisons of performance-tinted soft contact lenses and tinted spectacles [abstract]. *Optom Vis Sci*. 2004;81(Suppl):84.
221. Erickson GB, Horn FC, Barney T. Contrast discrimination with Nike MAXSIGHT contact lenses in natural light. *Optom Vis Sci*. 2006. E-abstract 060057.
222. Horn FC, Erickson GB, Karben B, Moore B. Comparison of low-contrast visual acuity between Eye Black and

Maxsight tinted contact lenses. *Eye Contact Lens.* 2011;37: 147–152.

223. Renzi-Hammond L, Buch JR, Cannon J, et al. A contra-lateral comparison of the visual effects of a photochromic vs. non-photochromic contact lens. *Contact Lens Anterior Eye.* 2020;43:250–255. https://doi.org/10.1016/j.clae.2019.10.138.

224. Hammond BR, Buch J, Hacker L, et al. The effects of light scatter when using a photochromic vs. non-photochromic contact lens. *J Optom.* 2020 (in press).

225. Buch JR, Toubouti Y, Cannon J. Randomized crossover trial evaluating the impact of senofilcon A photochromic lens on driving performance. *Optom Vis Sci.* 2020;97: 15–23.

226. Ozek D, Kemer OE, Altiaylik P. Visual performance of scleral lenses and their impact on quality of life in patients with irregular corneas. *Arq Bras Oftalmol.* 2018;81: 475–480.

227. Macedo-de-Araujo RJ, van der Worp E, Gonzalez-Meijorne JM. A one-year prospective study on scleral lens wear success. *Contact Lens Anterior Eye.* November 13, 2019. https://doi.org/10.1016/j.clae.2019.10.140 [Epub ahead of print]).

228. Vincent SJ, Fadel D. Optical considerations for scleral contact lenses: a review. *Contact Lens Anterior Eye.* 2019; 42:598–613.

229. Lipson MJ, Musch DC. SynergEyes versus soft toric lenses: vision related quality of life. *Optom Vis Sci.* 2007;84: 593–597.

230. Bennett ES. Rigid gas permeable contact lenses for athletes. *NASV Sports Vision Newsletter.* 1989;5:30.

231. Legerton JA. Large dynamic lenses for dynamic water sports. *Sports.* 1990;6:12.

232. Nagel C, Monical JB. The design and development of a contact lens for underwater seeing. *Am J Optom Arch Am Acad Optom.* 1954;31:468.

233. Grant AH. SCAL: skindivers contact air lens. *Opt J Rev Optom.* 1963;55:17.

234. Faust KJ, Beckman EL. Evaluation of a swimmer's contact air-water lens system. *Mil Med.* 1966;131:779.

235. Bayshore CA. Underwater contact lenses. *Contact.* 1968; 12:6.

236. Hurlock R, Malin AH. Case report: underwater contact lens correction. *Am J Optom Arch Am Acad Optom.* 1973; 50:653.

237. Hoelting C, Egan DJ, Bennett ES. The use of contact lenses in swimming and scuba diving. *Can J Optom.* 1984;46:12.

238. Shoji PJ, Yamane SJ. Surfing with soft lenses. *Contact Lens Forum.* 1985;15. Aug.

239. Cotter J. Soft contact lens testing on fresh water scuba divers. *Contact Intraocul Lens Med J.* 1981;7:324.

240. Josephson JE, Caffery BE. Contact lens considerations in surface and subsurface aqueous environments. *Optom Vis Sci.* 1991;68:2.

241. Mandell RB. Sticking of gel contact lenses. *Int Contact Lens Clin.* 1975;2:28.

242. Solomon J. Swimming with soft lenses. *South J Optom.* 1977;19:13.

243. Stein HA, Slatt BJ. Swimming with soft contact lenses. *Contact Intraocul Lens Med J.* 1977;3:24.

244. Solomon J. Hydrophilic lenses for swimming. *Contact Intraocul Lens Med J.* 1978;4:93.

245. Lovsund P, Nilsson SEG, Oberg PA. The use of contact lenses in wet or damp environments. *Acta Ophthalmol.* 1980;58:794.

246. Soni PS, Pence NA, DeLeon C, et al. Feasibility of extended wear lens use in chlorinated swimming pools. *Am J Optom Physiol Optic.* 1986;63:171.

247. Diefenbach CB, Soni PS, Gillespie BJ, et al. Extended wear contact lens movement under swimming pool conditions. *Am J Optom Physiol Optic.* 1988;65:710.

248. Galkin KA, Semes L. Risk of loss of Soflens during water skiing. *J Am Optom Assoc.* 1983;54:267.

249. Banks LD, Edwards GL. To swim or not to swim. *Contact Lens Spectr.* 1987;6:46.

250. Bennett QM. The use of contact lenses for diving (sport and commercial). *Contact Lens J.* 1988;16:171.

251. Peterson WL. Contact lenses and surfing. *Contact Lens Spectr.* 1989;8:59.

252. Vesaluoma M, Kalso S, Jokipii L, et al. Microbiological quality in Finnish public swimming pools and whirl-pools with special reference to free living amoebae: a risk factor for contact lens wearers? *Br J Ophthalmol.* 1995;79:178.

253. Simon DR, Bradley ME. Corneal edema in divers wearing hard contact lenses. *Am J Ophthalmol.* 1978;85:462.

254. Jessen G. Orthofocus techniques. *Contact.* 1962;6:200.

255. Lui W-O, Edwards MH, Cho P. Contact lenses in myopia reduction—from orthofocus to accelerated Orthokeratology. *Contact Lens Anterior Eye.* 2000;23:68.

256. Caroline PJ. Contemporary orthokeratology. *Contact Lens Anterior Eye.* 2001;24:41.

257. Barr JT, Rah MJ, Jackson JM, et al. Orthokeratology and corneal refractive therapy: a review and recent findings. *Eye Contact Lens.* 2003;29:S49.

258. Walline JJ, Rah MJ, Jones LA. The children's overnight orthokeratology investigation (COOKI) pilot study. *Optom Vis Sci.* 2004;81:407.

259. Sorbara L, Fonn D, Simpson T, et al. Reduction of myopia from corneal refractive therapy. *Optom Vis Sci.* 2005;82:512.

260. Walline JJ, Holden BA, Bullimore MA, et al. The current state of corneal reshaping. *Eye Contact Lens.* 2005;31:209.

261. Swarbrick HA. Orthokeratology review and update. *Clin Exp Optom.* 2006;89:124.

262. Jayakumar J, Swarbrick HA. The effect of age on short-term Orthokeratology. *Optom Vis Sci.* 2003;82:505.

263. Sorbara L, Kort R, Lu F, et al. Overnight refractive and keratometric effects of corneal refractive therapy. *Optom Vis Sci.* 2002;79(suppl):127.

264. Sridharan R, Swarbrick H. Corneal response to short-term orthokeratology lens wear. *Optom Vis Sci.* 2003;80:200.

265. Wang J, Fonn D, Simpson TL, et al. Topographical thickness of the epithelium and total cornea after overnight wear of reverse-geometry rigid contact lenses for myopia reduction. *Invest Ophthalmol Vis Sci.* 2003;44: 4742.

266. Choy CKM, Cho P, Benzie IFF, et al. Effect of one overnight wear of orthokeratology lenses on tear composition. *Optom Vis Sci.* 2004;81:414.

267. Mountford J. An analysis of the changes in corneal shape and refractive error induced by accelerated Orthokeratology. *Int Contact Lens Clin.* 1997;24:128.

268. Nichols JJ, Marsich MM, Nguyen M, et al. Overnight orthokeratology. *Optom Vis Sci.* 2000;77:252.

269. Rah MJ, Jackson JM, Jones LA, et al. Overnight orthokeratology: preliminary results of the Lenses and Overnight Orthokeratology (LOOK) study. *Optom Vis Sci.* 2002;79:598.

270. Lui W-O, Edwards MH. Orthokeratology in low myopia. Part 1: efficacy and predictability. *Contact Lens Anterior Eye.* 2000;23:77.

271. Walline JJ, Lindsley KB, Vedula SS, et al. Interventions to slow progression of myopia in children. *Cochrane Database Syst Rev.* 2020;1:CD004916.

272. Swarbrick HA, Wong G, O'Leary DJ. Corneal response to orthokeratology. *Optom Vis Sci.* 1998;75:791.

273. Lui W-O, Edwards MH. Orthokeratology in low myopia. Part 2: corneal topographic changes and safety over 100 days. *Contact Lens Anterior Eye.* 2000;23:90.

274. Alharbi A, Swarbrick HA. The effects of overnight orthokeratology lens wear on corneal thickness. *Invest Ophthalmol Vis Sci.* 2003;44:2518.

275. Owens H, Garner LF, Craig JP, et al. Posterior corneal changes with Orthokeratology. *Optom Vis Sci.* 2004;81:421.

276. Soni PS, Nguyen TT, Bonanno JA. Overnight orthokeratology: visual and corneal changes. *Eye Contact Lens.* 2003;29:137.

277. Soni PS, Nguyen TT, XO Overnight Orthokeratology Study Group. Overnight orthokeratology experience with XO material. *Eye Contact Lens.* 2006;32:39.

278. Kwok LS, Pierscionek BK, Bullimore M, et al. Orthokeratology for myopic children: wolf in sheep's clothing? *Clin Exp Ophthalmol.* 2005;33:343.

279. Cho P, Cheung SW, Mountford J, et al. Incidence of corneal pigmented arc and factors associated with its appearance in orthokeratology. *Ophthalmic Physiol Optic.* 2005;25:478.

280. Watt K, Swarbrick HA. Microbial keratitis in overnight orthokeratology: review of the first 50 cases. *Eye Contact Lens.* 2005;31:201.

281. Sun X, Zhao H, Deng S, et al. Infectious keratitis related to Orthokeratology. *Ophthalmic Physiol Optic.* 2006;26:133.

282. Liu YM, Xie P. The safety of orthokeratology - a systematic review. *Eye Contact Lens.* 2016;42:35–42.

283. Cheung SW, Cho P. Subjective and objective assessments of the effect of orthokeratology—a cross-sectional study. *Curr Eye Res.* 2004;28:121.

284. Joslin CE, Wu SM, McMahon TT, et al. Higher-order wavefront aberrations in corneal refractive therapy. *Optom Vis Sci.* 2003;80:805.

285. Berntsen DA, Barr JT, Mitchell GL. The effect of overnight contact lens corneal reshaping on higher-order aberrations and best-corrected visual acuity. *Optom Vis Sci.* 2005;82:490.

286. Laby DM, Kirschen DG, DeLand P. The effect of laser refractive surgery on the on-field performance of professional baseball players. *Optometry.* 2005;76:647.

287. Duffey RJ, Leaming D. US trends in refractive surgery: 2003 ISRS/AAO survey. *J Refract Surg.* 2005;21:87.

288. Beran RF, Stewart C, Doty J. Refractive surgery and the athlete. *J Ophthalmic Nurs Technol.* 1995;14:11.

289. Vinger PF, Mieler WF, Oestreicher JH, et al. Ruptured globes following radial and hexagonal keratotomy surgery. *Arch Ophthalmol.* 1996;114:129.

290. Dudenhoefer EJ, Vinger PF, Azar DT. Trauma after refractive surgery. *Int Ophthalmol Clin.* 2002;42:33.

291. Seiler T, Mrochen M, Kaemmerer M. Operative correction of ocular aberration to improve visual acuity. *J Refract Surg.* 2000;16:S619.

292. Mrochen M, Kaemmerer M, Seiler T. Clinical results of wavefront-guided laser in situ keratomileusis three months after surgery. *J Cataract Refract Surg.* 2001;27:201.

293. Racine L, Wang L, Koch DD. Size of corneal topographic effective optical zone: comparison of standard and customized myopic laser in situ keratomileusis. *Am J Ophthalmol.* 2006;142:227.

294. Aristeidou A, Taniguchi EV, Tsatsos M, et al. The evolution of corneal and refractive surgery with the femtosecond laser. *Eye Vis (London).* 2015;2:12.

295. Yan MK, Chang JSM, Chan TCY. Refractive regression after laser in situ keratomileusis. *Clin Exp Opthalmol.* 2018;46:934–944.

296. Reinstein DZ, Archer TJ, Gobbe M. Small incision lenticule extraction (SMILE) history, fundamentals of a new refractive surgery technique and clinical outcomes. *Eye Vis (London).* 2014;1:3.

297. Chansue E, Tanehsakdi M, Sawsdibutra S, McAlinden C. Safety and efficacy of VisuMax circle patterns for flap creation and enhancement following small incision lenticule extraction. *Eye Vis (London).* 2015;2:21.

298. Drum BA. Aberration analyses needed for FDA evaluation of safety and effectiveness of wavefront-guided refractive surgical devices. *J Refract Surg.* 2003;19:S588–S591.

299. Pesudovs K. Wavefront aberration outcomes of LASIK for high myopia and high hyperopia. *J Refract Surg.* 2005;21:S508–S512.

300. Buhren J, Pesudovs K, Martin T, et al. Comparison of optical quality metrics to predict subjective quality of vision after laser in situ keratomileusis. *J Cataract Refract Surg.* 2009;35:846–855.

301. MacRae S, Schwiegerling J, Snyder RW. Customized and low spherical aberration corneal ablation design. *J Refract Surg.* 1999;15:S246–S248.

302. Phusitphoykai N, Tungsiripat T, Siriboonkoom J, Vongthongsri A. Comparison of conventional versus wavefront-guided laser in situ keratomileusis in the same patient. *J Refract Surg.* 2003;19:S217–S220.

303. Kim TI, Yang SJ, Tchah H. Bilateral comparison of wavefront-guided versus conventional laser in situ

keratomileusis with Bausch and Lomb Zyoptix. *J Refract Surg.* 2004;20:432−438.

304. Myrowitz EH, Chuck RS. A comparison of wavefront-optimized and wavefront-guided ablations. *Curr Opin Ophthalmol.* 2009;20:247−250.

305. Schallhorn SC, Tanzer DJ, Kaupp SE, et al. Comparison of night driving performance after wavefront-guided and conventional LASIK for moderate myopia. *Ophthalmol Times.* 2009;116:702−709.

306. He L, Manche EE. Contralateral eye-to-eye comparison of wavefront-guided and wavefront-optimized photorefractive keratectomy: a randomized clinical trial. *JAMA Ophthalmol.* 2015;133:51−59.

307. Hoffman RS, Packer M, Fine IH. Contrast sensitivity and laser in situ keratomileusis. In: Packer M, Fine HI, Hoffman RS, eds. *International Ophthalmology Clinics.* Philadelphia, PA: Lippincott Williams & Wilkins; 2003: 93−100.

308. Lawless MA, Hodge C, Rogers CM, Sutton GL. Laser in situ keratomileusis with Alcon CustomCornea. *J Refract Surg.* 2003;19:S691−S696.

309. Ginsburg AP. Contrast sensitivity: determining the visual quality and function of cataract, intraocular lenses and refractive surgery. *Curr Opin Ophthalmol.* 2006;17:19−26.

310. Aras C, Ozdamar A, Bahcecioglu H, et al. Decreased tear secretion after laser in situ keratomileusis for high myopia. *J Refract Surg.* 2000;16:362.

311. Lee JB, Ryu CH, Kim J, et al. Comparison of tear secretion and tear film instability after photorefractive keratectomy and laser in situ keratomileusis. *J Cataract Refract Surg.* 2000;26:1326.

312. Battat L, Macri A, Dursun D, et al. Effects of laser in situ keratomileusis on tear production, clearance, and the ocular surface. *Ophthalmology.* 2001;108:1230.

313. Patel S, Perez-Santonja JJ, Alio JL, et al. Corneal sensitivity and some properties of the tear film after laser in situ keratomileusis. *J Refract Surg.* 2001;17:17.

314. Toda I, Asano-Kato N, Komai-Hori Y, et al. Dry eye after laser in situ keratomileusis. *Am J Ophthalmol.* 2001; 132(1).

315. Albietz JM, Lenton LM, McLennan SG. Effect of laser in situ keratomileusis for hyperopia on tear film and ocular surface. *J Refract Surg.* 2002;18:113.

316. Donnenfeld ED, Solomon K, Perry HD, et al. The effect of hinge position on corneal sensation and dry eye after LASIK. *Ophthalmology.* 2003;110:1023.

317. Goto T, Zheng X, Kylce SD, et al. Evaluation of the tear film stability after laser in situ keratomileusis using the tear film stability analysis system. *Am J Ophthalmol.* 2004;137:116.

318. Stern ME, Beuerman RW, Fox RI, et al. The pathology of dry eye: the interaction between the ocular surface and lacrimal glands. *Cornea.* 1998;17:584.

319. Sekundo W, Gertnere J, Bertelmann T, Solomatin I. One-year refractive results, contrast sensitivity, high-order aberrations and complications after myopic small-incision lenticule extraction (ReLEx SMILE). *Graefes Arch Clin Exp Ophthalmol.* 2014;252:837−843.

320. Vestergaard AH, Grauslund J, Ivarsen AR, Hjortdal JO. Efficacy, safety, predictability, contrast sensitivity, and aberrations after femtosecond laser lenticule extraction. *J Cataract Refract Surg.* 2014;40:403−411.

321. Moshirfar M, McCaughey MV, Reinstein DZ, et al. Small-incision lenticule extraction. *J Cataract Refract Surg.* 2015; 41:652−655.

322. Shen Z, Zhu Y, Song X, et al. Dry eye after small incision lenticule extraction (SMILE) versus femtosecond laser-assisted in situ keratomileusis (FS-LASIK) for myopia: a meta-analysis. *PloS One.* 2016;11(12):e0168081.

323. Brown SM, Bradley JC, Xu KT, et al. Visual field changes after laser in situ keratomileusis. *J Cataract Refract Surg.* 2005;31:687.

324. Nose W, Neves RA, Schanzlin DJ, et al. Intrastromal corneal ring: one-year results of first implants in humans: a preliminary nonfunctional eye study. *Refract Corneal Surg.* 1993;9:452.

325. Schanzlin DJ, Asbell AA, Buris TE, et al. The intrastromal corneal ring segments: phase II results for correction of myopia. *Ophthalmology.* 1997;104:1067.

326. Guell JL. Are intracorneal rings still useful in refractive surgery? *Curr Opin Ophthalmol.* 2005;16:260.

327. Bautista-Llamas MJ, Sanchez-Gonzalez MC, Lopez-Izquierdo I, et al. Complications and explanation reasons in intracorneal ring segments (IRCS) implantation: a systematic review. *J Refract Surg.* 2019;35:740−747.

328. Wen D, McAlinden C, Flitcroft I, et al. Postoperative efficacy, predictability, safety, and visual quality of laser corneal refractive surgery: a network meta-analysis. *Am J Ophthalmol.* 2017;178:65−78.

329. Ridder WH, Tomlinson A. Blink-induced temporal variations in contrast sensitivity. *Int Contact Lens Clin.* 1991; 18:231.

330. Efron N. *Contact Lenses A-Z.* Oxford: Butterworth-Heinemann; 2002:174−177.

331. Katz HD, Malin AH. A new lens for sports proves an excellent troubleshooter. *Contact Lens Spectr.* 1990;5:27.

CHAPTER 7

Management of Sport-Related Ocular Injuries and Concussion

Many reports have been published regarding the incidence of eye injuries occurring during sports and recreational activities.[1–34] A retrospective analysis of data from the Nationwide Emergency Department Sample (NEDS) utilizing data from over 900 hospitals across the United States over a 4-year period found more than 30,000 individuals per year presented to emergency departments with sport-related ocular trauma.[34] This sample represents only injuries serious enough to warrant attention at a hospital emergency department; the incidence of eye injuries incurred during sports and recreational activities is much greater than the NEDS data estimates because many athletes seek care outside hospitals, if care is sought at all.[27] A better estimate is 2.5 times higher than the amount reported in hospital emergency departments, indicating a more accurate incidence of approximately 75,000 sport-related eye injuries per year in the United States.[35] It was notable that more than 80% of the individuals in the NEDS data were men and that more than half were under the age of 18 years.[34]

PREPARTICIPATION PHYSICAL EXAMINATION

Each year athletes receive a preparticipation physical examination (PPPE) before the start of the sports season. The PPPE is performed to identify athletes at risk of sudden death; identify medical conditions that require further evaluation and treatment; identify at-risk individuals for substance abuse, sexually transmitted diseases, violence, and depression; and satisfy legal requirements of sport-governing bodies (e.g., state high-school athletic associations and the National Collegiate Athletic Association).[36] The Committee on Sports Medicine and Fitness recommends that all youths involved in organized sports should be encouraged to wear appropriate eye protection (Box 7.1). The committee strongly recommends that functionally one-eyed athletes wear appropriate eye protection during all sports, recreational, and work-related activities.[37,38]

A functionally one-eyed athlete is defined as an individual who has a best corrected visual acuity of worse than 20/40 in the poorer eye.[37–39] Athletes who have sustained eye trauma or have had eye surgery should also be evaluated by an ophthalmologist or optometrist.[37,38] Athletes who fall into this category may need eye protection or should be restricted from particular sports (see Box 7.1).[37,38] If the provider performing the PPPE fails to identify eye conditions requiring further evaluation, an athletic trainer who is familiar with an athlete's health history can serve as a backup by referring the athlete to an eye care specialist.

MANAGEMENT OF SPORT-RELATED OCULAR INJURIES

Medical and allied health professionals providing sports medicine care for sports teams (both on the field and in the clinic) may include the team physician, optometrist or ophthalmologist, athletic trainer, and sports physical therapist. The eye care practitioner may see athletes for initial triage and management of sports and recreational eye injuries. Often, an athletic trainer provides the initial triage and first aid for sports eye injuries, and guides follow-up care when necessary. The athlete may not present immediately for healthcare or vision care if an injury seems treatable with basic first-aid measures, so the practitioner may also see the results of long-standing trauma.

Immediate Management of Sport-Related Ocular Emergencies

The American Optometric Association has developed an emergency management protocol to be used by sports medicine professionals in the event a sport-related ocular injury is sustained in practice or during a game. Many sport-related eye injuries could be serious and require immediate medical attention. The sports medicine professional must recognize the signs of a severe eye injury, administer first aid, make return-to-play decisions, and refer the athlete for appropriate follow-up care.

Sports Vision. https://doi.org/10.1016/B978-0-323-75543-6.00003-6

BOX 7.1
Recommendations of the Committee on Sports Medicine and Fitness

1. All youths involved in organized sports should be encouraged to wear appropriate eye protection.
2. The recommended sport-protective eyewear should be prescribed. Proper fit is essential. Because some children have narrow facial features, they may be unable to wear even the smallest sports goggles. These children may be fitted with 3-mm polycarbonate lenses in American National Standards Institute (ANSI) standard Z87.1 frames designed for children. The parents should be informed that this protection is not optimal and the choice of eye-safe sports should be discussed.
3. Because contact lenses offer no protection, athletes who wear contact lenses should be strongly encouraged to also wear the appropriate eye protection.
4. An athlete who requires prescription spectacles has three options for eye protection: (1) polycarbonate lenses in a sports frame that passes American Society for Testing of Materials (ASTM) standard F803 for the specific sport, (2) contact lenses plus an appropriate protector, or (3) an over-the-glasses eye guard that conforms to the specifications of ASTM standard F803 for sports in which an ASTM standard F803 protector is sufficient.
5. All functionally one-eyed athletes should wear appropriate eye protection for all sports.
6. Functionally one-eyed athletes and those who have had an eye injury or surgery must not participate in boxing or full-contact martial arts (Eye protection is not practical in boxing or wrestling and is not allowed in full-contact martial arts.). Wrestling has a low incidence of eye injury. Although no standards exist, eye protectors that are firmly fixed to the head have been custom made. The wrestler who has a custom-made eye protector must be aware that the protector design may be insufficient to prevent injury.
7. For sports in which a face mask or helmet with an eye protector or shield must be worn, functionally one-eyed athletes are strongly encouraged to also wear sports goggles that conform to the requirements of ASTM standard F803 (for any selected sport). This is to maintain some level of protection if the face guard is elevated or removed, such as for hockey or football players on the bench. The helmet must fit properly and have a chinstrap for optimal protection.
8. Athletes should replace sports eye protectors that are damaged or yellowed with age because they may have become weakened and may no longer be protective.

An athlete who has sustained an apparent sport-related ocular injury should be evaluated first for a concussion, as many of the same injury mechanisms that cause eye trauma may also cause a concussion. Eye injuries and can share some similar signs and symptoms (Boxes 7.2 and 7.3). These include blurred vision; unequal, dilated, or nonreactive pupils; and headache or head-related pain. If an athlete has sustained a concussion, the National Athletic Trainers' Association guidelines should be followed.[40] If the athlete meets any of the criteria listed in Box 7.3, immediately refer the athlete to a local emergency department. A secondary assessment may be performed, including evaluation for any potential eye injuries, once the primary survey for a serious or life-threatening injury has been completed.

Clinical Management of Sport-Related Ocular Injuries

The eye care practitioner has a legal and ethical responsibility to provide a thorough evaluation of the eye and orbit to determine the extent of any damage. A thorough methodic evaluation of an eye injury facilitates appropriate management recommendations. Systematic approaches for assessment of ocular sports injuries have been summarized in the literature and include assessment of visual acuity, ocular motilities, pupillary function, external adnexa, intraocular pressure, and anterior and posterior segment structures.[41,42]

The practitioner should take a comprehensive case history to determine the nature of the injury and elicit any long-standing conditions that may be present. A detailed account of symptoms should be noted as well as a complete description of how the injury was treated after the incident. The ultimate goal of the patient history is to raise the index of suspicion for eye and vision effects from an injury. Although a thorough eye health evaluation should be performed on all athletes with a history of ocular trauma, an effective case history can be particularly valuable for selecting appropriate assessment procedures for the symptoms reported and the type of injury. For example, a basketball player who was struck with considerable force by an opponent's elbow presents with the potential for eyelid damage, hemorrhaging and damage to the orbital contents, orbital bone fractures, corneal trauma, angle recession, hyphema, uveal structure damage, vitreous detachment, and retinal and choroidal ruptures. If the athlete reports sudden onset of diplopia after the injury, the practitioner is further alerted to assess extraocular muscle (EOM) function and determine if orbital bone fractures are present.

Before proceeding with any other evaluation procedures, an assessment of visual acuity should be made. Visual acuity information is useful for differential diagnosis and management decisions, but it may also be crucial for medicolegal issues.[43] Practitioners commonly use an anterior-to-posterior approach to ocular health assessment; however, this chapter considers the types of eye injuries that commonly occur in sports. A trauma typically is classified as either a closed-globe or open-globe injury, and the Birmingham Eye Trauma Terminology System (BETTS) was developed to standardize descriptions of damage.[42] This chapter provides brief descriptions of common eye injury mechanisms by sport, followed by consideration of the cause of the injury—blunt trauma, penetrating trauma, or chemical trauma.

RISKS OF OCULAR INJURY BY SPORT TYPE

Table 7.1 shows sport-related eye injury estimates collected by Prevent Blindness for 2019 by age and sport category. The incidence of eye injuries by sport is influenced by the number of participants in the region or country combined with the risk of sustaining an eye injury in that sport.[44,45] Athletes most often at risk for blunt trauma injuries play collision team sports or sports involving projectiles moving at high velocities. For example, basketball is a leading cause of sport-related eye injuries in the United States because of the large number of participants combined with the physicality of the sport. Baseball players and those playing racquet sports are susceptible to direct trauma caused by fast-moving balls, and even balls larger than the bony orbit can cause significant injury.

Baseball and Softball

There is a high incidence of reported eye injuries from baseballs in the United States, and baseball has been reported as the leading cause of sport-related eye injuries in children.[1,22–24,30,33,34] The hardness of the baseball, combined with the forces at which it is thrown and hit, produce potentially devastating damage to the eye and orbit.[46] When the baseball is rotating at a high rate, additional tractional forces can be transferred to the ocular tissues by the raised seam on the ball.[29] Similar patterns of eye injury can be found in cricket.[29,47,48] The incidence of eye injuries with softballs is not well known.[30] The softness of the ball reduces the risk of injury, but the forces of a thrown or hit ball are significant enough to cause substantial damage to the eye.[49] Even a Wiffle ball has been reported to cause significant ocular damage.[50] The risk of ocular foreign body also exists from the playing field environment.

Basketball

Basketball accounts for a large percentage of eye injuries in sport because of the intense contact encountered during play[51–53] and the large number of people who play the game. It is commonly a leading cause of sport-related eye injury in the United States.[22–24,30,33,34,54,55] Common injuries include eyelid abrasions or lacerations, orbital contusions and fractures, and corneal abrasions.[21] Eye injuries are rarely caused by the ball, but rather by fingers or elbows.

TABLE 7.1
Prevent Blindness Table[35].

Activity	Est. Injuries[a]	Age 0–60	Age 7–12	Age 13–22	Age 23+
Basketball	4597	86	523	2263	1725
Pools & Water Sports	4565	927	1003	1113	1523
Non-Powder Guns, Darts, Arrows, Slingshots	3612	308	1109	1129	1066
Bicycles & Accessories	2495	369	282	192	1652
Exercise, Weight-Lifting	2385	104	97	261	1924
Baseball/Softball	2109	90	718	679	623
Soccer	1618	10	362	913	333
Playground Equipment	1195	409	519	139	127
Football	959	0	431	333	194
Other Sports & Recreational Activities	845	264	15	274	292
Racquet Sports	775	10	14	357	394
Golf	765	86	18	18	642
Ball Sports, Unspecified/Other	736	73	242	174	247
Boxing, Martial Arts, Wrestling	683	5	69	277	332
Trampolines	677	487	130	60	0
All-Terrain Vehicles (4 Wheels)	579	87	162	0	330
Fishing	556	5	27	101	423
Misc. Ball Games	535	5	112	286	131
Sports & Recreational Activity Not Elsewhere Classified	491	55	286	95	55
Volleyball	429	55	84	254	36
Scooters, Skateboards, Skating, Go Carts	380	204	19	84	73
Winter Sports	115	0	10	5	101
Total[a]	**31,101**	**3637**	**6234**	**9007**	**12,223**

[a] Totals may not equal because the injuries are not mutually exclusive.
Source: Prevent Blindness. Based on statistics provided by the U.S. Consumer Product Safety Commission, Directorate for Epidemiology; National Injury Information Clearinghouse; National Electronic Injury Surveillance System (NEISS). Product Summary Report—Eye Injuries Only—Calendar Year 2019.

Boxing

Ocular trauma is a common result of boxing, and the extensive nature of ocular injuries has been well documented in the literature.[56–68] Most of the ocular injuries are the result of contusion forces on the orbital and periorbital bones and ocular contents. Damage to the lids and soft tissues is common, and more extensive damage to internal ocular structures and EOMs can occur. The thumb is capable of transmitting the largest force to the globe and therefore can result in the most significant damage to the eye.[30] Although some studies have suggested that the prevalence of severe ocular trauma is lower than that reported by others,[67,68] most studies confirm the serious nature of ocular injuries in boxing.[56–66]

Fishing

Fishing is an activity pursued by many and injury is periodically expected. Although eye injuries do not occur with high frequency, the reported cases are often quite serious.[45,55,69-75] The fish hook presents a challenge to remove without increasing tissue damage, and several removal methods have been discussed.[55,70-73] The anterior segment structures are most commonly damaged by fish hook penetration, including the cornea, iris, and lens tissues. Bystanders are also at risk for injuries caused by whipped pole tips, lures, weights, and fishing spears.[74,75] The most common injuries include corneal laceration, hyphema, and globe ruptures.[74]

Football

The incidence of face and eye injuries in football was dramatically reduced with the mandate for face guards. However, standard face guards offer incomplete protection for the eyes; specifically, a finger can enter with enough force to cause significant ocular trauma.[76,77] The addition of a clear protective visor to the helmet may help reduce the risk of eye injury; however, there is currently no American Society for Testing of Materials (ASTM) standard for this form of sports protection. The risk of ocular foreign body from the playing field environment also exists.

Golf

The golf ball can be struck with considerable force, and this hard sphere can cause considerable ocular damage because it fits inside the bony orbit. Similarly, the golf clubhead is quite hard and can directly transmit a large amount of force to the globe. Golf-related ocular injuries are relatively rare; however, the results are often quite severe.[30,78-85] Blunt trauma from a golf ball or golf clubhead that results in a ruptured globe typically has a poor prognosis and the rate of enucleation is high.[80,82,84,85] A closed-globe blunt trauma has a better visual outcome potential than open-globe trauma.

Hockey

Because of the mandate for face protection at all levels of ice hockey, except the National Hockey League, eye injuries in hockey have been virtually eliminated. Eye injuries are typically incurred only during unsupervised play, from improper use of face protection, or in the National Hockey League.[86-89] Beginning with the 2013–14 season, all players who have fewer than 25 games of National Hockey League experience must wear a visor. Although visor use can be discontinued after 25 games, very few players elect to remove them. The most common cause of eye injury is from the hockey stick, followed by the puck or opponent.[39,86-95] The tip of the hockey stick can transmit considerable force to the ocular tissues because it fits inside the orbital rim and severe blunt trauma can result. Injuries from the puck and the aggressive play of opponents can also cause considerable damage. A similar risk profile exists for other forms of hockey, such as field hockey, floor hockey, and street hockey.[96-98]

Lacrosse

Lacrosse has risks for eye injury that are similar to hockey, in which the stick and ball present significant hazards. Men's lacrosse mandates head and face protector use, thereby minimizing the risk for ocular injury. Women's lacrosse did not mandate face protection until recently; the incidence and severity of eye injuries had been a contentious issue in the sport.[30,99-103] US lacrosse changed the rules to endorse and mandate the use of protective eyewear in 2004, resulting in a significant reduction in eye injuries.[104] Aggressive stick play and ball-related accidents can cause extensive blunt force trauma to the ocular tissues.

Mountaineering

When mountaineers make ascents above approximately 3000 m, high-altitude retinopathy risk increases as climbers become more susceptible to acute mountain sickness. The decrease in atmospheric pressure for those unaccustomed to such heights can lead to observable tortuosity and increases in the diameter of retinal arteries and veins as well as optic disc hyperemia.[105-112] A faster rate of ascent, a higher altitude reached, and a longer length of time at altitude typically will increase the incidence of retinal hemorrhage, retinal nerve fiber layer defects, and other retinal vasculature changes.[112] The coughing problems commonly experienced with high-altitude climbing and the physical exertion from carrying heavy loads have been suggested to play a role in triggering retinal hemorrhages in the compromised vasculature.[108] Most climbers do not notice any symptoms of altitude retinopathy, although the more severe vasculature problems can produce permanent vision loss.[109,112,113] Because the amount of ultraviolet radiation markedly increases at higher elevations, and snow reflects 85% of the ultraviolet radiation, additional risk of photokeratitis exists when appropriate filters are not used.[114]

Racquet Sports

A significant portion of sport-related eye injuries is caused by racquet sports.[4,9,11,23,29,30,115] Racquet sports include badminton, handball, racquetball, squash, and tennis. The ball or shuttlecock is hit with tremendous force and can travel at dramatic speeds (see Table 6.4). Even though the balls used in some racquet sports are larger than the average orbital opening, the compression forces can push the ball deep inside the orbit.[30] The shuttlecock has a diameter of 0.75 inches and easily penetrates the orbital opening. Ocular trauma usually results from severe blunt force trauma caused by the racquet or ball, including a high prevalence of hyphema, traumatic glaucoma, commotio retinae, and retinal detachment.[30,115–125] In tennis and badminton, doubles play significantly increases the risk of eye injury because of the proximity of the doubles partner. The ocular damage may be increased with inappropriate eyewear (see Chapter 6). Many of the ocular injuries require in-hospital care, and the ocular damage may cause permanent vision changes.[116,117,119–121,123–126] The retinal detachments from squash injuries have been reported to have a worse prognosis than other rhegmatogenous detachments.[124] The experience and expertise level of the athlete have not been shown to reduce the risk of eye injury during racquet sports.[119,122]

Scuba Diving

The increased ambient pressure encountered in scuba diving must be equalized by exhaling through the nose during descent to avoid mask barotrauma. The increased pressure of the mask pulls the eyes and surrounding tissues into the airspace of the mask unless it is equalized, potentially causing hemorrhaging and edema in the ocular tissues.[30,127–132] Fortunately most mask barotrauma is self-resolving, and the only treatment is supportive (e.g., ice packs) with patient reassurance.

Decompression sickness (DCS) can result from surfacing too quickly, causing the rapid release of gas accumulated in the body's tissues during the period of high compression. Many neurologic ocular manifestations of DCS have been reported in the literature, including nystagmus, diplopia, visual field defects, cortical blindness, central retinal artery occlusion, and optic neuropathy. The ocular manifestations of DCS are successfully managed with recompression therapy and hyperbaric oxygen.

If a diver wears contact lenses, soft lenses are preferred.[133–135] Rigid lenses, particularly polymethyl methacrylate lenses, can cause corneal edema from nitrogen gas bubble formation under the lens during outgassing of decompression. If a diver has had an ophthalmic surgical procedure, Butler[131] recommends minimal convalescent periods before clearing the patient for diving (Table 7.2). The main risk involves infection from the rich microbial environment of water during wound healing. The increased pressure associated with diving

TABLE 7.2
Recommended Minimum Convalescent Period Before Diving After Ophthalmic Surgery.

Procedure	Recommended Convalescent Period
ANTERIOR SEGMENT SURGERY	
Penetrating keratoplasty	6 months
Corneal laceration repair	6 months
Cataract surgery	
Noncorneal valve incision	3 months
Corneal valve incisions	
Clear corneal	2 months
Scleral tunnel	1 month
Radial keratotomy	3 months
Astigmatic keratotomy	3 months
Glaucoma filtering surgery	2 months (relative contraindication)
Photorefractive keratectomy	2 weeks
Pterygium excision	2 weeks
Conjunctival surgery	2 weeks
Corneal suture removal	1 week
Argon laser trabeculoplasty or iridectomy	No wait necessary
YAG laser capsulotomy	No wait necessary
VITREORETINAL SURGERY	
Vitrectomy	2 months (contraindicated until intraocular gas absorbed)
Retinal detachment repair	2 months
Pneumatic retinopexy	2 months (contraindicated until intraocular gas absorbed)
Retinal cryopexy or laser photocoagulation for breaks	2 weeks
OCULOPLASTIC SURGERY	
Sutured wound	2 weeks
Skin graft or granulating wound	Until epithelialization is complete
Enucleation	2 weeks (contraindicated with hollow orbital implants)
Strabismus Surgery	2 weeks

YAG, yttrium-aluminum-garnet.
Reprinted from Butler FK. Diving and hyperbaric ophthalmology. *Surv Ophthalmol.* 1995;39:347.

does not pose a significant risk for patients who have undergone corneal or refractive surgery, with glaucoma, or with vitreoretinal disorders.[131]

Soccer

The soccer ball is responsible for most ocular traumas in soccer, although the incidence of eye injuries is relatively low.[11,12,15,44,45,136−140] Although the soccer ball is significantly larger than the orbital opening, a portion of the ball will deform and enter the orbit during contact with the high velocities at which the ball is kicked.[139,140] A study found that, although the soccer ball did not penetrate the orbital opening as deeply as smaller sports balls (e.g., baseballs, golf balls, tennis balls, squash balls), the ball remains inside the orbital space considerably longer than the other ball types.[140] An appreciable rebound effect also occurs after the initial compression phase that produces a suction distortion to the globe, potentially increasing the severity of the blunt force trauma (see Fig. 7.1). The predilection for retinal lesions in the superotemporal quadrant is proposed to be caused by the more exposed temporal retina when the compression forces expand the globe equatorially; the nose offers some protection from the forces transmitted to the nasal retina.[140]

Swimming and Water Sports

Swimming and water sports do not present a significant risk of eye trauma; however, water sports can be a significant source of eye infections and chemical burns. Swimming goggles can potentially cause a blunt trauma injury if they slip during removal or when cleared. The elastic band can cause the goggles to snap back and cause severe injuries, including globe ruptures.[30] Water polo presents a risk of blunt trauma from fingers, elbows, or the ball to the improperly protected eye. Other risks include infections in soft contact lens wearers who are not adequately compliant with appropriate lens cleaning and pingueculae and pterygia in outdoor water sports (e.g., surfing, windsurfing, kiteboarding, kayaking).[30,141]

Paintball

War games with paintball guns present a tremendous risk for ocular injury when proper protection is not used. The paint pellet is shot with sufficient energy to cause severe eye trauma, including corneal lacerations, hyphema, traumatic cataract, and retinal pathology.[142−150]

OVERVIEW OF OCULAR INJURY MANAGEMENT

Blunt Trauma

Most eye injuries reported from sports and recreational activities result from objects larger than the orbit, producing blunt trauma, and objects smaller than the orbit, resulting in penetrating trauma.[29−32,43,151,152] Blunt trauma to the head can also result in damage to the visual pathway.[30,153] In cases in which only one eye is injured, the other eye should also be thoroughly assessed for either recent or long-standing damage.

Blunt trauma is produced by significant pressures exerted on the orbital contents. The ocular damage is usually produced by direct injury to the local site of the trauma (coup effects) or the forces transferred through the ocular tissues along the path of the shock waves (contrecoup effects).[43,154−156] Ocular damage may also result from the compression forces exerted when the orbital contents are compacted within the bony orbit.[29,43] In ocular compression injuries, the globe is compressed along the anteroposterior direction and must compensate by expanding equatorially or it will rupture (Fig. 7.2). Each of these mechanisms is capable of causing significant harm to the delicate orbital bones and ocular tissues. Most blunt eye trauma is caused by a ball, stick, finger, or other object or body part during sports participation, as previously described. The examination should also determine whether any penetrating intraocular foreign body injury occurred that was not reported in the trauma history.

Sideline management: When evaluating the athlete after a blunt trauma, the sports medicine professional must assess the following regarding the eye: Is the lid swollen shut? Is blood present inside the eye? Is the cornea white or hazy? Is the pupil irregularly shaped, fixed, dilated, or constricted? Is the athlete experiencing problems with vision (e.g., seeing stars, floaters, distortion)? If the athlete has any of these signs or symptoms, then apply a cold compress and immediately refer the athlete to an eye care professional. If eye pain is the only symptom, the injury sustained is usually not emergent. If an immediate referral is not required, then have the athlete apply ice for 15- to 20-minute periods during the first 24 h after injury. The athlete should be referred to an eye care professional within 24−36 h of the event (Table 7.3). Athletes who have sustained a blunt trauma injury should have a dilated fundus examination performed by an eye care professional within 96 h.

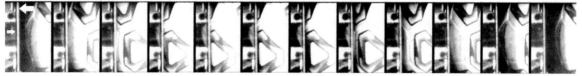

FIG. 7.1 Soccer ball impact on an artificial orbit. The orbit (anterior plane, *small arrow*) is penetrated 8.1 mm by the 18-m/s (40 mph) size 3 soccer ball, which compresses on the steel plate surrounding the orbital fixture (*large arrow*). The compression phase of the ball, which drives a small knuckle of the ball into the orbit (1–4 ms), is easily seen by studying the dark triangles on the ball. During rebound, the slow orbital exit of the ball compared with the rebound from the plate (5–10 ms) produces a secondary suction effect on the orbital contents. (Courtesy Paul Vinger, MD, Concord, Massachusetts.)

Eyelids

The eyelids should be assessed for any lacerations or limitation of lid movement or closure. Substantial lacerations typically require surgical repair, and a broad-spectrum topical antibiotic should be applied to prevent secondary infection if possible. Incomplete lid closure may necessitate treatment with ocular lubricants to prevent exposure keratitis until surgical lid repair can be performed. The lids should be specifically assessed for damage to cranial nerves III and VII, the levator muscle, the orbicularis muscle, and the lacrimal system.[43,157] A referral to an oculoplastic specialist may be indicated when lid involvement is substantial.

Sideline management: In the case of a superficial injury to the eyelid, gently apply direct pressure to stop the bleeding. Cleanse the wound and apply a sterile dressing taped in place or a bandage encircling head. Refer the athlete to an eye care professional for follow-up care of the injury. Mild lacerations sustained at a competition away from the athlete's hometown may wait to receive medical treatment until the athlete returns home.[161] The laceration should be bandaged and cleaned, with antibiotic coverage.

If a corneal abrasion is suspected or the pupil appears irregularly shaped, the athlete should immediately be referred to an ophthalmologist or optometrist. Place a protective pad or shield over the eye. Covering both eyes may be necessary to reduce bilateral eye movement. If the laceration crosses the margin of the lid, suturing by an eye expert is necessary. Lid deformities (ectropion) from scarring may result if the athlete does not receive proper care.

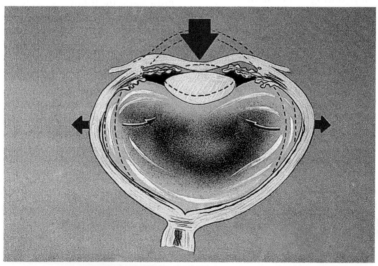

FIG. 7.2 Mechanism of ocular damage by blunt trauma. (Reprinted from Kanski JJ. *Clinical Ophthalmology*. 5th ed. Boston: Butterworth Heinemann; 2003.)

TABLE 7.3
Triage of Sport-Related Ocular Injuries.

Emergency Situation	Treatment
FOREIGN OBJECT IN EYE/EYE PAIN	
Visible object, not embedded	Lift object gently with tissue or cotton moistened with sterile eye solution. If solution is not available use water.
Object not visible	Gently grasp lashes of upper lid and pull lid forward and down. Allow tears to wash out foreign body.
Visible object that cannot be removed	See eye care professional the same day.
Possible penetration of the globe of the eye or surrounding tissue by the object	Do not attempt to remove object; see eye care professional the same day.
Blood seen in the eye	See eye care professional the same day.
Object possibly trapped behind the upper lid	See eye care professional the same day.
Vision problems	See eye care professional the same day.
Eye pain	See eye care professional the same day.
BLUNT TRAUMA	
Patient should have a dilated fundus examination performed by an eye care professional within 96 h of the event because serious internal eye injuries may have occurred. Apply cold compress for the first 24 h unless one of the signs below is present. If no improvement occurs see an eye care professional within 24–36 h of the traumatic event.	
Lid swollen shut	See eye care professional immediately.
Blood inside the eye	See eye care professional immediately.
Cornea (front of the eye) white or hazy	See eye care professional immediately.
Pupil irregularly shaped, fixed, dilated, or constricted	See eye care professional immediately.
Problem with vision (e.g., stars, floaters, distortion)	See eye care professional immediately.
Eye pain	See eye care professional the same day.
Superficial injury to eyelid	Gently apply direct pressure to stop bleeding. Cleanse wound and apply sterile dressing taped in place or apply a bandage encircling the head. See eye care professional immediately.
BURNS	
In the event of a chemical burn do not attempt to neutralize the acid or alkali. Do not use an eye cup. Do not bandage the eye. When irrigating ensure that the chemical does not wash into the other eye. If sterile eye solution is not available use water.	
Ultraviolet burn (most commonly occurs in water and snow sports)	See eye care professional the same day.
Chemical is a strong base (alkali; e.g., drain cleaner, lime, cement, plaster)	Irrigate 30 min with sterile eye solution and lids forced open. See eye care professional immediately.
Chemical is a strong acid (e.g., battery acid)	Irrigate at least 15 min with sterile eye solution and lids forced open. See eye care professional immediately.
Chemical is a mild acid or base (e.g., pool chlorine, bleach, gasoline)	Irrigate at least 15 min with sterile eye solution and lids forced open. See eye care professional the same day.

Laceration of the upper or lower lacrimal canaliculi (tear duct) also requires suturing by an ophthalmologist. If the tear duct is not repaired, the patient may have permanent epiphora (watering of the eye).

Orbital contents
The athlete may sustain orbital hemorrhaging, leading to ecchymosis, proptosis, and extraocular muscle (EOM) abnormalities.[151,152] A simple black eye should

be examined as if the eye had sustained serious trauma until proven otherwise.[32] Hematomas can have many ocular sequelae, necessitating a thorough internal health evaluation and assessment of intraocular pressure. Visual acuity, color vision, pupillary responses, and intraocular pressure should be carefully assessed. Additionally, severe proptosis can compromise the function of the optic nerve and retinal vasculature, requiring rapid diagnosis to determine whether orbital decompression or corticosteroid treatment is necessary. Many orbital hemorrhages completely resolve with no direct treatment, but closely monitoring the athlete throughout the recovery period is prudent.

Any head trauma can result in direct damage to the EOMs or cranial nerves III, IV, or VI. The practitioner needs to determine if the muscle abnormality is caused by hemorrhage or edema around the muscle or direct damage such as a muscle tear or disinsertion. Orbital fractures may also entrap EOMs and directly affect muscle function. These direct causes of muscle damage usually produce symptoms of pain, diplopia, and gaze restrictions.[153,157] If the damage has occurred to the cranial nerves, the patient will report the same symptoms but is less likely to report any pain. Cranial nerve damage is a sign of significant closed-head trauma or compression of an expanding intracranial hematoma and should immediately be treated.[32]

Differential diagnosis for concomitancy of EOM function is achieved with version testing, alternate cover testing in the diagnostic action fields, Hess-Lancaster test, red lens or Maddox rod testing in the diagnostic action fields, or the Park three-step test.[158–160] The diagnostic action fields are the gaze positions where the individual action of each EOM is isolated (Table 7.4). Passive and forced duction testing can help determine if mechanical damage of the muscle(s) has occurred or if the damage occurred in the innervation from the cranial nerves.[165,166] Management of EOM abnormalities includes monitoring for spontaneous resolution, prism prescriptions, occlusion (usually partial occlusion in the affected field), orthoptic vision therapy to assist recovery of muscle function, botulinum toxin therapy,[167–169] and surgical interventions.

Sideline management: The presence of a black eye is a cue to evaluate the eye and face further, with subsequent referral of the patient to an eye care professional. An orbital hemorrhage may present with proptosis (eyeball bulging) and decreased EOM motility.[170] Furthermore, visual loss may occur as a result of a compromised vascular supply to the retina and optic nerve.[170] Immediate management includes application of an ice pack and referral to an eye care professional.

TABLE 7.4 Diagnostic Action Fields of Extraocular Muscles.[162]		
Eye Position	**Right Eye**	**Left Eye**
Right gaze	Lateral rectus	Medial rectus
Left gaze	Medial rectus	Lateral rectus
25 degrees right gaze and up	Superior rectus	Inferior oblique
25 degrees left gaze and up	Inferior oblique	Superior rectus
25 degrees right gaze and down	Inferior rectus	Superior oblique
25 degrees left gaze and down	Superior oblique	Inferior rectus

Bone Structures

Blunt trauma to the bony orbit can cause external fractures to the orbital rim; however, the more fragile internal orbital walls are more prone to fractures.[29,151–153,157] Lang[171] was the first to postulate the mechanism for what would later be referred to as a blowout fracture.[172] The blunt trauma to the eye forces the globe back into the orbit, and the hydraulic pressure of the compressed globe can break through one or two orbital walls. The term blowout fracture is used to describe fractures of the internal orbital floor (separating the maxillary sinus) without fractures of the external orbital rim. The medial wall (lamina papyracea) separating the ethmoid sinus may also be fractured during a blowout fracture.[151,157] Medial wall fractures may also cause orbital emphysema from air forced into the orbit from the nasal sinuses (Fig. 7.3), most noticeable when blowing the nose or during a Valsalva maneuver. These fractures are confirmed by a computed tomographic scan or radiograph of the orbit (Fig. 7.4) and often produce pain, EOM restrictions, and eventual enophthalmos. Significant fractures necessitate surgical interventions to minimize enophthalmos and EOM restrictions.[151,157]

Jones[162] reported that one-third of orbital blowout fractures are the result of sports activities, with soccer being the most common sport involved in the United Kingdom. Aggressive play was identified as the most common cause of the fractures, typically through high-energy blows by an opponent's fingers, fists, elbows, knees, or boots.

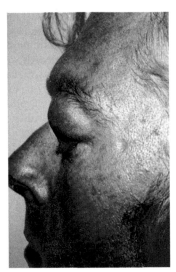

FIG. 7.3 Subcutaneous emphysema in a patient with a medial orbital wall blowout fracture. (Reprinted from Kanski JJ. *Clinical Ophthalmology*. 5th ed. Boston: Butterworth Heinemann; 2003.)

Sideline management: A blowout fracture can prevent concentric gaze and result in double vision. The athlete will report pain at the site of injury and with movement of the eye. Visual inspection often reveals hyphema, swelling, numbness of the ipsilateral cheek, a protruding or a sunken eye, vertical dystopia, and periorbital hematoma.[163,164,173] An athlete presenting with signs consistent with a

blowout fracture should have a sterile eye pad placed over the eye to prevent him or her from looking around. The athlete may require bilateral eye pads to further reduce the chance of eye movement. The use of ice will help with pain modulation while the athlete is transferred to the emergency department.

A retrospective review of National Football League players found the most common signs and symptoms experienced immediately after an orbital fracture included decreased visual acuity, decreased eye movements, hyphema, and infraorbital numbness.[161] The mechanism of injury was either a digital poke or a blunt facial trauma.[161] To highlight the seriousness of orbital fractures, 15 of the 19 cases reviewed required surgical reconstruction.[161] Two of the football players were unable to return to football because of residual visual impairment.[161]

Zygomatic fractures

A fracture of the zygomatic bone usually occurs from a powerful force directed at the cheek or from a fall.[163] Signs of a possible zygomatic bone fracture include epistaxis, periorbital ecchymosis, numbness about the cheek, enophthalmos, restriction of upward gaze and diplopia, subconjunctival hemorrhage, a depressed cheekbone, and inability to open the mouth.[163,173] Concomitant injury to the infraorbital nerve will cause hypesthesia or anesthesia of the ipsilateral upper lip, lower eyelid, lateral nose, and medial cheek.[163] Palpation of the area often reveals a bony discrepancy or step-off deformity. If a fracture is suspected apply ice to control edema and immediately refer the patient to a physician.

As with other fractures, healing will take a minimum of 6–8 weeks. The athlete should wear protective face equipment or eyewear when returning to sport.[173]

Frontal bone fracture

A frontal bone fracture can occur from a severe blow to the supraorbital region. An example of a potential mechanism for this type of injury is two heads colliding during a soccer match.[174] A visible or palpable depression superior to the frontal sinus should cue the sports medicine specialist to a possible fracture.[174] Crepitus or depression in the frontal sinus may be noted, as well as numbness in the supraorbital region.[164] Immediate management by a physician is necessary.

Conjunctival and Scleral injuries

Fingers commonly cause damage to the conjunctival tissue in contact sports. A simple subconjunctival hemorrhage often is the sole result of such contact, and the

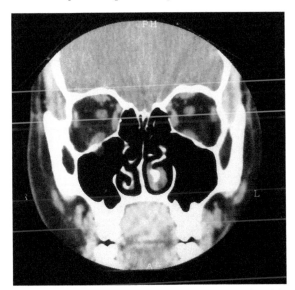

FIG. 7.4 Coronal computed tomographic scan of a right orbital floor blowout fracture. (Reprinted from Kanski JJ. *Clinical Ophthalmology*. 5th ed. Boston: Butterworth Heinemann; 2003.)

condition self-resolves with no long-term consequences. However, determination of whether more extensive scleral lacerations or ruptures may be hidden by the blood and chemosis is important. Small scleral lacerations may be managed with a prophylactic broad-spectrum antibiotic ointment, whereas larger lacerations may require suturing.[152] Examination of the athlete should entail a thorough assessment of the internal structures that may also have sustained damage, including Seidel testing with fluorescein to determine if a rupture or penetrating injury has occurred. Fluorescein leakage near the injury site indicates a rupture or penetrating wound,[175] and a surgical consultation is warranted. The limbus region and EOM insertion areas are most prone to scleral rupture,[43] and previous eye injuries or surgeries make the globe more vulnerable.[32]

Sideline management: A subconjunctival hemorrhage will present as a bright red region within the white conjunctiva. The "red eye" may make this form of injury appear serious in nature, but in many cases, this form of hemorrhage will not require medical attention. However, a subconjunctival hemorrhage often accompanies a contusion or corneal abrasion, so if visual impairments, photophobia, or extensive hemorrhaging is apparent, then the athlete should be referred to an eye care specialist.

Corneal injuries

The cornea is a frequent site of damage from both blunt and penetrating or foreign body trauma. Injuries to the corneal epithelium are particularly painful because of the high concentration of sensory nerve innervation, leading to photophobia and reflexive tearing. Athletes participating in contact sports are at particular risk for finger injuries, and a fingernail can cause significant harm to the corneal tissues. The practitioner must therefore perform a careful evaluation of the layers of the cornea with a biomicroscope to determine the depth and extent of the damage. Fortunately, epithelial wounds heal rather rapidly without sequelae unless the Bowman layer has been involved. Injuries to Bowman layer increase the incidence of residual scarring, which can affect visual clarity. Athletes whose corneal injuries involved vegetative matter should be carefully monitored for subsequent fungal infections. Corneal lacerations (Fig. 7.5) that are large and not self-sealing require protection with a Fox shield and referral for surgical consultation.

Pressure patching had been the standard approach for the management of corneal abrasions (Fig. 7.6); however, the reduction of oxygen to the epithelium and increased temperature produced by patching can retard healing and increase the risk of infection.[152,176] A Cochrane review in 2016 did not show any improvement in pain, symptoms, or healing when comparing patching with nonpatching for corneal abrasions.[177] The use of topical antibiotics without patching may yield faster healing rates while protecting from secondary infection.[178] Aggressive use of ocular lubricants can further improve patient comfort and promote healing, especially the use of lubricant ointments at bedtime. Because of the significant pain associated with epithelial injuries, oral nonsteroidal antiinflammatory agents are frequently prescribed.[179] A Cochrane review did not show clinically relevant pain reduction from the use of topical nonsteroidal antiinflammatory drugs in traumatic corneal abrasions, and because antiinflammatory agents can slow tissue healing, their use should be limited to twice daily.[180] The use of topical anesthetics to improve patient comfort is specifically

(A)

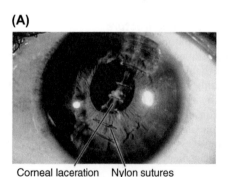

Corneal laceration   Nylon sutures

(B)

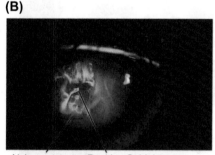

Nylon sutures   Positive Seidel test

FIG. 7.5 (A) Large corneal laceration through visual axis. Note the linear scar from the wound and around the multiple interrupted nylon sutures of various lengths used to repair the laceration. (B) Corneal laceration demonstrating positive Seidel test result (bright stream of fluorescein around the central suture). (Reprinted from Kaiser PK, Friedman, NJ. *The Massachusetts Eye and Ear Infirmary Illustrated Manual of Ophthalmology*. 2nd ed. Philadelphia: W.B. Saunders; 2004.)

(A)   **(B)**   **(C)**

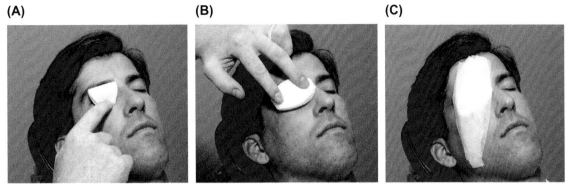

FIG. 7.6 Pressure patching to manage corneal abrasions. (A) The examiner applies an eye pad to the closed eyelids, either lengthwise or folded in half. (B) The examiner places a second patch lengthwise over the first patch. (C) Finally the examiner secures the patches with tape placed from the center of the forehead to the angle of the jaw across the patched eye. (Reprinted from Palay DA, Krachmer JH. *Primary Care Ophthalmology*. 2nd ed. St Louis: Mosby; 2005.)

contraindicated because of significant interference with corneal healing and increased risk of infection.[152]

A bandage contact lens can be an effective management tool for corneal injuries, although the lenses may also slow healing. The lens can protect the epithelium without significantly reducing the oxygen supply or increasing the corneal temperature like traditional pressure patching does. A contact lens offers the additional benefit to the athlete of allowing use of the eye during healing. For the athlete who is already a contact lens wearer, this is an excellent management approach. The athlete should be encouraged to use rewetting drops frequently to maintain good ocular lubrication.

A particular problem with corneal injuries inflicted by fingernails is the chance of recurrent corneal erosions. Most epithelial injuries heal well but 7%–8% of injuries result in recurrent erosions.[181,182] Management is designed to reestablish the adhesion complex between the epithelium and Bowman layer and includes sequential use of topical hyperosmotic agents, bandage contact lens wear, surgical debridement, stromal micropuncture, and excimer laser phototherapeutic keratectomy.[152,182–187] Newer therapies include oral matrix metalloproteinase inhibitors, blood-derived eye drops, amniotic membrane graft application, and topical corticosteroids.[188] However, a review concluded, "well-designed, masked, randomised controlled trials using standardised methods are needed to establish the benefits of new and existing prophylactic and treatment regimens for recurrent corneal erosion."[189]

The forces generated in many fast ball and contact sports can result in ruptures to all layers of the cornea. Damage to Descemet membrane or the endothelium results in considerable corneal edema and possibly corneal blood staining. The corneal edema and blood staining typically resolves spontaneously; however, the disruption in the endothelial cell junctions can be permanent.[43,190] Injuries with sufficient force to rupture the deeper corneal layers often result in damage to the adjoining sclera as well.[191,192] Athletes who have had corneal refractive surgery may be at higher risk for ruptures and should be strongly counseled regarding the use of appropriate protective eyewear.

Sideline management: If a foreign object injury is suspected and the athlete has been unable to remove the object on his or her own, the sports medicine professional may be able to assist with the removal. If an object is visible (and not embedded) then lift the object gently with tissue or cotton moistened with sterile eye solution (or water if solution is not available). If the object cannot be seen the eyelid must be everted (Fig. 7.7). Allow tears to wash out the foreign body. If the object is difficult to remove, if the athlete has vision problems or blood in the eye, or if the foreign object has penetrated the globe or surrounding tissue, immediately refer the patient to an eye care professional.

Immediate management of suspected corneal injury requires covering or patching the eye, instructing the athlete not to rub the eye, and referring the athlete to an eye care specialist. The use of fluorescein dye and illumination of the eye are necessary to ascertain the extent of damage.

Removing contact lenses. Contact lenses should be removed from the eye in the case of minor injuries such as a corneal abrasion.[36] In cases in which the eye

(A)   **(B)**

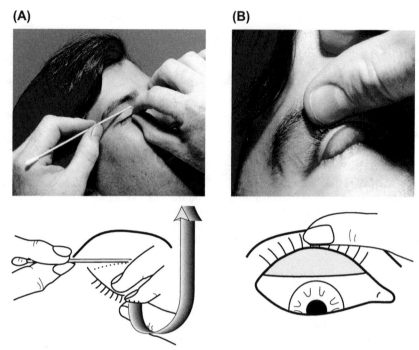

FIG. 7.7 Steps to evert the upper eyelid. (A) Ask the athlete to look down while keeping his or her eyes open. Grab the eyelash and the tarsal plate close to the edge of the eyelid and gently pull forward and down. The eyelid should not be pulled up or out (top). Place a cotton-tipped applicator or lid evertor just above the tarsal plate of the eyelid. While still holding the eyelashes evert the eyelid over the applicator (bottom). (B) The eye can then be examined with the eyelid held against the superior bony ridge of the orbit (top). Instruct the athlete to look upward and blink. This will return the lid to its normal position (bottom). (Reprinted from Palay DA, Krachmer JH. *Primary Care Ophthalmology*. 2nd ed. St Louis: Mosby; 2005.)

exhibits serious surface trauma, the contact lens should be left in place until the eye can be more thoroughly evaluated by a physician or an eye care specialist.

Anterior chamber and uvea

The pressure forces generated with blunt trauma in sports can result in damage to the iris or ciliary body tissues. Contusion pressure forces the cornea, iris-lens diaphragm, and ciliary body to rapidly expand posteriorly and circumferentially.[29,152,193,194] The resulting damage can lead to anterior chamber angle and pupillary effects and traumatic hyphema problems.

A relatively mild trauma may cause injury to the iris stroma, resulting in iritis that spontaneously recovers with time. Topical cycloplegic agents are prescribed to decrease the pain and photophobia produced by the iritis. The iris sphincter may rupture in one or more locations, causing characteristic triangular defects and notched pupillary borders that are permanent (Fig. 7.8). The iris and ciliary body may respond to blunt trauma with temporary miosis, mydriasis,

cycloplegia, or spasm of accommodation. More severe trauma may result in iridoschisis (detachment of an anterior mesodermal leaf) or iridodialysis (base of the iris separates from the ciliary body). Iridodialysis

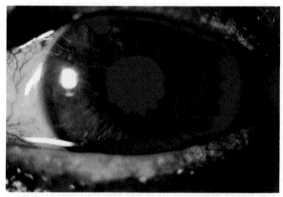

FIG. 7.8 Rupture of the iris sphincter. (Reprinted from Kanski JJ. *Clinical Ophthalmology*. 5th ed. Boston: Butterworth Heinemann; 2003.)

typically produces a substantial hyphema that makes the injury difficult to detect until the hyphema clears. Iridodialysis may not require treatment unless it has created monocular diplopia because of an accessory pupil.

The ciliary body is also at risk for damage from blunt trauma, usually producing a cleft in the anterior ciliary body and causing angle recession (Fig. 7.9).[29,43,152,193] Angle recession can occur with or without bleeding and affects anterior chamber drainage by damage to the trabecular meshwork. Gonioscopic studies suggest that most injuries that result in traumatic hyphema also produce angle recession.[195,196] Angle recession is responsible for glaucoma, often unilateral in cases when only one eye received the trauma. A secondary open-angle glaucoma can occur within 2 months to 2 years after the injury or even 10–15 years after the injury.[197] The incidence of secondary glaucoma with angle recession is estimated to be approximately 7%,[193,198] and eyes with angle recessions larger than 180 degrees are at greater risk of developing glaucoma.[197–199] Athletes who have angle recession injuries should be frequently monitored throughout life for development of glaucoma. Rarely, a 360-degree ciliary detachment can occur (cyclodialysis) and cause hypotony and phthisis bulbi, requiring surgical management.[152]

Damage to the iris and ciliary body tissues often results in bleeding in the anterior chamber, and the resulting hyphema presents a considerable diagnostic and management challenge. The hyphema can obscure the clinician's view of the internal ocular structures, making evaluation of the extent of damage quite difficult. Nevertheless, a thorough case history and evaluation should be performed to the degree possible. The extent of the hyphema should be carefully noted, including notation of the presence and location of a clot. A grading system for traumatic hyphema is useful for recording and communicating the extent of the bleeding (Box 7.4).[193]

Traumatic hyphema has many consequences, including elevated intraocular pressure during the acute phase of the hyphema, secondary hemorrhage, anterior and posterior synechiae formation, corneal blood staining, and optic atrophy. Sport-related injuries are a common cause of hyphema, with a study reporting almost 40% of traumatic hyphema seen in an outpatient clinical setting resulted from sporting injuries.[200] Transient elevated intraocular pressure is presumably caused by blockage of the trabecular meshwork and typically returns to normal quickly as the hyphema resolves. This mechanism is similar to the exercise-induced elevations in intraocular pressure found with pigmentary dispersion syndrome.[201] Athletes with sickle cell disease, and undiagnosed athletes of African or Hispanic descent, are at a higher risk for elevated intraocular pressure and subsequent central retinal artery obstruction because the sickled erythrocytes cannot pass through the trabecular meshwork.[202–206] Secondary bleeding presents a significantly worse prognosis for vision recovery[196,206,207] and secondary glaucoma.[206,208,209] Synechiae formation in traumatic hyphema is often caused by associated iritis and angle closure, and changes in pupillary responses may be noted.[196,207] Optic atrophy can result from the trauma itself or from prolonged periods of significantly elevated intraocular pressure.[196,207]

All these complications, along with the absence of a definitive treatment approach, present a complex and difficult clinical problem.[206,210] Many medical and surgical treatment options must be carefully considered. Conventional initial treatment of traumatic hyphema has included strict bed rest, bilateral patching, sedation, and hospitalization. Medical management is most appropriate for patients with grade 3 or less hyphema and surgical intervention is considered for grade 4

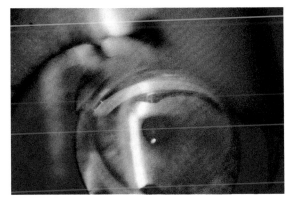

FIG. 7.9 Severe angle recession. (Reprinted from Kanski JJ. *Clinical Ophthalmology*. 5th ed. Boston: Butterworth Heinemann; 2003.)

BOX 7.4
Grading System for Hyphema[194]

Grade 1: Layered blood occupying less than one-third of the anterior chamber

Grade 2: Blood filling one-third to one half of the anterior chamber

Grade 3: Layered blood filling one half to less than total

Grade 4: Total clotted hyphema, often referred to as "black ball" or "eight ball" hyphema

hyphema that does not respond to medical management within approximately 4 days.[193]

Sideline management: Signs of a hyphema include a reddish tinge in the anterior chamber initially after the injury and visual acuity may be affected with a large bleed. Within a few hours the blood will settle in the inferior eye or fill the entire chamber.[211] The sports medicine professional should recognize the signs of a hyphema and immediately refer the athlete to an optometrist or ophthalmologist.[46] The patient should be transported to the emergency department in a sitting or upright position.[36] The athletic trainer should advise the family to avoid giving aspirin or other antiinflammatory medication, which may increase the bleeding.

Crystalline lens

The crystalline lens can be damaged from both coup and contrecoup effects of the trauma. If the globe is compressed enough to push the cornea posteriorly until it makes contact with the lens, a permanent Vossius ring may result from the contact between the iris pupillary ruff and anterior lens surface.[29,41,153] More significant force can produce a transient rosette cataract, although the cataract often remains and can become progressively worse. Removal of the cataract can be complicated by the presence of hyphema and damage to other structures, especially the zonules. If the lens capsule has been ruptured, further complications of uveitis and phacolytic glaucoma may result.

In more severe cases of ocular trauma, the lens can become subluxated or completely dislocated. The pressure of the injury may rupture the zonules and cause the lens to tilt anteriorly or posteriorly, potentially leading to fluctuations in vision and diplopia. If this patient requires dilation, care must be taken to preclude having the subluxated lens shift into the anterior chamber. If the displaced lens is in contact with the iris, or if the vitreous has prolapsed into the anterior chamber, surgical intervention is often required. In the rare occasion when the zonules have been completely severed, the lens can be dislocated internally into the anterior chamber or the vitreous, or suprachoroidally.[152,212–214] The lens may also dislocate externally in severe trauma, especially in globe rupture. In addition to the poor vision resulting from lens dislocation, the clinician may also observe iridodonesis (quivering of the iris).[41] A dislocated lens presents a poor prognosis, and the ensuing complications increase if the capsule has ruptured. The best treatment for lens dislocation is removal of the lens with a complete pars plana vitrectomy.[152]

Vitreous body

The vitreous body can be directly affected in ocular trauma by vitreous base avulsion or posterior vitreous detachment or indirectly affected by hemorrhaging into the vitreous. Many uveal and retinal sites of possible bleeding exist, which highlights the need for a thorough posterior segment evaluation. If the views of the retina are obscured by blood in the vitreous, B-scan ultrasonography may be necessary to evaluate the integrity of the retina. Vitreal hemorrhaging can spontaneously resolve after several weeks; however, indications for vitrectomy may be present. The cells of the hemorrhage can migrate into the anterior chamber to produce ghost cell glaucoma, often requiring treatment with a vitrectomy.[152,194,215]

Vitreous traction can produce tears from the locations where the vitreous is attached. Most commonly, the vitreous base can be torn away along the anterior retina and pars plana and is pathognomonic for blunt trauma.[43] The vitreous base avulsion can cause the vitreous base to hang over the peripheral retina, creating a "bucket handle" appearance.[29,152] The vitreous base avulsion can often cause detachment of the peripheral retina as well. The vitreous is also strongly attached to the retina around the optic nerve, macula, and retinal vessels. Traction from blunt trauma can produce posterior vitreous detachment and subsequent retinal detachment. Detachment of the anterior or posterior vitreous may be monitored unless the traction on the retina necessitates surgical intervention.[152]

Retinal injuries

The retina is often affected by ocular trauma. Many effects are possible, several of which cause permanent loss of visual function and require surgical treatment. Athletes with high myopia or otherwise compromised retinas are at particular risk of retinal damage from trauma.

Commotio retinae is a fairly common contrecoup injury first described by Berlin in 1873.[216] The contusion causes a white, opaque appearance to the damaged retina (Fig. 7.10) that often resolves without intervention unless permanent damage to the photoreceptors or retinal pigment epithelium occurs.[43,152,194,215] Commotio retinae can occur to peripheral retina or the central macular region (known as Berlin edema) and have varying effects on visual acuity. Considerable damage to the retinal pigment epithelium can occur, eventually leading to granular pigmentation and bone corpuscular appearance of the affected retina resembling retinitis pigmentosa.[217–219] The athlete should also be evaluated for serous retinal detachment, which also diminishes the prognosis for vision recovery.[220]

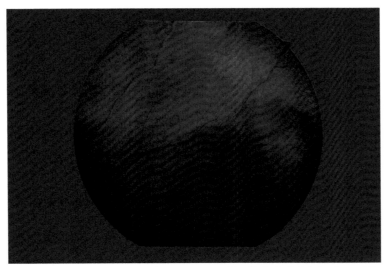

FIG. 7.10 Peripheral commotio retinae. (From Kanski JJ. *Clinical Ophthalmology*. 5th ed. Boston: Butterworth Heinemann; 2003.)

Traumatic macular holes are relatively common with blunt trauma, and the possible mechanisms include necrosis, vitreous traction, and subfoveal hemorrhage.[152,194,221,222] The vision is usually poor with a full-thickness macular hole, and it is frequently associated with injuries to other internal ocular tissues.[223] Traumatic macular holes may spontaneously resolve but surgical intervention may be necessary. Surgical success for recovering vision lost to traumatic macular holes, especially in younger patients, has recently improved.[222,224–234]

Retinal dialysis, a separation at the anterior edge of the ora serrata with the vitreous remaining attached to the posterior edge, is the most common traumatic retinal break.[235] The dialysis frequently occurs during the trauma,[236,237] and the vitreous attachment is most likely responsible for the gradual development of retinal detachment. Retinal dialysis may be difficult to observe and diagnose; however, prophylactic surgical treatment can prevent progression to retinal detachment.[152]

Many varieties of retinal tears and detachments can result from ocular trauma. The clinician should be skilled at identifying horseshoe tears, holes with operculum, stretch tears, giant retinal tears, necrotic tears, and rhegmatogenous retinal detachments.[43,152] Advances in retinal imaging technologies can significantly improve diagnostic accuracy. Retinal detachment may not present immediately after the trauma; therefore frequent monitoring and athlete education regarding detachment symptoms is strongly recommended after trauma. Most tears and detachments require surgical treatment to prevent progression of retinal damage; however, no evidence exists that surgically induced adhesions offer protection against retinal detachment in high-contact sports such as boxing or martial arts.[63]

Sideline management: Retinal detachment is a painless injury caused by blunt trauma to the eye.[211] The athlete may describe the symptoms as "a curtain falling in front of the eye" or as lights "flashing on and off."[161,211] The athlete may also see black specks floating across the eye. A detached retina is a serious eye injury requiring immediate referral to a physician. The athletic trainer should use a protective eye shield or the base of a paper cup to cover the eye.

Optic nerve

The optic nerve can be damaged by many direct and indirect causes. The most common form of optic nerve injury is from indirect contrecoup forces damaging the nerve itself or the supply vasculature for the nerve or through edematous compression (e.g., orbital emphysema).[43,153,238,239] In more rare cases, the optic nerve can be directly damaged by intraocular foreign bodies or bone fragments from orbital fractures, or a partial or complete avulsion of the optic nerve may occur from shearing or compression forces.[151,152,164,240,241] Athletes are at particular risk for finger injuries in the orbit, which have been reported to cause optic nerve avulsion.[242–244] As previously discussed, prolonged elevation of intraocular pressure can also produce damage to the optic nerve. Imaging is essential in trauma affecting the optic nerve to determine the nature of the damage.

Many treatment options have been promoted for traumatic optic neuropathy. High-dose corticosteroids and surgical decompression are the most common approaches, either separately or in combination.[151,152,157,245] Although vision recovery has been reported to occur spontaneously,[246] treatment is recommended to improve the chances of recovery. Optic nerve avulsion has a poor prognosis for visual recovery, although some suggest high-dose intravenous corticosteroid treatment.[152]

Choroid

Ruptures to the choroidal vasculature, Bruch membrane, or the overlying retinal pigment epithelium can result from blunt trauma. Choroidal ruptures most often occur as a contrecoup injury from compression in the posterior pole, and ruptures of the choriocapillaris often produce significant subretinal hemorrhages in the optic disc and macular areas (Fig. 7.11). Advances in retinal imaging technologies can significantly improve diagnostic accuracy. The hemorrhage may take weeks to resolve and a yellow-white scar may result (Fig. 7.12). The visual prognosis can be relatively good unless hemorrhaging has occurred under the fovea. If Bruch membrane has been ruptured, choroidal vessels can develop under the retina.[247−249] Photocoagulation therapy may be useful for the prevention of retinal detachments and subretinal neovascular membrane formation that can even occur many years after the choroidal rupture.[43,194]

Direct trauma to the choroid commonly produces damage more anteriorly and can affect the uveal structures as well. The location of anterior choroidal ruptures makes it difficult to visualize the damage; therefore the practitioner must be purposeful in the assessment of the posterior segment. If a large area of the choroid detaches, extreme secondary glaucoma can result that is resistant to treatment.[193]

Visual fields

The forces that cause eye injuries can also result in closed-head trauma.[153] Closed-head injuries involving cerebral edema, hemorrhaging, compression, or ischemia can damage the visual pathway. Visual field, pupillary reflex, visual acuity, and color testing can be useful adjunct information for other health professionals in determining the nature and extent of the damage.

Penetrating Trauma

A penetrating intraocular injury is relatively rare in sports, particularly when protective eyewear is worn by the athlete. Common penetrating objects include fish hooks, darts, weapon-related objects (e.g., BBs), and inappropriate spectacle lenses and frames.[250] Although glass is generally well tolerated inside the eye, the sharp edges of shattered glass can cause considerable secondary progressive damage.[250] A detailed case history is crucial for determining the exact nature of the injury and potential intraocular foreign object. In cases of small, fast objects such as BBs, signs of external damage may be limited. All ocular tissues should be thoroughly assessed and Seidel testing performed to help detect any entry points. A computed tomographic

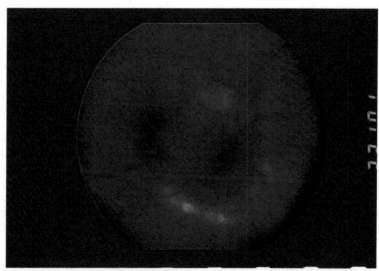

FIG. 7.11 Acute choroidal rupture with subretinal hemorrhage. (Reprinted from Kanski JJ. *Clinical Ophthalmology.* 5th ed. Boston: Butterworth Heinemann; 2003.)

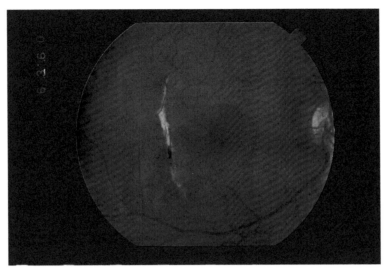

FIG. 7.12 Old choroidal rupture scar. (Reprinted from Kanski JJ. *Clinical Ophthalmology*. 5th ed. Boston: Butterworth Heinemann; 2003.)

scan is often essential for locating the presence and position of the foreign object. Penetration of the ocular tissues causes many complications; the cornea may remain scarred, the iris may remain partially impaired, the crystalline lens may need to be removed, the vitreous may need to be removed, and the retina may have long-term problems.[29,152]

Many metallic and organic foreign bodies have a high risk for causing intraocular infection and inflammation; prophylactic treatment with broad-spectrum antibiotics therefore is recommended for all foreign bodies.[151] The management of intraocular foreign bodies is determined by "the composition of the foreign body, the mechanical effect of the retained foreign body, and the presence of infection."[151] Foreign materials that are not well tolerated in the eye or have potential for causing secondary damage should be removed when possible. Infection, especially from organic foreign materials, is not successfully treated by antibiotics alone; removal of the object is often necessary. The surgeon must consider the location, composition, and infection issues when determining whether to remove the foreign object and how to accomplish the removal with minimal surgical damage to the ocular tissues.

Perforating injuries from blunt trauma often have a worse prognosis than nonperforating contusions or penetrating foreign objects. The extent of damage to ocular tissues and structures typically is significant when blunt trauma force has caused an open-globe injury. Additionally, the scarring from perforating injuries can cause even more extensive damage than the initial injury.[152] Management with vitrectomy and other medical and surgical options should be initiated as soon as possible.

Sideline management: Blunt trauma to the eye by a small object such as a racquetball can create pressure intense enough to rupture the globe. In this type of injury, the athlete complains of double vision (diplopia), decreased visual acuity, and intense pain.[211] Signs of a ruptured globe include leakage around the orbit and irregular pupils.[211] Immediately refer the athlete to the emergency department.

Chemical Injuries

Chemical burns (Fig. 7.13) are fairly rare in sports. Swimmers may present with chemosis and irritation from swimming pools that have been chemically treated improperly. Occasionally an athlete may get chalk in his or her eyes from field markings in sports such as football and baseball. These chemical injuries are almost always mild and meticulous irrigation with sterile saline or water may be the only treatment necessary. If the chemical agent is a solid, scrupulous examination of the fornices is recommended to remove any retained substance. If the corneal epithelium has been compromised, prophylactic treatment with a broad-spectrum antibiotic is advocated.[251] If iridocyclitis develops, usually from corneal epithelial damage, treatment with a cycloplegic agent is necessary to prevent posterior synechiae.[251]

Sideline management: In the event of a chemical burn do not attempt to neutralize acids or alkalis. In

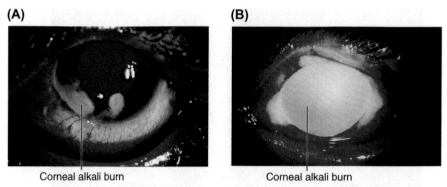

(A)

(B)

Corneal alkali burn

Corneal alkali burn

FIG. 7.13 Alkali burn demonstrating corneal burns and conjunctival injection on the day of the accident (A) and complete destruction 7 days after the burn (B). (Reprinted from Kaiser PK, Friedman, NJ. *The Massachusetts Eye and Ear Infirmary Illustrated Manual of Ophthalmology.* 2nd ed. Philadelphia: W.B. Saunders; 2004.)

addition, do not use an eyecup or bandage the eye. An alkali burn caused by contact with chalk line markings requires irrigation with sterile saline or water for at least 20 min, with the athlete then referred for medical attention.

FOLLOW-UP COMANAGEMENT

The athlete returning to sport after a sport-related ocular injury requires continued assessment and management by the entire sports medicine team to ensure an optimal outcome. After the eye care specialist has managed the athlete's injury, the athlete and the athletic trainer should receive detailed instructions regarding further treatment, indications for returning to the eye care specialist, and eyewear recommendations.

Communication between the eye care specialist and the on-site sports medicine provider (usually the certified athletic trainer) is paramount. This communication is most effective if it is delivered both in writing and verbally. Written communication should contain sufficient detail to enhance the potential for excellent compliance. Verbal communication allows the athlete and other professionals to ask specific questions regarding what needs to be done, where it needs to be done, when it should occur, who should carry out the recommendations, and why it needs to be done. Also, educating the family and the coaching staff will increase the athlete's compliance with the physician's orders.

The athletic trainer serves a valuable role in that he or she can assess the injury daily and refer the athlete to the physician if necessary. If the eye care specialist is unfamiliar with the athlete's sport, the athletic trainer can provide invaluable information about practice and game situations. The athletic trainer can also improve

compliance by ensuring that the athlete returns for recommended follow-up care.

MANAGEMENT OF SPORT-RELATED CONCUSSION

Sport-related concussion (SRC), often considered a subtype of traumatic brain injury (TBI), has been broadly defined as "a traumatic brain injury induced by biomechanical forces."[252] There are some common features in SRC, including an alteration in mental status and neurologic function that may or may not involve loss of consciousness. The neuropathologic disturbances in most SRCs reflect functional disturbances rather than structural injuries that are detectable with neuroimaging studies, requiring diagnosis and recovery decisions to be based on a clinical assessment of signs and symptoms. The clinical signs and symptoms of SRC cannot be attributed to drug, alcohol, or medication use; other injuries; or other comorbidities. The signs and symptoms of SRC often resolve spontaneously in a sequential manner over the course of 10—14 days,[253] although children and athletes with more severe presentations or other complicating factors may take longer to fully recover.[254,255] One of the significant challenges of SRC is determining a diagnosis with limited observation time and evaluation ability at the sporting venue, especially considering the intense pressure sports medicine practitioners face with regard to return to play decisions.

Pathophysiology of Sport-Related Concussion

SRC is often caused by a blunt head trauma that can involve acceleration or deceleration forces creating the initial tissue damage and resulting ischemia.

Mechanical damage can be localized to the areas of the brain that contacted the intracranial surface of the skull, often resulting in coup-contrecoup injuries to regions on opposite sides of the brain.[256] There can also be rotational or translational movement of the brain that can stretch or tear axons, causing diffuse axonal injury.[257–260] It is thought that diffuse axonal injury may induce neuronal degeneration or atrophy, which may lead to prolonged neuronal dysfunction.[261–263] The tissue damage in SRC can diminish brain metabolism and affect cerebral blood flow regulation, which is the initial phase in the pathophysiology of TBI.

The secondary phase of brain injury involves the development of cytotoxic (intracellular) and/or vasogenic (interstitial) edema, which can ultimately cause elevated intracranial pressure and further damage.[264] Edema in the brain is commonly worse 24–48 h following the injury,[265] with sustained inflammatory responses that affect metabolic regulation and disruption of cerebral vascular function.[266–271] There are myriad alterations in cerebral function and neuronal morphology produced by the neurochemical cascade of metabolic and pathophysiologic responses to brain trauma[264,271]; however, the details of these responses is beyond the scope of this chapter. The challenge with most mild TBIs is that traditional computed tomographic scans do not detect these alterations. Recent advances in neuroimaging (diffusion tensor imaging, positron emission tomography, functional magnetic resonance imaging, magnetic resonance spectroscopy, etc.) and the use of fluid biomarkers and genetic testing show potential for improving the clinical assessment and management of SRC, but further research is needed.[264,272]

Second impact syndrome, also referred to as repetitive head injury syndrome, is a condition where a second concussion occurs before symptoms from a prior concussion have resolved. It has been more commonly reported in children and young adult athletes, many occurring in American football.[273] A hallmark of this syndrome, first described by Saunders and Harbaugh in 1984, is diffuse cerebral edema that can have potentially lethal effects.[274] While there are differences in how this condition is defined and the associated mortality rate,[275] the potentially devastating consequences have profound effects on decisions regarding return to sport.

Chronic traumatic encephalopathy (CTE) is a progressive neurodegenerative disease that has been associated with a history of repetitive head impacts.[276] CTE is a serious concern for athletes in contact sports that involve repetitive head impacts, such as American football, boxing, and ice hockey.[277] Early descriptions of CTE focused on boxers,[278] and more recent

publications focused on professional athletes from American football, hockey, and wrestling.[279–283] Postmortem examinations of 111 former National Football League players found evidence of CTE in 110.[284] The diagnosis of CTE is based on the observation of hyperphosphorylated tau protein (seen as neurofibrillary tangles) during postmortem examination of cerebral cortex tissue.[285,286] A fluid biomarker, the chemokine protein CC11, has been found to be an important part of the neuroinflammatory and neurodegenerative disease processes.[287–289] This fluid biomarker level was found to be significantly elevated in former American football players with CTE compared with that in the brains of controls and individuals with Alzheimer disease and also correlated with the number of years playing football.[290] Advances in neuroimaging, such as positron emission tomography, combined with innovations in fluid biomarker utilization show promise for detecting the development of CTE at earlier stages.

Incidence of Sport-Related Concussion

The true incidence of SRC is difficult to determine due to several factors, including challenges of detection and diagnosis, lack of treatment sought, injuries sustained outside formal practice and competition, and reluctance to report symptoms. It has been estimated that about 300,000 SRCs occur annually in the United States,[291,292] with one study estimating 1.6 to 3.8 million SRCs when including those who did not seek medical care.[293] SRC has been found to account for approximately 20% of all TBIs.[294]

Two studies of concussion incidence in high-school sports found similar results, with American football accounting for the highest number and incidence rate and girls' soccer having the second highest incidence rate of all sports.[295,296] A historical review of the history of concussion in American football reveals the risks inherent in the game.[297] In a study of professional American football, most of the impacts that cause SRC are to the side of the helmet from another player or are caused from ground contact to the back of the helmet.[298] Similarly, in high-school sports, the most common mechanism for SRC was found to be player-to-player contact, followed by contact with the playing surface.[296] Although both studies found the majority of concussions occurred in boys' sports, they also found higher concussion rates in girls when comparing similar sports where both genders participate (e.g., soccer, basketball, baseball/softball). These results suggest that concussion risk may be higher in girls' sports and that SRC risk exists in sports not typically associated with a high risk of concussion. There is also an increased risk of prolonged symptoms in athletes with a history of mental health conditions, especially depression.[254,255]

Assessment of Sport-Related Concussion

The assessment and diagnosis of SRC can be complex and challenging because there are a variety of signs and effects. This challenge is often compounded by the need for quick assessment during a sporting event, and all the pressure surrounding decisions about the ability of the athlete to continue to compete. More thorough assessment should be conducted, when feasible, utilizing healthcare providers with extensive experience diagnosing, assessing, and managing SRC; a multidisciplinary team of professionals may be prudent in cases with prolonged or severe symptoms. SRC assessments should include a systematic review of symptoms, behavioral changes, physical signs, cognitive impairments, sleep disturbances, and vision/balance disorders.[252] There is potential to use helmet-based or body (mouthguard or behind the ear) sensors to assist in the diagnosis of SRC; however, at this time the technology may not have the sensitivity to measure the acceleration impact effects on the brain.[299]

Rapid assessment for potential SRC during a sporting event is an essential part of injury evaluation, and the Sport Concussion Assessment Tool (SCAT5 and Child SCAT5) is a well-developed and evidence-based instrument designed for use by physicians and licensed healthcare professionals for this purpose.[300–303] Similarly, the Concussion Recognition Tool (CRT5) was designed for use by nonmedically trained individuals.[252,304] A sideline evaluation comprises recognition of injury, followed by assessment of symptoms, cognitive and cranial nerve function, and balance. Computerized neurocognitive testing is also an option for evaluating cognitive function and symptoms of SRC; available programs include ImPACT (www.impacttest.com), HeadMinder (www.mybraintest.org), and Cognigram (www.cogstate.com/). More comprehensive assessments provide additional testing of reaction time, gait and balance, and oculomotor function. The modified BESS (Balance Error Scoring System) test is a balance assessment protocol specifically designed for SRC and is part of the SCAT5.[305] A baseline or pre-season neurocognitive assessment can be useful for interpreting postinjury performance but is not required to make decisions about return to play.[252] One challenge with baseline testing is that the athlete may provide invalid measures due to lack of motivation, attention, or ability to understand test instructions or to simply sabotage the test to ensure an artificially low baseline score. Some evaluation instruments, such as ImPACT, provide instructions for determining the validity of a baseline assessment. A review of sideline screening tools found high sensitivity and specificity for evaluations that included symptom assessment, multimodal assessment, and the use of the King-Devick test but had lower sensitivity for use of balance and cognitive tests.[306] Studies of sideline assessments were judged to be at high risk of bias, with the overall strength of evidence being very low.[306] These neurocognitive screening instruments are important for making rapid decisions at the time of injury but do not replace a comprehensive neurologic assessment.

The 22-question symptom evaluation on the SCAT5 is particularly useful for tracking changes in symptoms over time. For children and adolescents, the Post-Concussion Symptom Inventory provides a developmentally sensitive symptom questionnaire.[307] Common symptoms from SRC include loss of consciousness, amnesia, headache, confusion, disorientation, dizziness, fatigue, "fogginess," visual disturbance, sleep disturbance, and nausea.[308] A greater number and severity of symptoms, especially of prolonged headache or concentration problems, has been associated with a longer recovery period before returning to sport.[308] A history of multiple prior concussions is associated with athletes reporting a greater number and severity of symptoms, an increased risk of future concussions, and a longer time required for recovery.[309–315] The increased symptoms, risk, and delayed neurocognitive recovery may indicate that there is residual neuronal vulnerability to injury following concussive episodes. The cascade of metabolic and pathophysiologic responses in the brain likely contribute to this increased vulnerability.

An Overview of Sport-Related Concussion Management

There are many published guidelines to assist with the difficult process of providing proper assessment and decisions regarding return to play, including those by the international Concussion In Sport Group,[252] the American Academy of Neurology (www.aan.com), the National Athletic Trainers' Association,[316] the American Medical Society for Sports Medicine,[317] the Team Physician Consensus Statements,[318–320] and the neuropsychologists' Inter-Organizational Statement.[321] A review of some of these guidelines found significant similarity in the recommendations,[322] which is summarized here. When there is suspicion that an athlete may have sustained an SRC, the athlete should be immediately removed from sport participation to receive immediate assessment. Issues of first aid and assessment for cervical spinal injury should be conducted initially by a physician or other healthcare professional with appropriate training and expertise, followed by evaluation for SRC that should be conducted using a sideline assessment instrument. The medical decision of whether the athlete has sustained an SRC is based on the clinical judgment of the healthcare professional with support from assessment results. If the athlete is suspected of having an SRC, it is important that the athlete not be allowed to return to play or to be left alone for the first few hours after the injury. The athlete with an SRC should receive a comprehensive medical and neurologic evaluation within a reasonable timeframe following the injury (preferably within the first 24—48 h). Neuroimaging may be necessary to determine if there is more severe brain injury. Serial daily assessments may be needed to determine improvements or deterioration following the initial injury presentation.

Following the diagnosis of SRC, the gradual return-to-sport process begins when concussion symptoms have resolved. Following an SRC, a 24- to 48-h period of cognitive and physical rest is typically appropriate.[323] As stated previously, most symptoms of SRC resolve within 10—14 days, although recovery may take up to 4 weeks in younger athletes.[253,254] The amount of rest needed for optimal recovery has yet to be delineated.[323] It is important that all clinical signs and neurocognitive function has returned to preinjury levels before

initiating a process for returning to the sport. Once symptoms have resolved following a rest period, the athlete should be encouraged to gradually increase exertion activities. The Concussion In Sport Group has developed guidelines for gradually returning to activity (see Table 7.5).[252] It is important to note that the exertion progression should stay below the level that aggravates a return of symptoms or decline in neurocognitive performance; if so, the activity should be discontinued and a period of 24 h of rest is suggested before restarting.[324] It is common for athletes to only need 24 h between the exertion levels described in Table 7.5 but each athlete should proceed at an individualized pace.

For those with persistent SRC symptoms, appropriate activities and exercise are also recommended and have been shown to be safe and effective for supporting recovery.[325—327] It is important to note that physiologic anomalies may persist despite resolution of symptoms and neurocognitive performance so a gradual return to exercise and sport participation has merit.[328] While there is no predictable timeframe for SRC recovery, it appears that athletes with more severe symptoms have a more prolonged recovery period.[329] There is evidence supporting the use of multifaceted physiotherapy treatments and vestibular rehabilitation for the treatment of persistent symptoms resulting from TBIs.[330—334]

TABLE 7.5
Consensus Statement: Graduated Return-To-Sport Strategy.[252]

Stage	Aim	Activity	Goal of Each Step
1	Symptom-limited activity	Daily activities that do not provoke symptoms.	Gradual reintroduction of work/school activities
2	Light aerobic exercise	Walking or stationary cycling at slow to medium pace. No resistance training.	Increase heart rate
3	Sport-specific exercise	Running or skating drills. No head impact activities.	Add movement
4	Noncontact training drills	Harder training drills, e.g., passing drills. May start progressive resistance training.	Exercise, coordination, and increased thinking
5	Full-contact practice	Following medical clearance participate in normal training activities.	Restore confidence and assess functional skills by coaching staff
6	Return to sport	Normal game play	—

Note: An initial period of 24—48 h of both relative physical rest and cognitive rest is recommended before beginning the return-to-sport (RTS) progression. There should be at least 24 h (or longer) for each step of the progression. If any symptoms worsen during exercise, the athlete should go back to the previous step. Resistance training should be added only in the later stages (stage 3 or 4 at the earliest). If symptoms are persistent (e.g., more than 10—14 days in adults or more than 1 month in children), the athlete should be referred to a healthcare professional who is an expert in the management of concussion.

It is common for children and adolescents to have SRC, but separate guidelines for the management of SRC in children are limited. A review recommended that age modifications to the recovery timeframe be applied (the expected duration of symptoms is less than 4 weeks), the use of computerized neuropsychologic testing is discouraged, and a gradual approach to exercise and sport be employed.[335] In addition, schools should also have a concussion policy to guide the accommodations and support provided during the recovery phase. The Concussion In Sport Group has also developed guidelines for gradually returning to school (see Table 7.6).[252]

Management of Visual Sequelae With Sport-Related Concussion

It is common for those who have experienced a mild TBI to report a variety of vision-related symptoms.[336–340] Studies of hierarchic organization of the cerebral cortex estimate that approximately 40% of cortical pathways and connections are involved with vision, so it is not unexpected that visual symptoms are common in SRC.[341] The Brain Injury Vision Symptom Survey (BIVSS) is a 28-item scaled, self-administered questionnaire that was developed to provide a validated, reliable, comprehensive symptom assessment covering eight categories: eyesight clarity, visual comfort, doubling, light sensitivity, dry eyes, depth perception, peripheral vision, and reading (see Fig. 7.14).[342] The BIVSS has shown good test-retest reliability[343] and has validity for identifying TBI.[342] Use of the BIVSS or similar instrument may be helpful for identifying SRC-related vision problems, as well as for monitoring recovery and success of interventions.

The most common oculomotor conditions reported in TBI include convergence insufficiency, accommodative dysfunction, and saccadic dysfunction.[336–338,340,344,345] The prevalence reported for these oculomotor conditions is significantly higher in those with a history of TBI than that in the general population. While these conditions account for some of the visual symptoms, some of the common symptoms reported have perceptual characteristics. These symptoms include photosensitivity, sensitivity to peripheral motion, abnormal egocentric localization, balance problems, and deficits in visual information processing. Optometric or ophthalmologic examination of athletes who have vision symptoms related to an SRC should include careful evaluation of refractive status, oculomotor function (including vergence, accommodation, sensory fusion, and eye movements), and ocular health.[346,347] Quantitative pupillometry has shown measurable changes in the reactivity of the pupil following asymptomatic high-acceleration head impacts in American football.[348] In addition, perceptual symptoms should be assessed and managed to assist in daily function and recovery.

The frequency of visual symptoms in SRC stimulated the development of sideline assessment options that target elements of oculomotor performance. The King-

---

TABLE 7.6
Consensus Statement: Graduated Return-to-School Strategy.[252]

Stage	Aim	Activity	Goal of Each Step
1	Daily activities at home that do not give the child symptoms	Typical activities of the child during the day as long as they do not increase symptoms (e.g., reading, texting, screen time). Start with 5—15 min at a time and gradually build up.	Gradual return to typical activities
2	School activities	Homework, reading, or other cognitive activities outside the classroom.	Increase tolerance to cognitive work
3	Return to school part-time	Gradual introduction of schoolwork. May need to start with a partial school day or with increased breaks during the day.	Increase academic activities
4	Return to school full time	Gradually progress school activities until a full day can be tolerated.	Return to full academic activities and catch up on missed work

BIVSS CHECKLIST (Brain Injury Vision Symptom Survey)

Patient Name: _____ Today's date: _____

My brain injury was: _____ years ago   My age is: _____ years   today's date: _____
☐ I have had a medical diagnosis of brain injury (check box if true) Cause of injury: _____
☐ I sustained a brain injury without medical diagnosis (check box if true)   _____
☐ I have NOT ever sustained a brain injury (check box if true)

Please check the most appropriate box, or circle the item number that best matches your observations. All information will be held in confidence. Thank you for your help!

SYMPTOM CHECKLIST   *Circle a number below:*

Please rate each behavior. How often does each behavior occur? (circle a number)	Never	Seldom	Occasionally	Frequently	Always
EYESIGHT CLARITY					
Distance vision blurred and not clear -- even with lenses	0	1	2	3	4
Near vision blurred and not clear -- even with lenses	0	1	2	3	4
Clarity of vision changes or fluctuates during the day	0	1	2	3	4
Poor night vision / can't see well to drive at night	0	1	2	3	4
VISUAL COMFORT					
Eye discomfort / sore eyes / eyestrain	0	1	2	3	4
Headaches or dizziness after using eyes	0	1	2	3	4
Eye fatigue / very tired after using eyes all day	0	1	2	3	4
Feel "pulling" around the eyes	0	1	2	3	4
DOUBLING					
Double vision -- especially when tired	0	1	2	3	4
Have to close or cover one eye to see clearly	0	1	2	3	4
Print moves in and out of focus when reading	0	1	2	3	4
LIGHT SENSITIVITY					
Normal indoor lighting is uncomfortable – too much glare	0	1	2	3	4
Outdoor light too bright – have to use sunglasses	0	1	2	3	4
Indoors fluorescent lighting is bothersome or annoying	0	1	2	3	4
DRY EYES					
Eyes feel "dry" and sting	0	1	2	3	4
"Stare" into space without blinking	0	1	2	3	4
Have to rub the eyes a lot	0	1	2	3	4
DEPTH PERCEPTION					
Clumsiness / misjudge where objects really are	0	1	2	3	4
Lack of confidence walking / missing steps / stumbling	0	1	2	3	4
Poor handwriting (spacing, size, legibility)	0	1	2	3	4
PERIPHERAL VISION					
Side vision distorted / objects move or change position	0	1	2	3	4
What looks straight ahead--isn't always straight ahead	0	1	2	3	4
Avoid crowds / can't tolerate "visually-busy" places	0	1	2	3	4
READING					
Short attention span / easily distracted when reading	0	1	2	3	4
Difficulty / slowness with reading and writing	0	1	2	3	4
Poor reading comprehension / can't remember what was read	0	1	2	3	4
Confusion of words / skip words during reading	0	1	2	3	4
Lose place / have to use finger not to lose place when reading	0	1	2	3	4

BIVSS_28.item.clinical.use._[09/14_Hannu Laukkanen]   Predictive score = ≥ 31   **total score for all 28-items:** _____

FIG. 7.14 The Brain Injury Vision Symptom Survey (BIVSS).

Devick Test, an assessment task of rapid number naming with saccadic eye movement demands that simulate reading, has been studied and utilized as a rapid sideline assessment instrument for concussion.[349–356] The test generally shows good test-retest reliability, as well as good sensitivity and specificity for identifying concussion when the athlete demonstrates significant slowing in performance when compared to baseline measures.[357] There is some concern that athletes may purposely perform slowly during baseline assessment in order to avoid removal from play for SRC concerns and also there is the potential for a high false-positive rate at baseline.[358] The King-Devick test is also limited to oculomotor elements involving saccadic eye movements, and the inclusion of other oculomotor performance measures may improve the identification of SRC. The use of automated eye tracking instrumentation offers an objective method for potentially detecting oculomotor abnormalities following SRC and may be less prone to the challenges of assessments that rely on subjective responses.[359]

The vestibular/ocular motor screening (VOMS) assessment was designed to provide a more comprehensive evaluation of vestibular and oculomotor injuries and symptoms.[360] VOMS is composed of short assessments of smooth pursuit eye movements, horizontal and vertical saccadic eye movements, convergence, horizontal and vertical vestibular ocular reflex, and visual motion sensitivity. The SCAT5 and predecessors assess balance symptoms in SRC by using a modified BESS test, which addresses disruption of vestibulospinal function. The VOMS evaluates vestibuloocular function through a subjective rating of increases in symptoms of dizziness, nausea, and fogginess when performing each element of the assessment. The VOMS has shown good reliability and sensitivity in preliminary studies.[358,360–364] The portion of the VOMS that assesses convergence (near point of convergence repeated three times) appears to be particularly sensitive to detect concussion. Studies of football players have shown that even repetitive head impacts that do not cause concussion, or produce symptoms related to concussion, are associated with a linear receding of near point of convergence measurements.[365,366] In addition, symptom provocation when performing VOMS assessments may be associated with longer recovery times in SRC.[367,368]

A thorough review of the many treatment options for visual sequelae is beyond the scope of this book; however, the following is a brief overview of treatment considerations for athletes who have visual symptoms related to an SRC.

Refractive Care: An SRC may produce more sensitivity to small refractive errors or even cause refractive changes that may be transient. It is also likely that athletes with hyperopia may need more refractive compensation due to accommodative dysfunction. Added plus lenses at near may be indicated due to the increased likelihood of accommodative dysfunction following SRC. In some cases, it may be necessary to prescribe unequal near addition lenses due to unequal effects on accommodation. These modifications in refractive prescribing may be temporary during the recovery period.

Prism Options: An athlete may be more sensitive to small phorias following SRC, especially vertical phorias. Small prismatic correction may improve visual symptoms during the recovery period. In more severe head injury, there may be changes in cranial nerve function that affect EOM function, potentially causing strabismus with diplopia. Diplopia symptoms may be especially troubling for the athlete; therefore prism or occlusion to eliminate the diplopia may be necessary. There is some concern that prism may interfere with the recovery process, so occlusion or a monovision correction may be preferred to minimize the diplopia symptoms. A program of vision therapy designed to improve oculomotor function has been shown to be beneficial for assisting in the recovery from concussion and may be effective for reducing the need for prismatic correction.[345,369]

Yoked prism (i.e., prism with the bases in the same direction, such as bases right) may be useful for reducing some visual symptoms associated with concussion. In severe trauma, yoked prisms can be helpful for visual field defects, visual neglect/unilateral spatial inattention, or acquired nystagmus.[370,371] Yoked prism may also be beneficial for symptoms associated with abnormal egocentric localization, which is an alteration in the self-perception of the "straight-ahead" direction.[371] Yoked prism can modify the perceptual mismatch of spatial direction and reduce directional mobility and object localization symptoms.

Filter Options: Filter prescribing can be beneficial due to the high prevalence of photosensitivity symptoms following SRC. Photosensitivity may be caused by pupillary changes following concussion.[372–374] Filters of various colors and densities have been recommended to reduce photosensitivity symptoms, including use of red (rose), yellow (amber), blue, gray (neutral), and photochromic filters. Clinical experience suggests that, while there are some useful patterns in filter selection, it is often an individual preference that is best conducted using a trial-and-error approach. It is useful to start with tint color selection first and then proceed with determination of the optimal light transmission density. A retrospective study found that prescribing a lighter tint density (higher light transmission) may support adaptation to photosensitivity symptoms over a longer duration.[372] Filters may also help with symptoms of visual motion sensitivity, which are hypersensitivities to motion in the peripheral retina. Common symptoms of visual motion sensitivity following concussion include an inability to tolerate visually busy places, avoiding crowds, and nausea and instability when walking due to the flow of peripheral vision.

Binasal Occlusion: The use of binasal occlusion (see Fig. 7.15) has been shown to improve symptoms of visual motion sensitivity.[375,376] Specifically, binasal occlusion appears to produce an increase in visual evoked potential (VEP) amplitude in mild TBI, whereas it produces a decrease in amplitude in those who are visually normal. These changes in VEP responsivity correspond to improvements in symptoms.

Neurovisual Rehabilitation: This area of vision therapy includes all the treatment options described previously in addition to modifications in traditional oculomotor and visual information processing therapy. There have been several studies of efficacy of oculomotor therapy for the treatment of binocular vision conditions following TBI, and many aspects of oculomotor function show improvements using objective assessment measures.[369,377–383] The number of therapy sessions needed for effective treatment may be more than that typically required in those without SRC, and care should be taken to prevent exacerbation of symptoms when conducting the therapy, but this treatment option may provide meaningful improvements in visual function and relief of visual symptoms. Some have concluded that sports vision training in the preseason may reduce the incidence of SRC in American football[384]; however, others have not found a correlation between better visual abilities and head impact severity.[385]

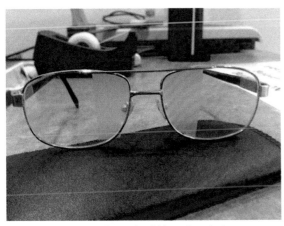

FIG. 7.15 Example of binasal occlusion.

Neurovisual rehabilitation may also be designed to address acquired deficits in visual information processing and perception. There are many potential areas that may be altered following SRC, and therapeutic approaches used for the treatment of developmental delays may also be beneficial for in this population.[386]

The eye care practitioner is a valuable resource for managing eye injuries and the visual effects of SRC in athletes. As a vital member of the sports medicine team, the eye care practitioner is uniquely positioned to diagnose and treat ocular injuries and assist in returning the athlete to sports participation. The eye care practitioner can also provide valuable training to the Athletic Training staff on sideline triage and management of sports eye injuries. Creating an eye injury triage kit with a triage card as shown in Table 7.3 is an excellent resource for the Athletic Training staff. The eye care practitioner is also a valuable team member in the diagnosis and management of SRC. Visual sequelae of SRC are common, and expertise in treating this element of SRC recovery is an important component of the multidisciplinary management of SRC.

REFERENCES

1. Vinger PF. The incidence of eye injuries in sports. In: Vinger PF, ed. *Ocular Sports Injuries*. Boston: Little, Brown; 1981:21−46.
2. Vinger PF. Sports eye injuries: a preventable disease. *Am Acad Ophthalmol*. 1981;88:108.
3. Diamond GR, Quinn GE, Pashby TJ, et al. Ophthalmologic injuries. *Clin Sports Med*. 1982;1:469.
4. Diamond GR, Quinn GE, Pashby TJ, et al. Ophthalmologic injuries. *Prim Care*. 1984;11:161.
5. Gregory PT. Sussex eye hospital sports injuries. *Br J Ophthalmol*. 1986;70:748.
6. Grove D. Study: eye injuries in varsity sports. *Physician Sportsmed*. 1987;15:64.
7. Jones NP. Eye injuries in sport: an increasing problem. *Br J Sports Med*. 1987;21:168.
8. MacEwen CJ. Sport associated eye injury: a casualty department survey. *Br J Ophthalmol*. 1987;71:701.
9. Jones NP. One year of severe eye injuries in sport. *Eye*. 1988;2:484.
10. LaRoche GR, McIntyre L, Shertzer RM. Epidemiology of severe eye injuries in childhood. *Ophthalmology*. 1988; 95:1603.
11. Jones NP. Eye injury in sport. *Sports Med*. 1989;7:163.
12. Larrison WI, Hersh PS, Kunzweiler T, et al. Sports-related ocular trauma. *Ophthalmology*. 1990;97:1265.
13. Pashby TJ. Eye injuries in Canadian sports and recreational activities. *Can J Ophthalmol*. 1992;27:226.
14. Zagelbaum BM, Tostanoski JR, Kerner DJ, et al. Urban eye trauma: a one-year prospective study. *Ophthalmology*. 1993;100:851.

15. Orlando RG. Soccer-related eye injuries in children and adolescents. *Phys Sportsmed.* 1988;16:103.

16. Capoferri C, Martorina M, Menga M, et al. Eye injuries from traditional sports in Aosta Valley. *Ophthalmologica.* 1994;208:15.

17. Fong LP. Sports-related eye injuries. *Med J Aust.* 1994; 160:743.

18. Fong LP. Eye injuries in Victoria, Australia. *Med J Aust.* 1995;162:64.

19. Pardhan S, Shacklock P, Weatherill J. Sport-related ocular trauma: a survey of the presentation of eye injuries to a casualty clinic and the use of protective eye-wear. *Eye.* 1995;9(pt. 6 suppl):50.

20. Ghosh F, Bauer B. Sports-related eye injuries. *Acta Ophthalmol Scand.* 1995;73:353.

21. Zagelbaum BM, Starkey C, Hersh PS, et al. The National Basketball Association eye injury study. *Arch Ophthalmol.* 1995;113:749.

22. Napier SM, Baker RS, Sanford DG, et al. Eye injuries in athletics and recreation. *Surv Ophthalmol.* 1996;41:229.

23. Orlando RG, Doty JH. Ocular sports trauma: a private practice study. *J Am Optom Assoc.* 1996;67:77.

24. Strahlman E, Elman M, Daub E, et al. Causes of pediatric eye injuries: a population-based study. *Arch Ophthalmol.* 1990;108:603.

25. Capao Filipe JA, Barros H, Castro-Correia J. Sports-related ocular injuries: a three-year follow-up study. *Ophthalmology.* 1997;104:313.

26. Barr A, Baines PS, Desai P, et al. Ocular sports injuries: the current picture. *Br J Sports Med.* 2000;34:456.

27. Vinger PF. A practical guide for sports eye protection. *Physician Sportsmed.* 2000;28:49.

28. Vinger PF. Understanding eye trauma through computer modeling. *Arch Ophthalmol.* 2005;123:833.

29. Jones NP. Eye injuries in sport. In: Loran DFC, MacEwen CJ, eds. *Sports Vision.* Oxford: Butterworth-Heinemann; 1995.

30. Vinger PF. The eye and sports medicine. In: Tasman W, Jaeger EA, eds. *Duane's Clinical Ophthalmology.* Philadelphia: J.B. Lippincott; 1985.

31. Pizzarello LD, Haik BG, eds. *Sports Ophthalmology.* Springfield, IL: Charles C. Thomas; 1999.

32. Pane A, Simcock P. *Practical Ophthalmology: A Survival Guide for Doctors and Optometrists.* Edinburgh: Elsevier Churchill Livingston; 2005:106–127.

33. Kim T, Nunes AP, Mello MJ, et al. Incidence of sports-related eye injuries in the United States: 2001–2009. *Graefes Arch Clin Exp Ophthalmol.* 2011;249:1743–1744.

34. Haring RS, Sheffield ID, Canner JK, et al. Epidemiology of sports-related eye injuries in the United States. *JAMA Ophthalmol.* 2016;134:1382–1390.

35. *Prevent Blindness America: Sports Eye Injuries by Type/Age (Detailed).* https://preventblindness.org/wp-content/uploads/2020/06/FS09_SportsInjuriesbyAge-detailed2020.pdf. Accessed 1 July 2020.

36. Landry GL, Bernhardt DT. *Essentials of Primary Care Sports Medicine.* Champaign, IL: Human Kinetics; 2003.

37. American Academy of Pediatrics Committee on Sports Medicine and Fitness. Protective eyewear for young athletes. Policy statement. *Pediatrics.* 2004;113:619.

38. American Academy of Pediatrics Committee on Sports Medicine and Fitness, American Academy of Ophthalmology, Eye Health and Public Information Task Force. Protective eyewear for young athletes. *Ophthalmology.* 2004;111:600.

39. Jeffers JB. An on-going tragedy: pediatric sports-related eye injuries. *Semin Ophthalmol.* 1990;5:21.

40. Guskiewicz KM, Bruce SL, Cantu RC, et al. National athletic trainers' position statement: management of sport related concussion. *J Athl Train.* 2004;39:280.

41. Fingeret M. The initial evaluation of ocular trauma in sports. *J Am Optom Assoc.* 1980;51:687.

42. Kuhn F, Morris R, Witherspoon CD, Mester V. The Birmingham Eye Trauma Terminology system (BETT). *J Fr Ophthalmol.* 2004;27:206–210.

43. Benson WE, Shakin J, Sarin LK. Blunt trauma. In: Tasman W, Jaeger EA, eds. *Duane's Clinical Ophthalmology.* Philadelphia: J.B. Lippincott; 1983.

44. Leivo T, Haavisto AK, Sahraravand A. Sports-related eye injuries: the current picture. *Acta Ophthalmol.* 2015;93: 224–231.

45. Hoskin AK, Yardley AM, Hanman K, et al. Sports-related eye and adnexal injuries in the Western Australian paediatric population. *Acta Ophthalmol.* 2016;94: e407–e410.

46. Stilger VG, Alt JM, Robinson TW. Traumatic hyphema in an intercollegiate baseball player: a case report. *J Athl Train.* 1999;34:25.

47. Jones NP, Tullo AB. Severe eye injuries in cricket. *Br J Sports Med.* 1986;20:178.

48. Aburn N. Eye injuries in indoor cricket at Wellington hospital: a survey January 1987 to June 1989. *NZ Med J.* 1990;103:454.

49. Vinger PF, Duma SM, Crandall J. Baseball hardness as a risk factor for eye injuries. *Arch Ophthalmol.* 1999;117: 354.

50. Sowka JW, Kabat AG. A pop fly straight to the eye. *Rev Optom.* 2017:98–100.

51. Abrams JH. Sports related ocular trauma. *Athl Ther Today.* 1996;1:31.

52. Marton K, Wilson D, McKeag D. Ocular trauma in college varsity sports. *Med Sci Sports Exerc.* 1987;19:S53.

53. Meeuwisse WH, Sellmer R, Hagel BE. Rates and risks of injury during intercollegiate basketball. *Am J Sports Med.* 2003;31:379.

54. Witherspoon CD, Kuhn F, Morris R, et al. Epidemiology of general and sports eye injuries. *Ophthalmol Clin N Am.* 1999;12:333.

55. Mandelcorn MS, Crichton A. Fish-hook removal from vitreous and retina. *Arch Ophthalmol.* 1989;107:493.

56. Doggart JH. The impact of boxing on the visual apparatus. *Arch Ophthalmol.* 1955;54:161.

57. Palmer E, Lieberman TW, Burns S. Contusion angle deformity in prizefighters. *Arch Ophthalmol.* 1976;94:225.

58. Maguire JI, Benson WE. Retinal injury and detachment in boxers. *J Am Med Assoc.* 1986;255:2451.

59. Giovinazzo VJ, Yannuzzi LA, Sorenson JA, et al. The ocular complications of boxing. *Ophthalmology.* 1987; 94:587.

60. Smith DJ. Ocular injuries in boxing. *Int Ophthalmol Clin.* 1988;28:242.

61. Enzenauer RW, Mauldin WM. Boxing-related ocular injuries in the United States Army, 1980 to 1985. *South Med J.* 1989;82:547.

62. Leach A, McGalliard J, Dwyer MH, et al. Ocular injuries from boxing. *Br Med J.* 1992;304:839.

63. McLeod D. Ocular injuries from boxing: what about prophylactic laser coagulation of boxers' retinas? *Br Med J.* 1992;304:197.

64. Whiteson A. Ocular injuries from boxing. *Br Med J.* 1992; 304:574.

65. Wedrich A, Velikay M, Binder S, et al. Ocular findings in asymptomatic amateur boxers. *Retina.* 1993;13:114.

66. Vadala G, Mollo M, Roberto S, et al. Boxing and the eyes: morphological aspects of the ocular system in boxers. *Eur J Ophthalmol.* 1997;7:174.

67. Hazar M, Beyleroglu M, Subasi M, et al. Ophthalmological findings in elite amateur Turkish boxers. *Br J Sports Med.* 2002;36:428.

68. Bianco M, Vaiano AS, Colella F, et al. Ocular complications of boxing. *Br J Sports Med.* 2005;39:70.

69. Bartholomew RS, MacDonald M. Fish-hook injuries of the eye. *Br J Ophthalmol.* 1980;64:531.

70. Grand GM, Lobes LA. Technique for removing a fishhook from the posterior segment of the eye. *Arch Ophthalmol.* 1980;98:152.

71. Aiello LP, Iwamoto M, Guyer DR. Penetrating ocular fishhook injuries. *Ophthalmology.* 1992;99:862.

72. Aiello LP, Iwamoto M, Taylor HR. Perforating ocular fishhook injuries. *Arch Ophthalmol.* 1992;110:1316.

73. Yuksel N, Elibol O, Caglar Y. Penetrating corneal fishhook injury. *Ophthalmologica.* 1994;208:112.

74. Alfaro DV 3d, Jablon EP, Rodriguez FM, et al. Fishing-related ocular trauma. *Am J Ophthalmol.* 2005;139:488.

75. Tanton JH, Elliott DC. Fishing-spear injury of the orbit. *Am J Ophthalmol.* 1967;64:973.

76. Heinrichs EH, Willcockson JR. Catastrophic eye injury in a football player. *Phys Sportsmed.* 1982;10:71.

77. Sherwood DJ. Eye injuries to football players. *N Engl J Med.* 1989;320:742.

78. Millar GT. Golfing eye injuries. *Am J Ophthalmol.* 1967;64: 741.

79. Portis JM, Vassallo SA, Albert DM. Ocular sports injuries: a review of cases on file in the Massachusetts eye and ear infirmary pathology laboratory. *Int Ophthalmol Clin.* 1981;21:1.

80. Mieler WF, Nanda SK, Wolf MD, et al. Golf-related ocular injuries. *Arch Ophthalmol.* 1995;113:1410.

81. Burnstine MA, Elner VM. Golf-related ocular injuries. *Am J Ophthalmol.* 1996;121:437.

82. Pollack JS, Mieler WF, Mittra RA. Golf-related ocular injuries. *Curr Opin Ophthalmol.* 1997;8:15.

83. Jayasundera T, Vote B, Joondeph B. Golf-related ocular injuries. *Clin Exp Ophthalmol.* 2003;31:110.

84. Weitgasser U, Wackernagel W, Oetsch K. Visual outcome and ocular survival after sports ocular trauma in playing golf. *J Trauma.* 2004;56:648.

85. Park SJ, Park KH, Heo JW, Woo SJ. Visual and anatomic outcomes of golf ball-related ocular injuries. *Eye.* 2014; 28:312−317.

86. Devenyi RG, Pashby RC, Pashby J. The hockey eye safety program. *Ophthalmol Clin N Am.* 1999;12:359.

87. Stuart MJ, Smith AM, Malo-Ortiguera SA, et al. A comparison of facial protection and the incidence of head, neck, and facial injuries in junior a hockey players. *Am J Sports Med.* 2002;30:39.

88. Micieli JA, Zurakowski D, Ahmed IIK. Impact of visors on eye and orbital injuries in the National Hockey League. *Can J Ophthalmol.* 2014;49. 2014:243−248.

89. Pashby TJ, Pashby RC, Chisholm LD, et al. Eye injuries on Canadian hockey. *Can Med Assoc J.* 1975;113:663.

90. Vinger PF. Ocular injuries in hockey. *Arch Ophthalmol.* 1976;94:74.

91. Pashby TJ. Eye injuries in Canadian hockey. Phase II. *Can Med Assoc J.* 1977;117:677.

92. Pashby TJ. Eye injuries in Canadian amateur hockey. *Am J Sports Med.* 1979;7:254.

93. Pashby TJ. Eye injuries in Canadian hockey. Phase III. *Can Med Assoc J.* 1979;121:643.

94. Pashby TJ. Ocular injuries in hockey. *Int Ophthalmol Clin.* 1988;28:228.

95. . Benson B, Meeuwisse W, Ice hockey injuries. In: Maffulli N, Caine DJ, eds. *Epidemiology of Pediatric Sports Injuries: Team Sports, Med Sport Sci* 49; 2005:86.

96. Kriz PK, Comstock RD, Zurakowski D, et al. Effectiveness of protective eyewear in reducing eye injuries among high school field hockey players. *Pediatrics.* 2012;130: 1069−1075.

97. Kriz PK, Zurakowski D, Almquist JL, et al. Eye protection and risk of eye injuries in high school field hockey. *Pediatrics.* 2015;136:521−527.

98. Gardner EC. Head, face and eye injuries in collegiate women's field hockey. *Am J Sports Med.* 2015;43: 2027−2034.

99. Lapidus CS, Nelson LB, Jeffers JB, et al. Eye injuries in lacrosse: women need their vision less than men? *J Trauma.* 1992;32:555.

100. Livingston LA, Forbes SL. Eye injuries in women's lacrosse: strict rule enforcement and mandatory eyewear required. *J Trauma.* 1996;40:144.

101. Webster DA, Bayliss GV, Spadaro JA. Head and face injuries in scholastic women's lacrosse with and without eyewear. *Med Sci Sports Exerc.* 1999;31:938.

102. Waicus KM, Smith BW. Eye injuries in women's lacrosse players. *Clin J Sport Med.* 2002;12:24.

103. Mantz SO, Nibbelink G. Injuries in intercollegiate women's lacrosse. *Am J Sports Med.* 2004;32:608.

104. Lincoln AE, Caswell SV, Almquist JL, et al. Effectiveness of the women's lacrosse protective eyewear mandate in the

reduction of eye injuries. *Am J Sports Med.* 2012;40: 611–614.

105. Singh I, Khanna PK, Srivastava MC, et al. Acute mountain sickness. *N Engl J Med.* 1969;280:175.

106. Frayser R, Houston CS, Gray GW, et al. Retinal hemorrhage at high altitude. *N Engl J Med.* 1970;282:1183.

107. Kobrick JL, Appleton B. Effect of extended hypoxia on visual performance and retinal vascular state. *J Appl Physiol.* 1971;31:357.

108. Rennie D, Morrisey J. Retinal changes in Himalayan climbers. *Arch Ophthalmol.* 1975;93:395.

109. Wiedman M. High altitude retinal hemorrhage. *Arch Ophthalmol.* 1975;93:401.

110. Clarke C, Duff J. Mountain sickness, retinal haemorrhages, and acclimatisation on Mount Everest in 1975. *Br Med J.* 1976;2:495.

111. McFadden DM, Houston CM, Sutton JR, et al. High-altitude retinopathy. *J Am Med Assoc.* 1981;245:581.

112. Butler FK, Harris DJ, Reynolds RD. Altitude retinopathy on mount everest, 1989. *Ophthalmology.* 1992;99:739.

113. Shults WT, Swan KC. High altitude retinopathy in mountain climbers. *Arch Ophthalmol.* 1975;93:404.

114. Classe JG. Prescribing for noncontact sports. *Optom Clin.* 1993;3:111.

115. Easterbrook M. Ocular injuries in racquet sports. *Int Ophthalmol Clin.* 1988;28:232.

116. Ingram DV, Lewkonia I. Ocular hazards of playing squash rackets. *Br J Ophthalmol.* 1973;57:434.

117. Chandran S. Ocular hazards of playing badminton. *Br J Ophthalmol.* 1974;58:757.

118. Jones WL. Ocular manifestations of blunt racquetball injury. *Optom Mon.* 1978;69:968.

119. Easterbrook M. Eye injuries in squash: a preventable disease. *Can Med Assoc.* 1978;118:303.

120. Barrell GV, Cooper PJ, Elkington AR, et al. Squash ball to eye ball: the likelihood of squash players incurring an eye injury. *Br Med J.* 1981;283:893.

121. Genovese MT, Lenzo NP, Lim RK, et al. Eye injuries among pennant squash players and their attitudes towards protective eyewear. *Med J Aust.* 1990;153:655.

122. Loran D. Eye injuries in squash. *Optician.* 1992:18.

123. Holdeman NR. Courting disaster: racquetball injury triggers hyphema. *Rev Optom.* 1993;130:83.

124. Knorr HL, Jonas JB. Retinal detachments by squash ball accidents. *Am J Ophthalmol.* 1996;122:260.

125. Schuiteman M, Mangen R. A bloody mess. *Rev Optom.* 2018:18–20.

126. McWhae J. Badminton-related eye injuries [letter]. *Can J Ophthalmol.* 1990;25:170.

127. Becker GD. Barotrauma resulting from scuba diving: an otolaryngological perspective. *Physician Sportsmed.* 1985; 13:112.

128. Melamed Y, Shupak A, Bitterman H. Medical problems associated with underwater diving. *N Engl J Med.* 1992; 326:30.

129. Andenmatten R, Piguet B, Klainguti G. Orbital hemorrhage induced by barotrauma. *Am J Ophthalmol.* 1994; 118:536.

130. Kirby BS. In deep water: scuba diving mishap causes ocular barotrauma. *Rev Optom.* 1994;131:113.

131. Butler FK. Diving and hyperbaric ophthalmology. *Surv Ophthalmol.* 1995;39:347.

132. Carkeet A. Mask barotrauma leading to subconjunctival haemorrhage in a scuba diver. *Clin Exp Optom.* 1995;78:18.

133. Hoelting C, Egan DJ, Bennett ES. The use of contact lenses in swimming and scuba diving. *Can J Optom.* 1984;46:12.

134. Josephson JE, Caffery BE. Contact lens considerations in surface and subsurface aqueous environments. *Optom Vis Sci.* 1991;68:2.

135. Jurkus J, Colarusso MA. To see or not to see: a swimmer's dilemma. *Contact Lens Spectr.* 1996;11:44.

136. Burke MJ, Sanitato JJ, Vinger PF, et al. Soccerball-induced eye injuries. *J Am Med Assoc.* 1983;249:2682.

137. Horn EP, McDonald HR, Johnson RN, et al. Soccer ball-related retinal injuries: a report of 13 cases. *Retina.* 2000;20:604.

138. Capao-Filipe JA, Fernandes VL, Barros H, et al. Soccer-related ocular injuries. *Arch Ophthalmol.* 2003;121:687.

139. Capao-Filipe JA. Soccer (football) ocular injuries: an important eye health problem. *Br J Ophthalmol.* 2004;88:159.

140. Vinger PF, Capao-Filipe JA. The mechanism and prevention of soccer eye injuries. *Br J Ophthalmol.* 2004;88:167.

141. Renneker M. Medical aspects of surfing. *Physician Sportsmed.* 1987;15:96.

142. Easterbrook M, Pashby TJ. Eye injuries associated with war games. *Can Med Assoc J.* 1985;133:415.

143. Randall KA. War games: a new sport that can cause eye casualties. *Sightsaving.* 1985;54:2.

144. Ryan EH, Lissner G. Eye injuries during "war games". *Arch Ophthalmol.* 1986;104:1435.

145. Tardif D, Little J, Mercier M, et al. Ocular trauma in war games. *Phys Sportsmed.* 1986;14:90.

146. Martin PL, Magolian JJ. Eye injury during "war games" despite the use of goggles. *Arch Ophthalmol.* 1987;105:321.

147. Easterbrook M, Pashby TJ. Ocular injuries and war games. *Int Ophthalmol Clin.* 1988;28:222.

148. Wellington DP, Johnstone MA, Hopkins RJ. Bull's-eye corneal lesion resulting from war game injury. *Arch Ophthalmol.* 1989;107:1727.

149. Hargrave S, Weakley D, Wilson C. Complications of ocular paintball injuries in children. *J Pediatr Ophthalmol Strabismus.* 2003;37:338.

150. Fineman MS. Ocular paintball injuries. *Curr Opin Ophthalmol.* 2001;12:186.

151. Iwamoto MA, Iliff NT. Management of orbital trauma. In: Tasman W, Jaeger EA, eds. *Duane's Clinical Ophthalmology.* Philadelphia: J.B. Lippincott; 1993.

152. Kuhn F, Pieramici DJ. *Ocular Trauma Principles and Practice.* New York: Thieme; 2002.

153. Vogel MS. An overview of head trauma for the primary care practitioner: part II—ocular damage associated with head trauma. *J Am Optom Assoc.* 1992;63:542.

154. Courville CB. Coup-contrecoup mechanism of craniocerebral injuries. *Arch Surg.* 1942;45:19.

155. Courville CB. Forensic neuropathology. *J Forensic Sci.* 1962;7(1).
156. Wolter JR. Coup-Contrecoup mechanism of ocular injuries. *Am J Ophthalmol.* 1963;56:785.
157. Baker SM, Hurwitz JJ. Management of orbital and ocular adnexal trauma. *Ophthalmol Clin N Am.* 1999;12:435.
158. Griffin JR, Erickson GB. Binocular vision problems. In: Alexander KL, ed. *The Lippincott Manual of Primary Eye Care.* Philadelphia: J.B. Lippincott; 1995:378−421.
159. Caloroso EE, Rouse MW. *Clinical Management of Strabismus.* Boston: Butterworth-Heinemann; 1993:32−39.
160. Griffin JR, Grisham JD. *Binocular Anomalies.* Amsterdam: Butterworth-Heinemann; 2002:110−126.
161. Williams RJ, Marx RG, Barnes R, et al. Fractures about the orbit in professional American football players. *Am J Sports Med.* 2001;29:55.
162. Jones NP. Orbital blowout fractures in sport. *Br J Sports Med.* 1994;28:272.
163. Guyette RF. Facial injuries in basketball players. *Clin Sports Med.* 1993;12:247.
164. Kaufman BR, Heckler FR. Sports-related facial injuries. *Clin Sports Med.* 1997;16:543.
165. von Noorden GK. *Burian-von Noorden's Binocular Vision and Ocular Motility. Theory and Management of Strabismus.* St Louis: Mosby−Year Book; 1985:350−351.
166. Amos JF, ed. *Diagnosis and Management in Vision Care.* Boston: Butterworth-Heinemann; 1987:549−550.
167. Magoon EH, Botulin therapy in pediatric ophthalmology. In: Smolin G, Friedlaender MH, eds. *Pediatric Ophthalmology, Int Ophthalmol Clin* 29; 1989:30.
168. Scott AB, Magoon EH, McNeer KW, et al. Botulinum treatment of strabismus in children. *Trans Am Ophthalmol Soc.* 1989;87:174.
169. Metz HS, Mazow M. Botulinum toxin treatment of acute sixth and third nerve palsy. *Graefes Arch Clin Exp Ophthalmol.* 1988;226:141.
170. Reid DC. *Sports Injury Assessment and Rehabilitation.* New York: Churchill Livingstone; 1992.
171. Lang W. Traumatic enophthalmos with retention of perfect acuity of vision. *Trans Ophthalmol Soc U K.* 1889;9:41.
172. Smith B, Regan WF. Blow-out fracture of the orbit: mechanism and correction of internal orbital fracture. *Am J Ophthalmol.* 1957;44:733.
173. Schenck RC, Barnes RP, Behnke RP, et al., eds. *Athletic Training and Sports Medicine.* Sudbury, MA: Jones and Bartlett; 1999.
174. Bahr R, Maehlum S. *Clinical Guide to Sports Injuries.* Champaign, IL: Human Kinetics; 2004.
175. Carter JH. Diagnosis of pupillary anomalies. *J Am Optom Assoc.* 1979;50:671.
176. Parris CM, Chandler JW. Corneal trauma. In: Kaufman HE, Barron BA, McDonald MB, et al., eds. *The Cornea.* New York: Churchill Livingstone; 1988:619.
177. Lim CHL, Turner A, Lim BX. Patching for corneal abrasion. In: *The Cochrane Database of Systematic Reviews [Internet].* Indianapolis (IN): John Wiley and Sons; 2016.
178. Kirkpatrick JNP, Hoh HB, Cook SD. No eye pad for corneal abrasion. *Eye.* 1993;7:468.
179. Thiel B, Sarau A, Ng D. Efficacy of topical analgesics in pain control for corneal abrasions: a systematic review. *Cureus.* 2017;9(3):e1121.
180. Wakai A, Lawrenson JG, Lawrenson AL, et al. Topical non-steroidal anti-inflammatory drugs for analgesia in traumatic corneal abrasions. In: *Cochrane Database of Systematic Reviews [Internet].* Indianapolis (IN): John Wiley and Sons, LTD; 2017.
181. Weene LE. Recurrent corneal erosion after trauma: a statistical study. *Ann Ophthalmol.* 1983;17:521.
182. Kenyon KR. Recurrent corneal erosion: pathogenesis and therapy. *Int Ophthalmol Clin.* 1979;19:169.
183. McLean EN, MacRae SM, Rich LF. Recurrent erosion: treatment by anterior stromal puncture. *Ophthalmology.* 1986;93:784.
184. Rubinfeld RS, Laibson PR, Cohen EJ, et al. Anterior stromal puncture for recurrent erosion: further experience and new instrumentation. *Ophthalmic Surg.* 1990;21:318.
185. Dausch D, Landesz M, Klein R, et al. Phototherapeutic keratectomy in recurrent corneal epithelial erosion. *Refract Corneal Surg.* 1993;9:419.
186. John ME, Van der Karr MA, Noblitt RL, et al. Excimer laser phototherapeutic keratectomy for treatment of recurrent corneal erosion. *J Cataract Refract Surg.* 1994;20:179.
187. Fountain TR, de la Cruz Z, Green WR, et al. Reassembly of corneal epithelial adhesion structures after excimer keratectomy in humans. *Arch Ophthalmol.* 1994;112:967.
188. Miller DD, Hasan SA, Simmons NL, et al. Recurrent corneal erosion: a comprehensive review. *Clin Ophthalmol.* 2019;13:325−335.
189. Watson SL, Leung V. Interventions for recurrent corneal erosions. *Cochrane Database Syst Rev.* 2018;7:CD001861.
190. Slingsby JG, Forstot SL. Effect of blunt trauma on corneal endothelium. *Arch Ophthalmol.* 1981;99:1041.
191. Cherry PMH. Rupture of the globe. *Arch Ophthalmol.* 1972;88:498.
192. Cherry PMH. Indirect traumatic rupture of the globe. *Arch Ophthalmol.* 1978;96:252.
193. Crouch ER, Williams PB. Trauma: ruptures and bleeding. In: Tasman W, Jaeger EA, eds. *Duane's Clinical Ophthalmology.* Philadelphia: J.B. Lippincott; 1983.
194. Reppucci VS, Movshovich A. Current concepts in the treatment of traumatic injury to the posterior segment. *Ophthalmol Clin N Am.* 1999;12:465.
195. Rakusin W. Traumatic hyphema. *Am J Ophthalmol.* 1972;74:284.
196. Read JE, Goldberg MF. Comparison of medical treatment for traumatic hyphema. *Trans Am Acad Ophthalmol Otolaryngol.* 1974;78:799.
197. Blanton FM. Anterior chamber angle recession and secondary glaucoma: a study of the after effects of traumatic hyphemas. *Arch Ophthalmol.* 1964;72:39.
198. Ng DS, Ching RH, Chan CW. Angle-recession glaucoma: long-term clinical outcomes over a 10-year period in traumatic microhyphema. *Int Ophthalmol.* 2015;35:107−113.
199. Milauskas AT, Fueger GF. Serious ocular complications associated with blowout fractures of the orbit. *Am J Ophthalmol.* 1966;62:670.

200. Kearns P. Traumatic hyphaema: a retrospective study of 314 cases. *Br J Ophthalmol.* 1991;75(3):137–141.

201. Haynes WL, Johnson AT, Alward WLM. Effects of jogging exercise on patients with pigmentary dispersion syndrome and pigmentary glaucoma. *Ophthalmology.* 1992;99:1096.

202. Goldberg MF. The diagnosis and treatment of secondary glaucoma after hyphema in sickle cell patients. *Am J Ophthalmol.* 1979;87:43.

203. Michaelson PE, Pfaffenbach D. Retinal arterial occlusion following ocular trauma in youths with sickle-trait hemoglobinopathy. *Am J Ophthalmol.* 1972;74:494.

204. Sorr EM, Goldberg RE. Traumatic central artery occlusion with sickle cell trait. *Am J Ophthalmol.* 1975;80:648.

205. Wax MB, Ridley ME, Magargal LE. Reversal of retinal and optic disc ischemia in a patient with sickle cell trait and glaucoma secondary to traumatic hyphema. *Ophthalmology.* 1982;89:845.

206. Hamill MB. Current concepts in the treatment of traumatic injury to the anterior segment. *Ophthalmol Clin N Am.* 1999;12:457.

207. Crouch ER, Frenkel M. Aminocaproic acid in the treatment of traumatic hyphema. *Am J Ophthalmol.* 1976;81:355.

208. Darr JL, Passmore JW. Management of traumatic hyphema: a review of 109 cases. *Am J Ophthalmol.* 1967;63:134.

209. Crouch ER. Traumatic hyphema. *J Pediatr Ophthalmol Strabismus.* 1986;23:95.

210. Kennedy RH, Brubaker RF. Traumatic hyphema in a defined population. *Am J Ophthamol.* 1988;106:123.

211. Arnheim DD, Prentice WE. *Principles of Athletic Training.* 10th ed. Boston: McGraw Hill; 2000.

212. Sneed S, Weingeist T. Suprachoroidal dislocation of a posterior chamber intraocular lens. *Am J Ophthalmol.* 1990;109:731.

213. Lam D, Chua J, Kwok A. Combined surgery for severe eye trauma with extensive iridodialysis, posterior lens dislocation, and intractable glaucoma. *J Cataract Refract Surg.* 1999;25:285.

214. Netland K, Martinez J, LaCour OR, et al. Traumatic anterior lens dislocation: a case report. *J Emerg Med.* 1999;17:637.

215. Shingleton BJ, Hersh PS, Kenyon KR, eds. *Eye Trauma.* St Louis: Mosby–Year Book; 1991.

216. Berlin R. Zur sogenannten commotio retinae. *Klin Monatsbl Augenheilkd.* 1873;1:42.

217. Cogan DG. Pseudoretinitis pigmentosa. *Arch Ophthalmol.* 1969;81:45.

218. Crouch ER, Apple DJ. Posttraumatic migration of retinal pigment epithelial melanin. *Am J Ophthalmol.* 1974;78:251.

219. Bastek JV, Foos RY, Heckenlively J. Traumatic pigmentary retinopathy. *Am J Ophthalmol.* 1981;92:621.

220. Friberg TR. Traumatic retinal pigment epithelial edema. *Am J Ophthalmol.* 1979;88:18.

221. Gass JDM. *Stereoscopic Atlas of Macular Diseases: Diagnosis and Treatment.* 4th ed. St Louis: Mosby–Year Book; 1997.

222. Kuhn F, Morris R, Mester V, et al. Internal limiting membrane removal for traumatic macular holes. *Ophthalmic Surg Laser.* 2001;32:308.

223. Yanagiya N, Akiba J, Takahashi M, et al. Clinical characteristics of traumatic macular holes. *Jpn J Ophthalmol.* 1996;40:544.

224. Kelly NE, Wendel RT. Vitreous surgery for idiopathic macular holes: results of a pilot study. *Arch Ophthalmol.* 1991;109:654.

225. Rubin JS, Glaser BM, Thompson JT, et al. Vitrectomy, fluid-gas exchange and transforming growth factor-beta-2 for the treatment of traumatic macular holes. *Ophthalmology.* 1995;102:1840.

226. de Bustros S. Vitreous surgery for traumatic macular hole. *Retina.* 1996;12:451.

227. Ciulla TA, Topping TM. Surgical treatment of a macular hole secondary to accidental laser burn. *Arch Ophthalmol.* 1997;115:929.

228. Garcia-Arumi J, Corcostegui B, Cavero L, et al. The role of vitreoretinal surgery in the treatment of posttraumatic macular hole. *Retina.* 1997;17:372.

229. Madreperla SA, Benetz BA. Formation and treatment of a traumatic macular hole. *Arch Ophthalmol.* 1997;115:1210.

230. Margherio AR, Margherio RR, Hartzer M, et al. Plasmin enzyme-assisted vitrectomy in traumatic pediatric macular holes. *Ophthalmology.* 1998;105:1617.

231. Sheidow TG, Gonder JR. Macular hole secondary to retrobulbar needle perforation. *Retina.* 1998;18:178.

232. Amari F, Ogino N, Matsumura M, et al. Vitreous surgery for traumatic macular holes. *Retina.* 1999;19:410.

233. Chow DR, Williams GA, Trese MT, al. Successful closure of traumatic macular holes. *Retina.* 1999;l9:405.

234. Budoff G, Bhagat N, Zarbin MA. Traumatic macular hole: diagnosis, natural history, and management. *J Ophthalmol.* 2019. Article:5837832.

235. Goffstein R, Burton TC. Differentiating traumatic from nontraumatic retinal detachment. *Ophthalmology.* 1982;89:361.

236. Weidenthal DT, Schepens CL. Peripheral fundus changes associated with ocular contusion. *Am J Ophthalmol.* 1966;62:465.

237. Tasman W. Peripheral retinal changes following blunt trauma. *Trans Am Ophthalmol Soc.* 1972;70:190.

238. Steinsaper KD, Goldberg RA. Traumatic optic neuropathy. *Surv Ophthalmol.* 1994;38:487.

239. Frenkel REP, Spoor TC. Diagnosis and management of traumatic optic neuropathies. *Adv Ophthalmic Plast Reconstr Surg.* 1987;6:71.

240. Sanborn GE, Gonder JR, Goldberg RE, et al. Evulsion of the optic nerve: a clinicopathological study. *Can J Ophthalmol.* 1984;19:10.

241. Steinsaper KD, Goldberg RA. *Traumatic Optic Neuropathy.* 5th ed. Baltimore: Williams & Wilkins; 1998:5.

242. Park JH, Frenkel M, Dobbie JG, et al. Evulsion of the optic nerve. *Am J Ophthalmol.* 1971;72:969.

243. Chow AY, Goldberg MF, Frenkel M. Evulsion of the optic nerve in association with basketball injuries. *Ann Ophthalmol.* 1984;16:35.

244. Rosenberg PN, Stasior OB. Optic nerve evulsion and transection. *Adv Ophthalmic Plast Reconstr Surg*. 1987;6:63.

245. Jang SY. Traumatic optic neuropathy. *Korean J Nutr*. 2018; 14:1−5.

246. Wolin MJ, Lavin PJM. Spontaneous visual recovery from traumatic optic neuropathy after blunt head injury. *Am J Ophthalmol*. 1990;109:430.

247. Fuller B, Gitter K. Traumatic choroidal rupture with late serous detachment of the macula. *Arch Ophthalmol*. 1973;89:354.

248. Smith RE, Kelley JS, Harbin TS. Late macular complications of choroidal ruptures. *Am J Ophthalmol*. 1974;77:650.

249. Hilton GF. Late serosanguineous detachment of the macula after traumatic choroidal rupture. *Am J Ophthalmol*. 1975;79:997.

250. Saar I, Raniel J, Neumann E. Recurrent corneal oedema following late migration of intraocular glass. *Br J Ophthalmol*. 1991;75:188.

251. Ralph RA. Chemical burns of the eye. In: Tasman W, Jaeger EA, eds. *Duane's Clinical Ophthalmology*. Philadelphia: J.B. Lippincott; 1983.

252. McCrory P, Meeuwisse W, Dvorak J, et al. Consensus statement on concussion in sport − the 5th international conference on concussion in sport held in Berlin, October 2016. *Br J Sports Med*. 2017;51:838−847.

253. McCrea M, Guskiewicz K, Randolph C, et al. Incidence, clinical course, and predictors of prolonged recovery time following sport-related concussion in high school and college athletes. *J Int Neuropsychol Soc*. 2013;19:22−33.

254. Zemek R, Barrowman N, Freedman SB, et al. Clinical risk score for persistent postconcussion symptoms among children with acute concussion in the ED. *J Am Med Assoc*. 2016;315:1014−1025.

255. Eisenberg MA, Andrea J, Meehan W, et al. Time interval between concussions and symptom duration. *Pediatrics*. 2013;132:8−17.

256. Hellewell SC, Ziebell JM, Lifshitz J, et al. Impact acceleration model of diffuse traumatic brain injury. In: Kobeissy FH, Dixon CE, Hayes RL, Mondello S, eds. *Injury Models of the Central Nervous System: Methods and Protocols. Methods in Molecular Biology*. 2016:253−266, 1462.

257. Topal NB, Hakyemez B, Erdogan C, et al. MR imaging in the detection of diffuse axonal injury with mild traumatic brain injury. *Neurol Res*. 2008;30:974−978.

258. Browne KD, Chen XH, Meaney DF, et al. Mild traumatic brain injury and diffuse axonal injury in swine. *J Neurotrauma*. 2011;28:1747−1755.

259. Lafrenaye AD, Todani M, Walker SA, et al. Microglia processes associate with diffusely injured axons following mild traumatic brain injury in the micro pig. *J Neuroinflammation*. 2015;12:186.

260. Hill CS, Coleman MP, Menon DK. Traumatic axonal injury: mechanisms and translational opportunities. *Trends Neurosci*. 2016;39:311−324.

261. Greer JE, McGinn MJ, Povlishock JT. Diffuse traumatic axonal injury in the mouse induces atrophy, c-Jun activation, and axonal outgrowth in the axotomized neuronal population. *J Neurosci*. 2011;31:5089−5105.

262. Greer JE, Povlishock JT, Jacobs KM. Electrophysiological abnormalities in both axotomized and nonaxotomized pyramidal neurons following mild traumatic brain injury. *J Neurosci*. 2012;32:6682−6687.

263. Rachmany L, Tweedie D, Rubovitch V, et al. Cognitive impairments accompanying rodent mild traumatic brain injury involve p53-dependent neuronal cell death and are ameliorated by the tetrahydrobenzothiazole PFT-alpha. *PLoS One*. 2013;8:e79837.

264. Kaur P, Sharma S. Recent advances in pathophysiology of traumatic brain injury. *Curr Neuropharmacol*. 2018;16: 1224−1238.

265. Unterberg AW, Stover J, Kress B, Kiening KL. Edema and brain trauma. *Neuroscience*. 2004;129:1021−1029.

266. McQuire JC, Sutcliffe JC, Coats TJ. Early changes in middle cerebral artery blood flow velocity after head injury. *J Neurosurg*. 1998;89:526−532.

267. Golding EM, Robertson CS, Bryan RM. The consequences of traumatic brain injury on cerebral blood flow and autoregulation: a review. *Clin Exp Hypertens*. 1999;21: 299−332.

268. DeWitt DS, Prough DS. Traumatic cerebral vascular injury: the effects of concussive brain injury on the cerebral vasculature. *J Neurotrauma*. 2003;20:795−825.

269. Pasco A, Lemaire L, Franconi F, et al. Perfusional deficit and the dynamics of cerebral edemas in experimental traumatic brain injury using perfusion and diffusion-weighted magnetic resonance imaging. *J Neurotrauma*. 2007;24:1321−1330.

270. Mouzon BC, Bachmeier C, Ferro A, et al. Chronic neuropathological and neurobehavioral changes in a repetitive mild traumatic brain injury model. *Ann Neurol*. 2014;75: 241−254.

271. MacFarlane MP, Glenn TC. Neurochemical cascade of concussion. *Brain Inj*. 2015;29:139−153.

272. McCrea M, Meier T, Huber D, et al. Role of advanced neuroimaging, fluid biomarkers and genetic testing in the assessment of sport-related concussion: a systematic review. *Br J Sports Med*. 2017;51:919−929.

273. McLendon LA, Kralik SF, Grayson PA, Golomb MR. The controversial second impact syndrome: a review of the literature. *Pediatr Neurol*. 2016;62:9−17.

274. Saunders RL, Harbaugh RE. The second impact in catastrophic contact sports head trauma. *J Am Med Assoc*. 1984;252:538−539.

275. Stovitz SD, Weseman JD, Hooks MC, et al. What definition is used to describe second impact syndrome in sports? A systematic and critical review. *Curr Sports Med Rep*. 2017;16:50−55.

276. Stern RA, Riley DO, Daneshvar DH, et al. Long-term consequences of repetitive brain trauma: chronic traumatic encephalopathy. *Pharm Manag R*. 2011;3(10 Suppl 2): S460−S467.

277. McKee AC, Daneshvar DH, Alvarez VE, Stein TD. The neuropathology of sport. *Acta Neuropathol*. 2014;127: 29−51.

278. Martland H. Punch drunk syndrome. *J Am Med Assoc*. 1928;91:1103−1107.

279. Omalu B, DeKosky S, Minster R, et al. Chronic traumatic encephalopathy in a National football league player. *Neurosurgery.* 2005;57:128−134.

280. Omalu B, DeKosky S, Hamilton R, et al. Chronic traumatic encephalopathy in a National football league player: Part II. *Neurosurgery.* 2006;59:1086−1093.

281. McKee A, Cantu R, Nowinski C, et al. Chronic traumatic encephalopathy in athletes: progressive tauopathy after repetitive head injury. *J Neuropathol Exp Neurol.* 2009; 68:709−735.

282. Omalu B, Fitzsimmons R, Hammers J, Bailes J. Chronic traumatic encephalopathy in a professional American wrestler. *J Forensic Nurs.* 2010;6:130−136.

283. McKee A, Stein T, Nowinski C, et al. The spectrum of disease in chronic traumatic encephalopathy. *Brain.* 2012;135:1−22.

284. Mez J, Daneshvar DH, Kiernan PT, et al. Clinicopathological evaluation of chronic traumatic encephalopathy in players of American football. *J Am Med Assoc.* 2017;318: 360−370.

285. McKee AC, Cairns NJ, Dickson DW, et al. The first NINDS/NIBIB consensus meeting to define neuropathological criteria for the diagnosis of chronic traumatic encephalopathy. *Acta Neuropathol.* 2015;131:75−86.

286. Solomon GS, Zuckerman SL. Chronic traumatic encephalopathy in professional sports: retrospective and prospective views. *Brain Inj.* 2015;29:164−170.

287. Wild E, Magnusson A, Lahiri N, et al. Abnormal peripheral chemokine profile in Huntington's disease. *PLoS Curr.* 2011;3:RRN1231.

288. Huber AK, Wang L, Han P, et al. Dysregulation of the IL-23/IL-17 axis and myeloid factors in secondary progressive MS. *Neurology.* 2014;83:1500−1507.

289. Furukawa T, Matsui N, Fujita K, et al. CSF cytokine profile distinguishes multifocal motor neuropathy from progressive muscular atrophy. *Neurol Neuroimmunol Neuroinflamm.* 2015;2(5):e138.

290. Cherry JD, Stein TD, Tripodis Y, et al. CCL11 is increased in the CNS in chronic traumatic encephalopathy but not in Alzheimer's disease. *PLoS One.* 2017;12(9):e0185541.

291. Patel DR, Shivdasani V, Baker RJ. Management of sport-related concussion in young athletes. *Sports Med.* 2005; 35:671−684.

292. Gessel LM, Fields SK, Collins CL, et al. Concussions among United States high school and collegiate athletes. *J Athl Train.* 2007;42:495−503.

293. Langlois JA, Rutland-Brown W, Wald MM. The epidemiology and impact of traumatic brain injury: a brief overview. *J Head Trauma Rehabil.* 2006;21:375−378.

294. Langlois JA, Sattin RW. Traumatic brain injury in the United States: research and programs of the centers for disease control and prevention (CDC). *J Head Trauma Rehabil.* 2005;20:187−188.

295. Lincoln AE, Caswell SV, Almquist JL, et al. Trends in concussion incidence in high school sports: a prospective 11-year study. *Am J Sports Med.* 2011;39:958−963.

296. Marar M, McIlvain NM, Fields SK, Comstock RD. Epidemiology of concussions among United States high school athletes in 20 sports. *Am J Sports Med.* 2012;40:747−755.

297. Harrison EA. The first concussion crisis: head injury and evidence in early American football. *Am J Publ Health.* 2014;104:822−833.

298. Pellman EJ, Viano DC, Tucker AM, Committee on Mild Traumatic Brain Injury NFL, et al. Concussion in professional football: location and direction of helmet impacts-Part 2. *Neurosurgery.* 2003;53:1328−1340.

299. O'Connor KL, Rowson S, Duma SM, Broglio SP. Head-impact-measurement devices: a systemic review. *J Athl Train.* 2017;52:206−227.

300. Davis GA, et al. Child sport concussion assessment tool 5th edition. *Br J Sports Med.* 2017;51:862−869.

301. Davis GA, Purcell L, Schneider KJ, et al. The child sport concussion assessment tool 5th edition (Child SCAT5): background and rationale. *Br J Sports Med.* 2017;51: 859−861.

302. Sport concussion assessment tool − 5th edition. *Br J Sports Med.* 2017;51:851−858.

303. Echemendia RJ, Meeuwisse W, McCrory P, et al. The sport concussion assessment tool 5th edition (SCAT5): background and rationale. *Br J Sports Med.* 2017;51:848−850.

304. Echemendia RJ, Meeuwisse W, McCrory P, et al. The concussion recognition tool 5th edition (CRT5): background and rationale. *Br J Sports Med.* 2017;51:870−871.

305. Linder S, Ozinga SJ, Koop MM, et al. Normative performance on the balance error scoring system by youth, high school, and collegiate athletes. *J Athl Train.* 2018; 53:636−645.

306. Patricios J, Fuller GW, Ellenbogen R, et al. What are the critical elements of sideline screening that can be used to establish the diagnosis of concussion? A systematic review. *Br J Sports Med.* 2017;51:888−894.

307. Sady MD, Vaughan CG, Gioia GA. Psychometric characteristics of the post-concussion symptom inventory (PCSI) in children and adolescents. *Arch Clin Neuropsychol.* 2014;29:348−363.

308. Makdissi M, Darby D, Maruff P, et al. Natural history of concussion in sport: markers of severity and implications for management. *Am J Sports Med.* 2010;38:464−471.

309. Guskiewicz KM, McCrea M, Marshall SW, et al. Cumulative effects associated with recurrent concussion in collegiate football players: the NCAA Concussion Study. *J Am Med Assoc.* 2003;290:2549−2555.

310. Zemper ED. Two-year prospective study of relative risk of a second cerebral concussion. *Am J Phys Med Rehabil.* 2003;82:653−659.

311. Iverson GL, Gaetz M, Lovell MR, Collins MW. Cumulative effects of concussion in amateur athletes. *Brain Inj.* 2004;18:433−443.

312. Slobounov S, Slobounov E, Sebastianelli W, et al. Differential rate of recovery in athletes after first and second concussion episodes. *Neurosurgery.* 2007;61:338−344.

313. Schatz P, Moser R, Covassin T, Karpf R. Early indicators of enduring symptoms in high school athletes with multiple previous concussions. *Neurosurgery.* 2011;68: 1562−1567.

314. Covassin T, Moran R, Wilhelm K. Concussion symptoms and neurocognitive performance of high school and

college athletes who incur multiple concussions. *Am J Sports Med*. 2013;41:2885–2889.

315. Mannix R, Iverson GL, Maxwell B, et al. Multiple prior concussions are associated with symptoms in high school athletes. *Ann Clin Translational Neurol*. 2014;1:433–438.

316. Broglio SP, Cantu RC, Gioia GA, et al. National Athletic Trainers' Association position statement: management of sport concussion. *J Athl Train*. 2014;49:245–265.

317. Harmon KG, Clugston JR, Dec K, et al. American Medical Society for Sports Medicine position statement on concussion in sport. *Br J Sports Med*. 2019;53:213–225.

318. Herring SA, Cantu RC, Guskiewicz KM, et al. Concussion (mild traumatic brain injury) and the team physician: a consensus statement–2011 update. *Med Sci Sports Exerc*. 2011;43:2412–2422.

319. Herring SA, Kibler WB, Putukian M. The team physician and the return-to-play decision: a consensus statement-2012 update. *Med Sci Sports Exerc*. 2012;44:2446–2448.

320. Herring SA, Kibler WB, Putukian M. Team physician consensus statement: 2013 update. *Med Sci Sports Exerc*. 2013;45:1618–1622.

321. Echemendia RJ, Iverson G, McCrea M, et al. Role of neuropsychologists in the evaluation and management of sports-related concussion: an interorganization position statement. *Arch Clin Neuropsychol*. 2011;25:1289–1294.

322. Echemendia RJ, Giza CC, Kutcher JS. Developing guidelines for return to play: consensus and evidence-based approaches. *Brain Inj*. 2015;29:185–194.

323. Schneider KJ, Leddy JJ, Guskiewicz KM, et al. Rest and treatment/rehabilitation following sport-related concussion: a systematic review. *Br J Sports Med*. 2017;51:930–934.

324. McGrath N, Dinn WM, Collins MW, et al. Post-exertion neurocognitive test failure among student-athletes following concussion. *Brain Inj*. 2013;27:103–113.

325. Leddy JJ, Kozlowski K, Donnelly JP, et al. A preliminary study of subsymptom threshold exercise training for refractory post-concussion syndrome. *Clin J Sport Med*. 2010;20:21–27.

326. Leddy JJ, Baker JG, Kozlowski K, et al. Reliability of a graded exercise test for assessing recovery from concussion. *Clin J Sport Med*. 2011;21:89–94.

327. Ellis MJ, Leddy J, Willer B. Multi-disciplinary management of athletes with postconcussion syndrome: an evolving pathophysiological approach. *Front Neurol*. 2016;7:136.

328. Kamins J, Bigler E, Covassin T, et al. What is the physiological time to recovery after concussion? A systematic review. *Br J Sports Med*. 2017;51:935–940.

329. Iverson GL, Gardner AJ, Terry DP, et al. Predictors of clinical recovery from concussion: a systematic review. *Br J Sports Med*. 2017;51:941–948.

330. Alsalaheen BA, Mucha A, Morris LO, et al. Vestibular rehabilitation for dizziness and balance disorders after concussion. *J Neurol Phys Ther*. 2010;34:87–93.

331. Gottshall K. Vestibular rehabilitation after mild traumatic brain injury with vestibular pathology. *NeuroRehabilitation*. 2011;29:167–171.

332. Hugentobler JA, Vegh M, Janiszewski B, et al. Physical therapy intervention strategies for patients with prolonged mild traumatic brain injury symptoms: a case series. *Int J Sports Phys Ther*. 2015;10:676–689.

333. Grabowski P, Wilson J, Walker A, et al. Multimodal impairment-based physical therapy for the treatment of patients with post-concussion syndrome: a retrospective analysis on safety and feasibility. *Phys Ther Sport*. 2017;23:22–30.

334. Makdissi M, Schneider KJ, Feddermann-Demont N, et al. Approach to investigation and treatment of persistent symptoms following sport-related concussion: a systematic review. *Br J Sports Med*. 2017;51:958–968.

335. Davis GA, Anderson V, Babl FE, et al. What is the difference in concussion management in children as compared to adults? A systematic review. *Br J Sports Med*. 2017;51:949–957.

336. Ciuffreda KJ, Kapoor N, Rutner D, et al. Occurrence of oculomotor dysfunctions in acquired brain injury: a retrospective analysis. *Optometry*. 2007;78:155–161.

337. Goodrich GL, Kirby J, Cockerham G, et al. Visual function in patients of a polytrauma rehabilitation center: a descriptive study. *J Rehabil Res Dev*. 2007;44:929–936.

338. Thiagarajan P, Ciuffreda KJ, Ludlam DP. Vergence dysfunction in mild traumatic brain injury (mTBI): a review. *Ophthalmic Physiol Optic*. 2011;31:456–468.

339. 0Kontos AP, Elbin RJ, Schatz P, et al. A revised factor structure for the Post-Concussion Symptom Scale: baseline and post-concussion factors. *Am J Sports Med*. 2012;40:2375–2384.

340. Master CL, Scheiman M, Gallaway M, et al. Vision diagnoses are common after concussion in adolescents. *Clin Pediatr*. 2016;55:260–267.

341. Felleman DJ, Van Essen DC. Distributed hierarchical processing in the primate cerebral cortex. *Cerebr Cortex*. 1991;1:1–47.

342. Laukkanen H, Scheiman M, Hayes JR. Brain injury vision symptom survey (BIVSS) questionnaire. *Optom Vis Sci*. 2016;93:43–50.

343. Weimer A, Jensen C, Laukkanen H, et al. Test-retest reliability of the brain injury vision symptom survey. *Vis Dev Rehabil*. 2018;4:177–185.

344. Cohen M, Groswasser Z, Barchadski R, Appel A. Convergence insufficiency in brain-injured patients. *Brain Inj*. 1989;3:187–191.

345. Gallaway M, Scheiman, Mitchell GL. Vision therapy for post-concussion vision disorders. *Optom Vis Sci*. 2017;94:68–73.

346. Peters M, Price J. The Peters/Price (see to play) vision concussion protocol: diagnosis and treatment. *Optom Vis Perf*. 2015;3:126–138.

347. Ciuffreda KJ, Tannen B, Ludlam D, Yadav NK. Basic neuro-optometric diagnostic tests for mild traumatic brain injury/concussion: a narrative review, perspective, proposed techniques and protocols. *Vis Dev Rehab*. 2018;4:159–171.

348. Joseph JR, Swallow JS, Willsey K, et al. Pupillary changes after clinically asymptomatic high-acceleration head im-

pacts in high school football athletes. *J Neurosurg.* 2019. https://doi.org/10.3171/2019.7.JNS191272.

349. Galetta KM, Barrett J, Allen M, et al. The King-Devick test as a determinant of head trauma and concussion in boxers and MMA fighters. *Neurology.* 2011;76:1456–1462.

350. Galetta KM, Brandes LE, Maki K, et al. The King-Devick test and sports-related concussion: study of a rapid visual screening tool in a collegiate cohort. *J Neurol Sci.* 2011; 309:34–39.

351. Galetta MS, Galetta KM, McCrossin, et al. Saccades and memory: baseline associations of the King–Devick and SCAT2 SAC tests in professional ice hockey players. *J Neurosci.* 2013;328:28–31.

352. King D, Brughelli M, Hume P, Gissane C. Concussions in amateur rugby union identified with the use of a rapid visual screening tool. *J Neurol Sci.* 2013;326(1–2):59–63.

353. Dhawan P, Starling A, Tapsell L, et al. King-Devick test identifies symptomatic concussion in real-time and asymptomatic concussion over time. *J Optom.* 2015;8:131–139.

354. King D, Hume P, Gissane C, Clark T. Use of the King-Devick test for sideline concussion screening in junior rugby league. *J Neurosci.* 2015;357:75–79.

355. Leong DF, Balcer LJ, Galetta SL, et al. The King-Devick test for sideline concussion screening in collegiate football. *J Optom.* 2015;8:131–139.

356. Seidman DH, Burlingame J, Yousif LR, et al. Evaluation of the King-Devick test as a concussion screening tool in high school football player. *J Neurosci.* 2015;356:97–101.

357. Galetta KM, Liu M, Leong DF, et al. The King-Devick test of rapid number naming for concussion detection: meta-analysis and systematic review of the literature. *Concussion.* 2015;1:CNC8.

358. Worts PR, Schatz P, Burkhart SO. Test performance and test-re-test reliability of the vestibular/ocular motor screening and King-Devick test in adolescent athletes during a competitive sport season. *Am J Sports Med.* 2018;46: 2004–2010.

359. Zahid AB, Hubbard ME, Lockyer J, et al. Eye tracking as a biomarker for concussion in children. *Clin J Sport Med.* 2018;00:1–11.

360. Mucha A, Collins MW, Elbin RJ, et al. A brief vestibular/ocular motor screening (VOMS) assessment to evaluate concussions: preliminary findings. *Am J Sports Med.* 2014;42:2479–2486.

361. Yorke AM, Smith L, Babcock M, Alsalaheen B. Validity and reliability of the vestibular/ocular motor screening and associations with common concussion screening tools. *Sport Health.* 2017;9:174–180.

362. Moran RN, Covassin T, Elbin RJ, et al. Reliability and normative reference values for the vestibular/ocular motor screening (VOMS) tool in youth athletes. *Am J Sports Med.* 2018;46:1475–1480.

363. Alkathiry AA, Kontos AP, Furman JM, et al. Vestibulo-ocular reflex function in adolescents with sport-related concussion: a preliminary report. *Sport Health.* 2019;11:479–485.

364. Iverson GL, Cook NE, Howell DR, et al. Preseason vestibular ocular motor screening in children and adolescents.

Clin J Sport Med. 2019:1–5. https://doi.org/10.1097/JSM.0000000000000767.

365. Kawata K, Rubin LH, Lee JH, et al. Association of football subconcussive head impacts with ocular near point of convergence. *JAMA Ophthalmol.* 2016;134:763–769.

366. Zonner SW, Ejima K, Fulgar CC, et al. Oculomotor response to cumulative subconcussive head impacts in US high school football players: a longitudinal study. *JAMA Ophthalmol.* 2019;137:265–270.

367. Anzalone AJ, Blueitt D, Case T, et al. A positive vestibular/ocular motor screening (VOMS) is associated with increased recovery time after sports-related concussion in youth and adolescent athletes. *Am J Sports Med.* 2017;45:474–479.

368. Sinnott AM, Elbin RJ, Collins MW, et al. Persistent vestibular-ocular impairment following concussion in adolescents. *J Sci Med Sport.* 2019;22:1292–1297.

369. Thiagarajan P, Ciuffreda KJ, et al. Effect of oculomotor rehabilitation on vergence responsivity in mild traumatic brain injury. *J Rehabil Res Dev.* 2013;50, 1223-140.

370. Kapoor N, Ciuffreda KJ. Vision disturbances following traumatic brain injury. *Curr Treat Options Neurol.* 2002; 4:271–280.

371. Bansal S, Han E, Ciuffreda KJ. Use of yoked prisms in patients with acquired brain injury: a retrospective analysis. *Brain Inj.* 2014;28:1441–1446.

372. Truong JQ, Ciuffreda KJ, Han MH, et al. Photosensitivity in mild traumatic brain injury (mTBI): a retrospective analysis. *Brain Inj.* 2014;28:1283–1287.

373. Thiagarajan P, Ciuffreda KJ. Pupillary responses to light in chronic non-blast-induced mTBI. *Brain Inj.* 2015;29: 1420–1425.

374. Capo-Aponte JE, Beltran TA, Walsh DV, et al. Validation of visual objective biomarkers for acute concussion. *Mil Med.* 2018;183(supplement 1):9–17.

375. Ciuffreda KJ, Yadav NK, Ludlam DP. Effect of binasal occlusion (BNO) on the visual-evoked potential (VEP) in mild traumatic brain injury (mTBI). *Brain Inj.* 2013;27: 41–47.

376. Yadav NK, Ciuffreda KJ. Effect of binasal occlusion (BNO) and base-in prisms on the visual-evoked potential (VEP) in mild traumatic brain injury (mTBI). *Brain Inj.* 2014;28:1568–1580.

377. Thiagarajan P, Ciuffreda KJ. Effect of oculomotor rehabilitation on accommodative responsivity in mild traumatic brain injury. *J Rehabil Res Dev.* 2014;51:175–192.

378. Thiagarajan P, Ciuffreda KJ. Versional eye tracking in mild traumatic brain injury (mTBI): effects of oculomotor training (OMT). *Brain Inj.* 2014;28:930–943.

379. Thiagarajan P, Ciuffreda KJ, Capo-Aponte JE, et al. Oculomotor neurorehabilitation for reading in mild traumatic brain injury (mTBI): an integrative approach. *NeuroRehabilitation.* 2014;34:129–146.

380. Yadav NK, Thiagarajan P, Ciuffreda KJ. Effect of oculomotor vision rehabilitation on the visual-evoked potential and visual attention in mild traumatic brain injury. *Brain Inj.* 2014;28:922–929.

381. Thiagarajan P, Ciuffreda KJ. Short-term persistence of oc-ulomotor rehabilitative changes in mild traumatic brain injury (mTBI): a pilot study of clinical effects. *Brain Inj.* 2015;29:1475−1479.

382. Scheiman MM, Talasan H, Mitchell GL, Alvarez TL. Objective assessment of vergence after treatment of concussion-related CI: a pilot study. *Optom Vis Sci.* 2017;94:74−88.

383. Conrad JS, Mitchell GL, Kulp MT. Vision therapy for binocular dysfunction post brain injury. *Optom Vis Sci.* 2017;94:101−107.

384. Clark JF, Graman P, Ellis JK, et al. An exploratory study of the potential effects of vision training on concussion inci-dence in football. *Optom Vis Perf.* 2015;3:116−125.

385. Schmidt JD, Guskiewicz KM, Mihalik JP, et al. Does visual performance influence head impact severity among high school football athletes? *Clin J Sport Med.* 2015;25:494−501.

386. Scheiman MM, Rouse MW. *Optometric Management of Learning-Related Vision Problems.* 2nd ed. Elsevier-Mosby; 2005.

CHAPTER 8

Sports Vision Training

There is significant interest in improving sports performance by using training procedures to enhance vision because visual skills are readily identified as a critical element to most sports performance. Chapter 4 provides support for the contention that athletes typically have better visual abilities than nonathletes and that top athletes benefit from visual abilities that often are superior to lower level athletes. Sports vision training (SVT) has similar goals of transferring improvements in function to athletic performance as do other areas of performance training, such as strength training, conditioning, speed and agility training, nutritional regimens, and sports psychology.[1] The relevant questions are whether visual abilities can indeed be trained and whether any improvements in visual skills transfer to improved sports performance by the athlete.

Many of the visual attributes identified as important in sports are amenable to training. This chapter presents SVT procedures for each of the visual skill areas, including any relevant laboratory and clinical research regarding skill improvement for these visual skills. Although few studies have attempted to demonstrate the transfer of visual skill improvement to actual sport performance, isolating one area of intervention as solely responsible for any changes in performance is quite difficult. Many of the reports in the literature are anecdotal, and many studies have significant flaws in the research design that preclude a definitive conclusion. Although there is a growing body of evidence supporting SVT approaches, the incomplete information regarding the efficacy of SVT clearly illuminates the need for more conclusive evidence.

AREAS OF SPORTS VISION TRAINING

SVT procedures can be selected to accomplish the following potential goals of training:

1. Remediation of vision inefficiencies that may have a negative impact on performance consistency.
2. Enhancement of vision skills deemed important to optimal sports task performance.
3. Enhancement of visual information processing skills to facilitate rapid utilization of critical visual information.
4. Enhancement of visuomotor proficiency, when indicated, for sports task performance.
5. Enhancement of cognitive functions that are critical for visual decision-making during competition.[2]

To determine the appropriate goals for an individual athlete, a thorough case history and sports vision evaluation must be completed. As discussed in Chapters 2 and 4, the sports vision practitioner must identify the vision factors essential to performance of the tasks critical for success in the sport and evaluate the quality of those skills in the most appropriate, accurate, and repeatable manner. A vision skill performance profile is recommended to communicate the relative strengths and "opportunities" demonstrated by the athlete from the sports vision evaluation, as described in Chapter 5. The vision skill performance profile can be used to develop readily measurable specific goals for the SVT program to determine skill improvement. These goals should be consistent with the information processing model of skilled motor performance discussed in Chapter 3, and each training procedure should be scrutinized to determine any impact on the three central cortical processing mechanisms: the perceptual mechanism, the decision mechanism, and the effector mechanism (see Fig. 3.1).

The athlete with identified visual deficiencies should logically expect improvement in affected aspects of sports performance if those deficient skills are improved to average performance levels. A review of the literature in 1988 concluded, "it is evident from the research presented that there is sufficient scientific support for the efficacy of vision therapy in modifying and improving oculomotor, accommodative, and binocular system disorders, as measured by standardized clinical and laboratory testing methods, in the majority of patients of all ages for whom it is properly undertaken and employed."[3] This conclusion was further supported by Ciuffreda in 2002.[4] Therefore vision therapy designed to remediate vision deficits is an essential element in the comprehensive vision care of an athlete, and a successful result should improve the function of the perceptual mechanism.

The athlete who possesses average, or even above-average, vision skills presents a compelling and controversial challenge. Can the vision skills of this athlete be

Sports Vision. https://doi.org/10.1016/B978-0-323-75543-6.00002-4

enhanced above the current level, and would this perceptual mechanism skill enhancement result in demonstrable improvements in sports task performance? A review of the literature concluded that most normal visual functions can be improved by specific training paradigms, although thousands of trials may be required to demonstrate enhancement.[5] Several studies have reported positive effects of vision training programs on sport-specific tasks[6-23] and some have not found improvement in performance.[24-26] The differences in study results are speculated to be caused by varying athlete skill levels (novice vs. expert subjects), the use of general versus specific SVT programs, the lack of control or placebo training groups, and the lack of a sport-specific transfer test (referred to as perception-action coupling). Additionally, a variety of research design factors in many of these studies weakened the results and conclusions, indicating the need for further study in this area of sports vision.

Many SVT programs attempt to improve overall processing of visual information. Ultimately, the goal of the training procedures is to improve the speed and efficiency of the decision mechanism. This mechanism requires the athlete to know where crucial visual information exists, be able to direct attention to those crucial elements, select the best information from all that is available, organize and interpret the information in the most appropriate manner based on experience and memory of similar situations and information, and select the most accurate response with consideration of an anticipated action plan. Many studies have demonstrated that experienced athletes develop an organization of common sport situations into a knowledge architecture that offers many advantages, including the ability to process larger quantities of information in a short amount of time and the possibility of priming the perceptual and effector mechanisms for subsequent information.[27-33] Recent advances in perceptual learning paradigms coupled with new digital technologies provide potentially useful platforms for SVT approaches that develop sport-specific visual-cognitive abilities.

Many sports require the translation of visual information into motor responses. For example, a tennis player must identify the anticipated trajectory of the opponent's serve when the ball is struck and initiate the appropriate motor sequence to respond to that serve. SVT procedures that provide feedback regarding eye-hand, eye-foot, balance, and/or eye-body responses may assist the athlete in developing improved speed, efficiency, and automaticity of visuomotor response. This type of motor learning is thought to be the result of

improved synaptic efficiency,[34] and performance feedback is considered a critical element of enhancing performance of the perceptual and effector mechanisms.[34,35]

The ability to modulate attention appropriately, and often split attention among multiple stimuli,[36] is another valuable function of the decision mechanism in the information processing model. Many SVT procedures provide the opportunity for feedback to the athlete to facilitate development and control of visual attention. Additionally, as expertise is developed in a sport, the complex knowledge structures acquired facilitate expanded and enhanced use of mental imagery strategies. Mental rehearsal is the act of constructing mental images of an event, commonly used by elite athletes in preparation for performance.[33-41] Studies have demonstrated that mental imagery may share the same types of neural processes as visual perception, which has significant implications in sports.[42] Sport psychologists, and some sports vision practitioners, use methods designed to improve the mental imagery capacity and application by athletes,[42-45] although only anecdotal evidence supports the validity of this approach.

Many goals are possible for an SVT program; some are hierarchic and necessitate a sequential strategy for use of specific procedures. The information processing model detailed in Chapter 3 can provide a framework for understanding the connection between the specific procedures and visual performance factors and ultimately sports performance.

OVERVIEW OF SPORTS VISION TRAINING

Once a visual performance profile has been completed and specific training goals have been established, specialized training procedures can be selected to accomplish those goals. Many idiosyncratic approaches to the selection of training procedures are available, from generalized programs administered to every athlete to precise, diagnosis-specific and task-specific individualized programs that are largely unique to the exact needs of each athlete. Each sports vision practitioner develops the approach that best suits his or her mode of practice; however, universal guidelines exist for SVT that should be heeded.

Training Hierarchy for Procedures

The development of an SVT program requires the practitioner to establish a series of procedures designed to improve, and progressively challenge, the visual skill(s) targeted for enhancement. The most important requirement of selecting training procedures is that the activity being performed must directly relate to specific task demands of the sport. The athlete will rarely invest the requisite effort needed for vision skill enhancement if the purpose of the procedure is not understood and correlated with sports performance.

Basic skill development procedures should be performed before challenging the athlete with more multifaceted demands. The visual skill targeted for enhancement should initially be isolated to allow the athlete to become aware of the visual response. With awareness of a visual response, strategies to improve the quality of the visual response should be discussed and practiced. An additional benefit of visual response awareness is the salutary effect on locus of attention; athletes can develop better control over modulation of attention during performance. Once a high quality of visual response is consistently demonstrated, the athlete should be pushed to increase the speed of the response while maintaining quality. Perceptual learning research has shown better training efficacy when participants understand the accuracy of their responses, use highly motivating tasks, and receive consistent reinforcement about the stimuli that are to be learned.[46-48] The actual visual demands of the sport tasks should be considered when prescribing the training procedures; most visual demands encountered in sports occur well beyond arm's length and in nonprimary gaze positions. Therefore many SVT procedures are designed to have viewing distances greater than 3 m, and the gaze position is adjusted to match the ecologic demands of the sport. For example, training activities for a volleyball player would be modified to have the targets presented at far and in upgaze positions to simulate the demands frequently encountered in volleyball.

The ultimate goal of the training program is to achieve an effortless, reflexive level of performance excellence in the targeted visual response ability—a level sometimes referred to as automaticity of response.[49-51] The amount of attention that an individual must devote to accomplishing a task is a key variable in determining how automatic the response process is. A high level of automaticity allows the athlete to allocate attentional resources from visual performance factors to other important aspects of performance. Many methods are used in an effort to build automaticity of visual responses in a training program, most of which attempt to simulate the sport tasks ecologically and divert attention to additional tasks.

Many sports require the athlete to process visual information that is in motion and/or while the athlete is in motion. Training procedures that may initially be performed under static conditions therefore can be altered to add dynamic elements, such as incorporating movement of the target or athlete during performance. Automaticity of a visual skill response is often encouraged by modifying the training procedure from a paradigm of skill isolation to integration of additional visual skill demands. For example, the athlete attempts to maintain fixation on a swinging Marsden ball while balancing on a balance board and catching beanbags tossed from their peripheral visual field. Incorporating additional sensory demands is also common while performing a training procedure to more closely match the ecologic demands encountered in the sport situation and to build automaticity of the visual response. Common sensory integration demands include adding balance activities, auditory processing tasks, and increasing the levels of cognitive processing and distractions. These sensory integration demands serve to increase the stress experienced by the athlete and require the reallocation of attentional resources. Specific examples of all these automaticity variables are presented throughout this chapter.

The ultimate goal of SVT is to transfer visual skill improvements to the field of play. The practitioner should discuss strategies to facilitate skill transfer with the athlete. Recent perceptual learning research has demonstrated that learning is improved when individuals are presented with information from multiple sensory modalities, leading to better encoding and retrieval of perceptual information.[52] Similarly, training on a diverse set of stimuli can assist in the transfer of learning to untrained conditions.[53] Many of the approaches discussed for increasing automaticity of visual performance skills also provide a means of assisting transfer. For example, when an athlete can perform a visual task at a superior level despite many sensory integration demands, distractions, and stress loaded onto the activity, the more likely the athlete's visual system will continue to perform at an optimal level during high-stress moments of competition and despite significant physical fatigue. Furthermore, some "naturalistic" SVT procedures have the athlete practice actual or simulated sporting activities with the addition of specific training elements that alter or augment the visual demands.[54] Athletes, athletic trainers, coaches, and other ancillary personnel can be invaluable resources for assisting in the development of on-field modifications to training procedures, thereby providing additional support for the transfer of skill improvements.

Taxonomy of Sports Vision Training

This overview of SVT, as well as many of the published studies utilizing SVT, represents a predominantly component skill training approach. Component skill training is based on the construct of skilled motor performance as the outcome of many visual subprocesses. This type of SVT is designed to eliminate obstacles in the visual information processing pathway in order to optimize performance. In a review article, four types of component skill training approaches were identified: "*Low-Level Visual Instruments* that target foundational visual skills, *Perceptual-Cognitive Training Instruments* that target generalizable visual-cognitive abilities, *Visual-Motor Reaction Training* that targets neuromuscular function, and *Integrated Sensorimotor Batteries* that bridge all these domains."[54] Studies have demonstrated improvements in fundamental visual abilities when applying perceptual learning approaches to component skill training, showing that practice can produce substantial improvements that can last for months or years.[55] More importantly for SVT, perceptual learning benefits have been shown to transfer to new untrained contexts.[56,57]

As mentioned previously, some SVT approaches have the athlete practice actual or simulated sporting activities with the addition of specific training elements that alter or augment the visual demands. These approaches have been called naturalistic SVT approaches in contrast to component skill training because they do not reduce the training context to the foundational elements of visual information processing.[54] Naturalistic SVT procedures provide the athlete with a natural performance environment while facilitating manipulations that can accelerate skill development. In a review article, three types of naturalistic training approaches were highlighted: "*Stroboscopic Visual Training* that uses eyewear to interrupt normal visual input, *Eye Tracking* interventions that train gaze behavior, and *Simulations* that recreate the sporting environment in virtual reality contexts."[54] The perceptual learning literature suggests that transfer of a training effect is facilitated by the training and transfer tasks involving overlapping cognitive processes.[58] These principles of naturalistic training highlight perception-action coupling encompassing a high level of similarity between training and real-life performance.[59] Many SVT programs provide elements of both component skills training and naturalistic training approaches to maximize the benefits of the program.

Athlete/Patient Selection

An SVT program provides the athlete with the conditions and opportunity for the improvement of critical visual skills; the equipment or activities themself do not cause the changes in performance. A baseball player can spend many hours in batting practice to develop the requisite skills for success, but if proper coaching is not available the athlete may simply reinforce inefficient or ineffective skills. Similarly, an innovative new bicycle does not allow an athlete to win the Tour de France; the effective use of that bicycle, unflagging motivation, and many other intangibles culminate in success. Therefore athletes should be thoroughly counseled regarding the commitment required for a successful outcome from an SVT program. A typical program will require frequent training sessions and many hours of quality practice to enhance visual performance successfully, and the athlete needs to fully understand the nature of this commitment. If the practitioner is not convinced that the athlete possesses the essential resources of motivation, time, and support for success with an SVT program, the athlete should seek other approaches for enhancing sports performance.

Similar to most physical and psychologic enhancement programs, the more quality effort the athlete invests in the program, the greater the potential impact on sports performance. The athlete must have the motivation to devote sufficient time and energy into developing the targeted visual skills to achieve a successful outcome. A dedicated support network (e.g., coaches, parents, teammates, family, friends) is an invaluable asset for sustaining the motivation of an athlete throughout the course of the SVT program. Members of the support network can also serve as training partners for the athlete when practicing visual performance activities between training sessions. One of the best methods of generating motivation is excellent education regarding the connection between visual skill performance and sports performance. For example, the better the golfer understands how reduced depth judgment ability affects putting performance, the better the motivation will be to improve that visual skill. This also applies to the athlete's support network because coaches, trainers, and teammates can provide valuable performance feedback and reinforcement of proper skills during practice and competition.

Specific training goals should be established before initiating an SVT program and measurable outcomes are desirable in determining program success. Training goals must be as task specific as possible. For example, rather than the point guard in basketball setting a goal of being a better playmaker, the point guard can establish a goal of improving his or her ability to process more peripheral visual information when bringing the ball up the court. These specific sports goals should be matched with goals of improving the requisite, and measurable, visual performance skills necessary for success. Once the specific goals have been determined, more global competitive aspirations can be recognized to assist in motivating the athlete. For example, the basketball player may wish to be the starting point guard on the team, garner a college scholarship, or be drafted by a professional team. No matter what level of competition the athlete is in, visual performance goals can be established to provide a potentially critical competitive edge for peak performance.

Delivery of Sports Vision Training

Many approaches can be used for the delivery of SVT. Most practitioners use one-on-one training sessions to assess the athletes' current visual skill performance and push the demand level of those skills to a higher level. These sessions are typically conducted by the eye care practitioner or a trained assistant. Others develop training programs to be delivered to a team or group of athletes simultaneously, although this approach reduces the ability to adjust the training program to each athlete's individual visual performance needs. Once the threshold of performance ability is determined during a training session, activities are customarily prescribed to allow the athlete to practice at that high demand level until the next session. A regular schedule of progress evaluations should be established to periodically assess both subjective changes in sports performance and changes in objective visual performance skills. These progress evaluations serve to reinforce training goals, maintain athlete motivation, and determine when specific goals have been achieved.

When an SVT program is recommended to an athlete, an estimated treatment period should be determined. The practitioner and the athlete can then agree on the appropriate frequency of one-on-one training sessions, the length of time for each session, and the location for the sessions. Depending on the intensity of the training program and the availability of the athlete, training sessions may occur two to three times per week or every 2−3 weeks. Each training session usually lasts at least 30 min and may be scheduled for up to 90 min if needed. The practitioner typically delivers the training program at his or her office, where equipment and supplies are located; however, receiving the training at the athlete's sports training facility may be more convenient for the athlete. A candid discussion of the advantages and disadvantages of the available location options should occur and an agreeable solution reached before initiating the training program. Prescribed out-of-office training activities typically require an average of 30 min each day of dedicated practice and should be integrated with any existing training programs (e.g., weight training, speed training, skills practice) if possible. The incorporation of visual skills training with other training programs can help with compliance and transfer of skill improvements to sports performance. This is also an efficient approach because there are often periods of recovery during a program of strength and conditioning activities and the athlete can work on SVT procedures during these recovery periods. The athlete should understand that the quality and frequency of out-of-office practice produce the greatest impact on skill development, and the athlete should not assume that the one-on-one training sessions alone will improve performance.

Expectations of Sports Vision Training

As previously mentioned, specific training goals should be established before initiating an SVT program and training goals should be as task specific as possible. If these goals are reasonable and the potential outcomes of the training program are clear, the athlete is more likely to have a realistic expectation of the benefits of committing to the training program. If the athlete has unrealistically high expectations or the practitioner makes unrealistic promises, disappointing results are inevitable. The practitioner and athlete should acknowledge that the training program is designed to improve only one aspect of sports performance. Even though vision may be a critical factor for successful sports performance, many other aspects may hinder performance. If the practitioner makes unrealistic promises and is not successful in achieving those goals, the program will not be perceived as successful by the athlete and his or her support network. If the athlete perceives that SVT is unsuccessful, that perception will be difficult for the practitioner to overcome when it is communicated to others in the sporting community. The old adage that it is better to underpromise and overdeliver is particularly relevant when setting goals and promising outcomes from SVT programs.

VISION SKILL REMEDIATION AND ENHANCEMENT

Over the years, many practitioners have contributed suggestions and ideas for visual performance enhancement procedures to the collective community of sports vision practitioners. The origins of each procedure or modifications of a procedure are often hard to identify, making proper credit difficult. The following suggested procedures have been culled from publications, lectures, and professional interactions, which makes identification of individual sources even more difficult. Although the following procedures do not represent all training procedures that have been developed, they have all been found to be effective by the author in clinical practice.

Perceptual Mechanism

Visual sensitivity: acuity and contrast sensitivity

The primary goal of training is to improve the athlete's ability to discriminate subtle details in the sport environment. Many examples in sports exist in which an athlete must judge finely detailed information to determine the most appropriate response. For example, the more sensitive a golfer is to the subtle contours of the green, the better his or her judgment will be of the optimal putt trajectory. This example of putting includes resolution of the details of the green as well as any muted contrast changes induced by the surface contours and variations in the grass. Several procedures encourage interpretation of blurred images, which may also help extract detailed information from a rapidly moving object.

Ample evidence shows that the ability to resolve detail can be enhanced with practice, both for foveal detail[60-70] and parafoveal information.[71-77] Most of the studies have involved blur interpretation in subjects with myopia; however, most studies did not find a change in refractive status from the training.[60,70,78-80] Contrast sensitivity function has also been shown to be amenable to enhancement with practice,[66-68] as has vernier acuity.[77,81,82]

Lens sensitivity. This procedure introduces lenses of varying powers that the athlete must classify while viewing a distant target. This procedure is performed monocularly to eliminate the interaction with the vergence system, and the choice of fixation targets should relate to the task demands of the sport. For example, having a golfer fixate a golf ball positioned 3–6 m away rather than a chart of letters is preferable to simulate the visual task demands of golf. The athlete is asked to distinguish how the lens affected his or her view of the target. The athlete is encouraged to notice induced changes in size, location, and clarity of the target. Improved sensitivity to lens-induced changes of spatial information is theorized to have a salutary impact on depth discrimination because these monocular cues to depth are abundant in many sports tasks (e.g., catching a fly ball in baseball). An athlete may also notice a difference in the amount of effort required to achieve clarity with minus lenses, and this additional information should provide enough cues to discriminate a 0.25 D difference in lens powers. To promote improved sensitivity to retinal image size without the feedback from the accommodative system, iseikonic lenses can be substituted. Iseikonic lenses allow comparison of small changes in image size without changing the focusing demand for the target. Ultimately, sensitivity to 0.12 D and 0.5% magnification or minification changes should be the goal for sports requiring detail discrimination or precise depth judgments. Targets can also be presented in the athlete's periphery to stimulate improved sensitivity to peripheral discrimination, which may be valuable in sports such as downhill skiing.

As discussed in Chapter 3, the perception of motion in depth is partially produced by a changing retinal image size information system that operates relatively independent of the changing retinal disparity system.[83-85] Human beings possess cortical neurons that are selectively sensitive to changing image size, and these "looming" detectors provide a significant amount of information for judging time to contact even under monocular viewing conditions.[86-88] Binocular viewing has been shown to offer advantages in catching or hitting a ball[89-91]; however, monocular catching ability can be trained to similar skill levels as binocular viewing.[92] For sports that require an athlete to make rapid depth judgments of approaching objects (e.g., a tennis ball), sensitivity to subtle changes in image size may provide a valuable advantage.

Howard-Dolman sensitivity. A Howard-Dolman apparatus can be used to enhance sensitivity to monocular cues to depth. A traditional Howard-Dolman device is a modification of the apparatus designed to measure the empirical longitudinal horopter and uses two rods of equal size and color to be viewed in primary gaze position through an aperture in a rectangular box of a homogeneous color (see Fig. 4.4).[93-95] The athlete makes depth judgments concerning the apparent location of the two rods under monocular viewing conditions instead of the traditional binocular method. This procedure can be further modified for sports purposes by substituting two identical balls or objects, such as golf balls, tennis balls, or shooting clays.[1] The initial goal of training is to refine the athlete's sensitivity to subtle monocular cues to depth. The athlete is then obligated to make the depth judgments in progressively shorter periods (tachistoscopic presentation).

Prism sensitivity. Low amounts of prism are used to increase visual sensitivity to target movement in a similar manner as lens sensitivity. A prism is introduced monocularly, with a random orientation of the prism base, while the athlete views a fixation target such as a golf ball, soccer ball, or shooting target. The initial goal for the athlete is to detect the direction of the target movement induced by the prism. As the athlete becomes more accurate in identifying spatial shifts stimulated with very small amounts of prism (e.g., $0.5-1^\Delta$), the athlete is encouraged to make those fine judgments in progressively shorter time intervals.

Haidinger brush fixation. In sports that require steadiness of fixation, such as target shooting, the visual biofeedback provided by the entoptic phenomenon of a Haidinger brush can be valuable. The perception of the Haidinger brush is generated by variable absorption of plane-polarized light by Henle fiber layer of the macular retina.[96] The athlete learns to maintain accurate and steady fixation of the Haidinger brush and achieves a proper state of concentration, reducing the tendency for fixation to drift off target. Di Russo et al.[97] demonstrated that elite shooters possess better fixational ability than novice shooters and can maintain the accuracy of fixation despite the presence of distractions. The Bernell Macula Integrity Tester 2 (www.bernell.com) is a commercially available device that produces the entopic phenomenon; many slides are available that contain various fixation targets (Fig. 8.1). The athlete should become aware of the feeling required for the proper concentration needed to maintain accurate and steady fixation in order to reproduce that level of concentration during sport practice and competition. As the accuracy and steadiness of fixation improve, distractions should be introduced during Haidinger brush training to simulate competition conditions and build automaticity of concentration and fixation.

Blur interpretation activities. Many studies have successfully demonstrated the ability to improve the threshold visual acuity level in subjects after a course of training.[15,60-69] The procedures used to improve acuity generally involve the reduction of target size or clarity to a level that is barely subthreshold for the subject and then guessing is encouraged as the targets are changed. Ample feedback is provided with each guess until the accuracy of target discrimination improves to a satisfactory level, at which time the target size or clarity is further reduced to a subthreshold level. When using this paradigm with athletes, the ability to discriminate subtle details from blurred or minuscule targets is enhanced. In sports that require rapid discrimination, such as batting in baseball, tachistoscopic presentation of stimuli is introduced as each level of performance is mastered.

Many targets and methods for reducing image clarity can be used to enhance the sensitivity of visual discrimination (Box 8.1). Random sequences of letters and numbers can be printed from a computer by using progressively smaller font sizes, and those targets can be held at increasing distances from the athlete as he or she attempts to discriminate the targets. The targets can be further degraded by having the subject view through filters that decrease the amount of visible light transmission or by reducing the light levels on the targets, thereby increasing the demand on contrast sensitivity to discriminate the targets. The athlete can also wear lenses that induce blur, such as lenses that overplus the athlete or lenses with degraded optics (e.g., stippled lenses). Bangerter foils can also be used to provide a graded reduction in acuity through the lenses (Fig. 8.2). These same acuity-degrading lenses can be worn during practice sessions of the athlete's sport (e.g., during putting practice in golf), and the athlete can experience the perceived enhancement of visual discrimination when the lenses are removed. The steps for this type of SVT procedure are (1) practice the activity without the foil goggles for a short period (e.g., 2-5 min); (2) repeat the activity with the foil goggles for 5-10 min, work to increasing foil density (change

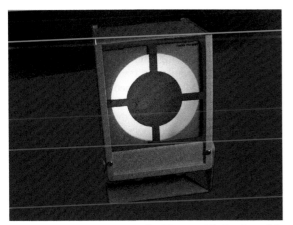

FIG. 8.1 The Macula Integrity Tester with fixation slide (www.bernell.com).

> **BOX 8.1**
> **Visual Discrimination Demands**
>
> Threshold acuity targets or increasing distance
> Bangerter foils
> Degraded optics (e.g., stippled lenses)
> Lenses with excessive plus power
> Lenses with excessive minus power (minification)
> Iseikonic lenses
> Dark filters
> Reduced light levels

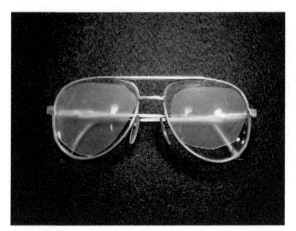

FIG. 8.2 Bangerter foils to reduce vision through a patient's spectacles.

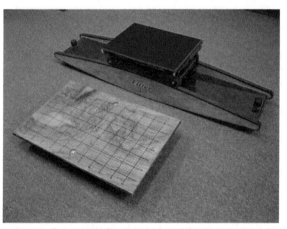

FIG. 8.3 Two types of commonly available balance boards.

foils after three to five successes at a level); and (3) remove the foil goggles and repeat activity for at least 5 min to maximize retention of improved performance. The safety of the athlete must be preserved during this activity, especially when a risk to the athlete is present, such as during batting practice in baseball. The use of sports protective eyewear for the training is recommended when there is any perceived risk to the athlete. As described with the other visual sensitivity training activities, tachistoscopic presentation of stimuli is another important step for enhancing the speed of visual discrimination.

Ultimeyes (www.ultimeyesvision.com) is a custom video application incorporating diverse stimuli, adaptive near-threshold training with learning-optimized flickering stimuli, and multisensory feedback in a digital training program designed to improve foundational aspects of visual sensitivity by applying the tenets of perceptual learning. In a series of studies, the Ultimeyes app has demonstrated improvements in visual acuity and contrast sensitivity in both nonathletes and athletes, as well as improved batting performance in collegiate baseball players.[15,98] There are other computer-based applications that are available to train visual acuity and contrast sensitivity, but these are not constructed for sport-specific purposes.

As previously discussed, incorporating additional sensory demands while performing these visual sensitivity training procedures is essential to more closely match the ecologic demands encountered in the sport situation and to build automaticity of the visual response. Many of these procedures allow the practitioner to include the addition of balance activities, auditory processing tasks, and increased levels of cognitive

processing and distractions in order to increase the stress experienced by the athlete (Box 8.2). Cognitive demands can be included in two principle approaches: questions that the athlete must attempt to answer while performing the task or verbal distractions that the athlete must ignore. The choice of cognitive demands is based on the task demands of the sport. Balance activities typically entail the use of balance boards (Fig. 8.3) or walking rails (Fig. 8.4). The training effect from these types of procedures has been shown to transfer to stimuli not used during training[63–65,69] and to improvements in contrast sensitivity function.[66–68] Evidence also exists that the training effect is produced at a level beyond the retina because the training effect has been shown to transfer to an untrained eye.[63,70] Training with sport-specific stimuli, such as baseball pitches, has also been shown to improve dynamic visual acuity and batting ability.[22]

Dynamic visual acuity

Many sports require the athlete to discriminate visual information that is moving, such as judging the speed and trajectory of a tennis serve. Traditional static visual acuity training may not fully address the visual demands encountered in some types of sports. Athlete

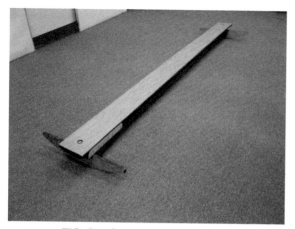

FIG. 8.4 An adjustable walking rail.

attributes that can affect dynamic visual acuity (DVA) include the resolving power of the retina (visual sensitivity), peripheral awareness, oculomotor abilities (pursuit and saccadic eye movements), and psychologic functions that affect interpretation of visual information.[99–122] DVA has been shown to be improvable with training,[123,124] with the training effect being most evident for the most challenging stimuli and tasks used in the studies.[124] Enhancement training for DVA is frequently recommended for athletes.[1,5,51,125–130] However, the nature of the training varies tremendously and few instruments are available to generate the necessary targets. Some practitioners recommend using targets that move toward the athlete[125] and some advocate for rotational targets.[1,125] Incorporation of a tachistoscopic presentation of the moving stimuli is valuable in sports for which the athlete must quickly fixate critical visual information and discriminate vital details, as in judging the trail contours when mountain biking. A study with collegiate softball players found that a program of SVT improved performance on the Target Capture (DVA) assessment of the Senaptec Sensory Station.[21]

Rotators with disks and charts. Target size is selected at a level that is at threshold for the athlete, and the target is placed on a rotating disk (see Fig. 4.1) and rotated at a speed that is too fast for the athlete to discriminate the target. Many targets can be used to enhance the sensitivity of visual discrimination while the targets are in motion. The athlete is encouraged to guess what the target is as the speed is slowly reduced to the point where accurate discrimination is achieved. Ample feedback is provided with each guess until the accuracy of target discrimination improves to

a satisfactory level, at which time the target size is further reduced to a new threshold level or the athlete is moved further from the target. When using this modified paradigm of method of limits, the ability to discriminate subtle details from rapidly moving targets is enhanced. This approach is meaningful for sports in which the movement of the target is mainly predictable (e.g., a baseball pitch); however, it may have a limited benefit in unpredictable sports (e.g., downhill skiing). Additional visual discrimination demands and sensory integration burdens can be added to this task, as previously described with blur interpretation activities.

Wayne tachistoscope rotator activities. The Wayne Tachistoscope Rotator Scanner was composed of two prisms that could be rotated in front of a Perceptamatic tachistoscope lens (Fig. 8.5). The speed at which each prism rotated could be adjusted between 20 and 240 rpm, allowing a projected image to move in a variety of directions. A variety of slide reels were available with images of numbers, arrows, patterns, and sports images (e.g., football, baseball pitches). These images could be presented for durations between 1 and 0.01 s, facilitating the training of short-exposure dynamic visual acuity. The product is no longer available and there is currently no similar product available. It is possible to program a computer-based application to replicate the vision demands created by this instrument and repeatability could be improved with a digital version. The use of ecologically appropriate targets or real-time videos would be preferred in order to produce a better simulation of the DVA demands encountered in a sport; however, gathering a suitable library of sport-specific images or

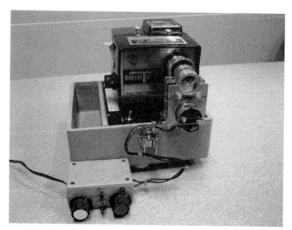

FIG. 8.5 The Wayne Tachistoscope rotator scanner.

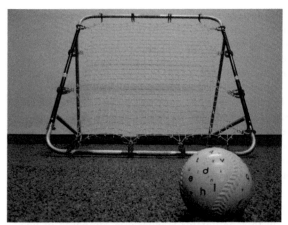

FIG. 8.6 A rubber baseball with letter stickers in front of a pitchback.

videos from the athletes' perspective would require considerable resources.

Pitchback or ball machine with ball and letters. A rubber or soft baseball with letter stickers placed randomly around the ball is commonly used for the pitchback procedure (Fig. 8.6). The athlete throws the ball into a pitchback net and attempts to locate and fixate one of the letters on the ball during the return flight. As the athlete's ability to discriminate the letters improves, the ball is thrown faster into the net; more spin can be induced by the athlete during the throw. To add a level of unpredictability to the task, the ball can be thrown by another person, thereby requiring the athlete to rapidly judge the speed and trajectory of the ball during flight. Once the athlete can demonstrate consistently accurate ability in this task, additional visual discrimination demands and sensory integration burdens can be added. If a pitchback is not available, the athlete can have someone throw the ball back, bounce the ball against a wall, or throw the ball high in the air to simulate the sport demands.

A variation in this procedure is the use of a ball machine rather than a pitchback. The distance and speed of the ball machine can be set for the preferred demand level. The machine is loaded with balls containing images to be discerned by the athlete, such as colors, shapes, numbers, or letters. The athlete is instructed to respond to a specific target (e.g., balls with a green dot or letter) and inhibit response to other targets (e.g., balls with a red dot or numbers). This modification can be done with tennis and baseball, softball, or cricket batting.

Accommodation and vergence facility

Accommodative and vergence facility training procedures aspire to improve the ability to rapidly adjust focus and eye alignment for the variety of fixation distances encountered in sports. Two principal methods are used to change accommodative and vergence demands: the use of lenses or prisms to alter the accommodative and vergence demands at a fixed distance and the use of charts or targets at different distances, with fixation being rapidly alternated between the targets. When lenses are introduced, the accommodative system must adjust ciliary muscle tonus to regain image clarity; however, the vergence system must remain aligned with the plane of the target to prevent diplopia. This separation of accommodation and vergence is a common method to improve relative accommodative facility binocularly at near in patients with asthenopia during near work.[131–133] However, it is not generally representative of the visual task demands experienced in sports. Charts or targets placed at different distances allow the accommodative and vergence responses to remain paired. Therefore procedures that use targets at a variety of different distances may be more appropriate for enhancing the strength and flexibility of focusing and eye alignment in athletes. A study with collegiate softball players found that a program of SVT that included distance rock activities improved performance on the Near-Far Quickness assessment of the Senaptec Sensory Station.[21] If a student athlete has symptoms of asthenopia during near work, the more traditional use of lenses and prisms may be warranted to alleviate those symptoms. A study of female ball sports athletes at a university found that some aspects of vergence function were effectively improved by an SVT program and that the effects were retained after 4 weeks.[20]

Distance rock. Charts with random letters (Fig. 8.7) are placed at a relatively far distance from the athlete, usually more than 10 feet, and at a near distance, usually within 50 cm. The athlete stands as far away from the distant chart as possible while still being able to read the letters. The athlete should start by holding the near chart at arm's length and slowly move it closer until the letters are too blurred to recognize. The athlete should take 2–3 s to try to clear the letters before adjusting the chart to a slightly further distance, where the letters can again be cleared. The task requires the athlete to then clear and call out successive letters on each chart alternately as rapidly as possible, making sure to achieve maximal visual clarity with each fixation. This procedure initially can be performed monocularly to equalize accommodative facility in each eye

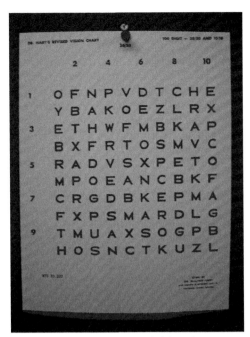

FIG. 8.7 Hart's revised vision chart.

Lens rock procedures are usually performed monocularly at first, and binocular lens rock procedures are introduced once an acceptable level of performance is achieved monocularly. Lens flippers of various powers are used for binocular training; one side of the flippers contains minus lenses and the other side has plus lenses. Once the athlete can demonstrate consistently accurate precision and speed on this procedure, additional visual discrimination demands and sensory integration burdens can be added.

The goal of lens rock training is to increase the speed and accuracy of the accommodative response induced by the lenses. Although remedial vision therapy for accommodative dysfunctions emphasizes development of the ability to clear relatively large lens powers rapidly (e.g., +2.50/−2.50 D), this may not offer a significant advantage for an athlete during sports performance. As previously mentioned with lens sensitivity procedures, sensitivity to subtle changes in image size may provide a valuable advantage through enhanced sensitivity to monocular cues to depth. Therefore awareness of image size changes with brisk accommodative changes may yield supplementary performance benefits above the traditional goal of extending the range of accommodation.

Prism rock. Prism sensitivity should be performed before initiating training with prism rock procedures to ensure that the athlete can accurately identify spatial shifts stimulated with very small amounts of prism (e.g., $0.5-1^{\Delta}$). Prism flippers of various powers are used for vergence facility training; one side of the flippers contains base-out prisms and the other side has base-in prisms. A threshold acuity target is placed at an appropriate distance based on the task demands of the sport. One side of the prism flippers is placed in front of the athlete's eyes and the athlete is instructed to make the target single and clear again as rapidly as possible. The athlete should be able to feel the difference between a positive and negative fusional vergence demand. Once the athlete can demonstrate consistently accurate precision and speed on this procedure, additional visual discrimination demands and sensory integration burdens can be added.

The goal of prism rock training is to increase the speed and accuracy of the vergence response induced by the prisms. Although remedial vision therapy for vergence anomalies emphasizes development of ability to rapidly fuse relatively large prism powers (e.g., 10^{Δ} base out/10^{Δ} base in), this may not offer a significant advantage for an athlete during sports performance. Similar to lens rock procedures, awareness of image size changes

individually, and the choice of viewing distance and positions of gaze should be based on the task demands of the sport. Once the athlete can demonstrate consistently accurate precision and speed on this task, additional visual discrimination demands and sensory integration burdens can be added.

Lens rock. A chart with random letters or words (e.g., reduced Hart chart, accommodative rock cards) is placed at a near distance, usually 40 cm. Lenses of various powers are placed in front of the athlete's eyes and the athlete is instructed to make the letters or words clear again as rapidly as possible. The athlete should be able to feel the difference between when accommodation is stimulated and when accommodation is released. Monocular lens sorting is a useful procedure for developing awareness of accommodative effort. Lens sorting requires the athlete to organize a variety of loose lenses into a sequence based on power. For example, a series of minus lenses is provided, ranging from −0.50 D to −4.00 D in 0.50-D steps. The athlete is instructed to clear a designated target through each lens; based on the apparent changes in image size and the accompanying feeling of accommodative effort, the athlete arranges the lenses from the weakest to the strongest power. A typical goal is sensitivity to differences of 0.25 D.

and apparent spatial localization shifts induced by brisk vergence changes may yield supplementary performance benefits beyond the traditional goal of extending the range of fusional vergence. The athlete is encouraged to localize the perceived location of the target through each prism power to provide feedback regarding spatial judgments.

Eye movements

The ability to maintain fixation of a rapidly moving object is frequently a critical aspect for allowing visual processing of crucial information in sports. The ability to change fixation from one location to another rapidly and accurately is also an essential aspect of many sports tasks. In nondynamic sports such as precision target shooting, the ability to maintain steady fixation is a vital aspect of successful performance. Many training procedures have been developed to provide feedback regarding performance accuracy and speed of eye movements. Most of these procedures applied to athletes are modified therapy procedures originally designed to improve deficient eye movements in children, and the primary goal for these procedures is to improve eye movement efficiency for reading-type tasks.[131–133] The Haidinger brush fixation activity previously described can be used to enhance control of fixation steadiness by providing direct visual feedback. A task analysis of the specific eye movement demands involved in an athlete's sport gives the practitioner essential insight that can be used to modify therapy procedures to target specific sport-related eye movement skill development.

Poor eye movement control is difficult to find in a successful athlete; this deficiency is more commonly found in the emerging youth athlete who is attempting to acquire performance skills. These young athletes are more apt to yield significant benefits from training procedures directed at improving eye movement efficiency. For the more seasoned athlete, the goal is often enhancement of performance capacity during high-stress situations in which accurate and rapid eye movement control is a critical factor. Ultimately the goal of enhancement training is to improve automaticity of eye movement performance so that minimal attention is required for skilled performance.[49–51] The work of Hebb[134] and others[135–137] supports the concept that development of visual performance skills should be elevated to a level that requires minimal attention so that attention can be selectively distributed to other crucial aspects of performance. Eye movement training must involve additional sensory integration burdens and cognitive processing demands to elevate the athlete's automaticity of accurate eye movement control and ability to modulate attention during performance.

Pursuit eye movements. The Marsden ball is commonly used to provide feedback regarding pursuit eye movement accuracy. The Marsden ball is a soft baseball with random letters placed around the sphere that is suspended from the ceiling with a string that allows it to swing in various trajectories (Fig. 8.8). The athlete is challenged to maintain fixation on specific letters on the ball while it is swung in various patterns. The exercise typically begins with the ball swinging on a plane perpendicular to the athlete's line of sight so the relative depth of the ball does not change while it is swinging. The athlete is encouraged to maintain a steady head position with instructions to only follow the ball with his or her eyes. When performance becomes smooth and efficient, the ball is swung in elliptical trajectories that induce changes in relative depth throughout the course the ball travels.

The athlete should be given verbal feedback regarding the accuracy of smooth pursuit eye movement performance during this activity so that he or she becomes aware when pursuit eye movements break down into saccades. A visual afterimage can be used to improve the feedback for the athlete when he or she has difficulty elevating the awareness of pursuit eye movement accuracy. An afterimage can be generated with a masked camera flash or similar commercially available device (Fig. 8.9). The athlete is asked to fixate a central spot monocularly on the flash unit held with the light portion oriented vertically approximately 25 cm from the eyes and the light is flashed. The athlete should

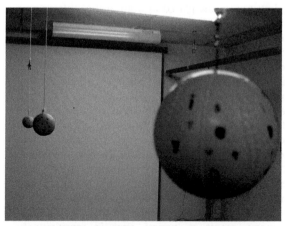

FIG. 8.8 Marsden balls suspended from the ceiling.

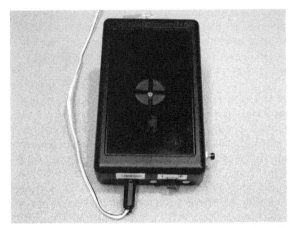

FIG. 8.9 The Bernell after image generator (www.bernell. com).

then see a vertical streak of light wherever fixation is directed so that fixation accuracy can be monitored while pursuing the Marsden ball. If the athlete is having difficulty seeing the afterimage, rapid blinking and dimming the room lights should enhance the appearance of the image.

Once the athlete has achieved accurate pursuit eye movement performance with the Marsden ball, sensory integration activities are incorporated. A motor response is commonly added to the task by asking the athlete to locate and point at letters on the ball as an index finger pokes the letter on the ball hard enough to make it swing in an arc away from the athlete. Each time the ball swings back toward the athlete, he or she is instructed to locate and track a different letter until he or she can alternately poke it with the right or left index finger. Another motor element that can be added to the Marsden ball procedure is to have the athlete hold a stringless racquet (tennis, squash, racquetball) under the ball while it is swinging. The athlete is further instructed to raise the racquet on command and encircle, or hoop, the swinging ball without touching either the ball or the string.

Because many sports require the athlete to track a moving object or person while maintaining balance, adding a balance demand to the Marsden ball activity is particularly beneficial. The athlete is instructed to stand on a balance board and achieve steady balance while fixating a motionless Marsden ball. Once the athlete has attained steady balance, the ball is swung while the athlete attempts to maintain balance and fixation with smooth pursuit eye movements. Pursuit eye movements will induce vestibular responses that the athlete must override to maintain steady balance. The

athlete can be further challenged with the elliptical trajectories and motor response activities previously described. Additionally, if the athlete competes in a sport that requires awareness of peripheral information while processing central visual information, the trainer can randomly toss beanbags at the athlete from a peripheral location that the athlete must either catch or block during performance. This is also an excellent activity to add cognitive challenges to the task demand. The athlete can be instructed to either answer questions that are asked at random intervals during performance or ignore the distracting chatter in the background.

Saccadic eye movements. Charts with random letters (see Fig. 8.7) are placed at a relatively far distance from the athlete, usually 10 feet or more. The task requires the athlete to find and call out successive letters on the chart as rapidly as possible, making sure to achieve visual clarity with each fixation. The athlete is instructed to call out the first letter and last letter of each row (O, E, Y, X, etc.) until the bottom of the chart is reached. With successful execution of this task, the athlete is instructed to call out the second letter and the next-to-last letter of each row, the third letter and the third-from-last letter of each row, or other challenging saccade patterns. Multiple charts can also be used, with fixations moving either in a predetermined sequence between charts or at the command of the trainer. Accuracy of saccadic performance can be monitored through observation by the trainer and verbal feedback provided to the athlete regarding any overshooting or undershooting of saccadic eye movements. Further visual feedback can be provided with a visual afterimage, as previously described. The goal is smooth, quick performance with each pattern of saccadic eye movements.

Once the athlete can demonstrate consistently accurate precision and speed on this task, additional visual discrimination demands and sensory integration burdens can be added. The use of a metronome is a particularly effective method for enhancing auditory-visual integration, and increasing the pace of the metronome can generate performance stress similar to athletic competition. When adding a metronome to this procedure, the athlete is challenged to correctly call out a letter on each successive chart with the beat from the metronome. Polarizing filters also can be worn to increase the contrast demand of the task, or lenses with degraded optics can be used to simultaneously enhance blur interpretation. Because many sports require the athlete to make rapid saccadic eye movements while maintaining balance, adding a balance demand to this activity is particularly beneficial. The athlete is instructed to stand on a balance board and maintain steady balance while performing the saccadic task. Additionally, if the athlete competes in a sport that requires awareness of peripheral information while processing central visual information, the trainer can randomly toss beanbags at the athlete from a peripheral location that the athlete must either catch or block during performance.

A chart with arrows pointing in random directions can be substituted for a letter chart (Fig. 8.10). The arrow chart provides a method for adding a motor performance feature to the saccadic eye movement tasks. For example, the athlete can be instructed to move his or her feet in the direction of the arrow being named (right, forward, etc.) or move a balance board in the direction indicated by each arrow. This sensory integration activity can also be performed with the athlete's hands or while holding a racquet, bat, or hockey stick, for example. Computer programs also are available for saccadic eye movement training with an arrow stimulus in a random orientation presented in a random location of the computer monitor that the athlete must respond to as quickly as possible by moving a joystick (or arrow key) in the same direction as the arrow. This is also an excellent activity to add cognitive challenges to the task demand. The athlete can be instructed to either answer questions that are asked at random intervals during performance or ignore the distracting chatter in the background.

Eye tracking and quiet eye training. The advent of lightweight portable eye tracking technology has allowed for evaluation and feedback of eye movements in sporting activities that are carried out in natural settings. These systems typically consist of two cameras mounted on an eyeglass-type frame: one to monitor eye position and one to monitor the scene (point-of-view) with an external camera that is positioned to monitor motor performance characteristics. The data collected by the mobile eye tracker is then synchronized with the elements of motor performance using software programs that can operate in real time.

Studies with such mobile eye trackers have typically found that experts have a lower number of fixations that occur for longer durations than do novices during the viewing of specific sport situations (this is referred to as the quiet eye [QE]), especially when the subjects are required to move while gaze behaviors are recorded.[138,139] Furthermore, for expert performers, fixations are typically clustered on features that provide the most information about the task being viewed.[140] The exact neural mechanisms that direct gaze behavior during QE are still under investigation; however, it appears to show an advantageous period of cognitive processing allowing for computation of force, direction, and velocity that guide and fine-tune the motor response.[141]

QE training typically involves the use of feedback to educate athletes about the importance of maintaining a longer QE duration.[139] Understanding the optimal visual search pattern, fixation location, attentional control, and onset of the QE fixation for specific sport tasks are critical elements of the training. In addition, training of attentional control is typically accomplished by developing a preperformance routine.[142]

Abundant research provides support for QE training in several sport applications, with many studies reporting benefits that persist for days or weeks. For example, studies have found that QE training can improve accuracy in golf putting performance, even under simulated pressure.[143–146] In basketball, QE training has demonstrated improvements in free throw shooting percentage and jump shot performance in game situations.[147–149] QE training has resulted in improved accuracy and ability to cope with pressure when taking penalty kicks in soccer.[150] International-level skeet shooters demonstrated

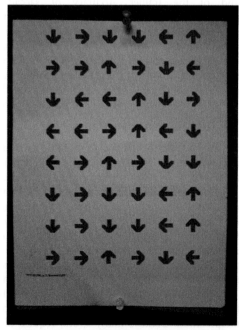

FIG. 8.10 A modified Kirschner arrows chart.

better shooting accuracy following three QE training sessions.[151] Furthermore, there is evidence that QE training has a positive effect on the development of ball throwing and catching in children with typical development, and also in those with developmental coordination disorder.[152] Collectively, these studies support the contention that the use of eye tracking technology can facilitate the development of improved visuomotor behaviors and control of attention and anxiety under pressure.

Several companies market complete mobile eye tracking systems for use with sport applications, such as SensoMotoric Instruments (www.smivision.com/en/gaze-and-eye-tracking-systems/applications/sports-professional-training-education.html), Tobii Pro (www.tobiipro.com/fields-of-use/human-performance/), and Arrington Research (www.arringtonresearch.com). There are also less expensive monitor-based systems, but these platforms may not provide the same benefits as training in the natural sport environment.

Speed and accuracy of depth perception

Many sport tasks require judgments of depth and spatial localization. In sports such as golf, precise localization is a critical factor in the short game, but the golfer is not required to make depth judgments rapidly. In contrast, spatial localization in American football can tolerate less precision, yet the athlete is required to make depth judgments very quickly. The amount of innervation exerted by each of the six extraocular muscles in each eye to align on a target or object provides some of the information necessary to judge depth, and significant heterophorias should be treated by traditional methods applied to nonathletes.[4,131–133] Strength and flexibility in vergence function should provide better stability of depth information to the athlete, particularly when the athlete must deal with excessive fatigue and psychologic stress. However, narrower vergence ranges have been found when comparing athlete to nonathlete populations, leading to the speculation that this may relate to more precise spatial judgment ability.[2,153,154] A study with collegiate ice hockey players found a program of SVT improved base-out vergence ranges.[18] Most SVT programs include procedures that provide feedback regarding depth judgments and many include feedback from changing vergence demands to stimulate sensitivity to alterations in relative depth. A program of SVT with collegiate baseball players was found to improve depth perception; however, the study design and method for measuring stereopsis contained significant shortcomings that curtail its conclusions.[155]

Brock string. The Brock string is a long white string of different colored beads (Fig. 8.11). One end of the

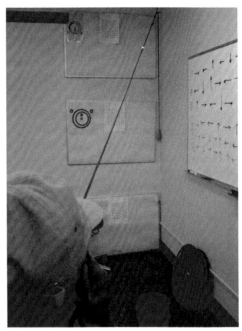

FIG. 8.11 A long brock string exercise being performed in the upgaze position.

string is held against the tip of the patient's nose and the other end can be either held by the clinician or tied to an object (e.g., a doorknob). The beads typically are placed in primary gaze position at near, intermediate, and far distances from the athlete. The athlete is instructed to look at a bead and report what is seen. Two strings should be seen in front of the bead and two strings seen emerging from behind the bead, with the strings forming an X at the bead. If the X appears to cross in front of or behind the bead, this represents an eso or exo fixation disparity, respectively. However, if the fixated bead is located beyond approximately 2 m, most patients will see the strings crossing in front of the bead because of the relative enlargement of Panum fusional area. If diplopic images of the string are not seen behind or in front of the bead, the athlete is likely cortically suppressing the information from one eye. The athlete should be instructed to blink his or her eyes rapidly to break the suppression or red/green filters may be worn to monitor any suppression more effectively.

The primary goal of the Brock string procedure is to provide visual feedback on the location of the visual axes when viewing an object. With practice, the athlete can learn to align the visual axes with the object, theoretically enhancing the precision of spatial localization provided by the extraocular muscles. The string can be moved from primary gaze position to other positions that simulate the task demands of the sport, such as viewing in baseball batting stance or golf putting stance. The athlete is assigned to practice alternately jumping from the far bead to the middle bead and then to the near bead. During practice, the athlete should be aware of the X pattern of the strings, and where it crosses, when fusing each bead so that quick, accurate alignment is reinforced. The athlete should be encouraged to become sensitive to the mental state that accompanies successful performance to facilitate transfer to the playing field.

Once the athlete can demonstrate consistently accurate precision and speed on this task, additional visual discrimination demands and sensory integration burdens can be added. Lenses and prisms can be introduced to add visual skill demands to the task. Because many sports require the athlete to shift eye alignment rapidly while maintaining balance, the addition of a balance demand to this activity is particularly beneficial. The athlete is instructed to stand on a balance board and maintain steady balance while performing the Brock string task. This is also an excellent activity to add cognitive challenges to the task demand.

Howard-Dolman training. A Howard-Dolman apparatus can be used to enhance sensitivity to binocular cues to depth. As previously described for monocular cues to depth, a traditional Howard-Dolman device uses two rods of equal size and color to be viewed in the primary gaze position (see Fig. 4.4).[93-95] The athlete makes depth judgments concerning the apparent location of the two rods under binocular viewing conditions in "real" space rather than simulated depth. This procedure can be further modified for sports purposes by substituting two identical balls or objects, such as golf balls, tennis balls, or shooting clays.[1] The initial goal of training is to refine the athlete's sensitivity to subtle cues to depth, and the athlete is subsequently obligated to make the depth judgments in progressively shorter periods (tachistoscopic presentation). The athlete can also move from primary gaze position to other positions that simulate the task demands of the sport, such as viewing in baseball batting stance or golf putting stance.

Simulated depth activities. Many therapy procedures are commonly used to treat anomalies of binocular vision with either polarizing or colored filters to simulate stereopsis. Vectograms are targets with oppositely polarized portions that allow the athlete to see some

portions with the right eye and some with the left eye when wearing polarizing filters with crossed axes. Tranaglyphs are examples of anaglyphic targets that use red and green targets to simulate depth when red/green filters are worn. Both systems provide feedback concerning suppression, although polarizing filters provide a closer approximation of natural conditions because no chromatic interval is induced by the filters.

Vectograms and tranaglyphs are typically used at near-viewing distances to increase positive and negative fusional vergence ranges (Fig. 8.12).[4,131-133] For athletes, training depth perception at far distances is often more appropriate, and large vergence ranges may only offer a benefit if the athlete has a significant heterophoria at far. The goal of SVT is development of accuracy of depth localization with vectogram or tranaglyph targets projected onto an appropriate screen. Tranaglyph targets can be projected onto a white screen; however, vectograms require a silverized screen to preserve the polarization. A small amount of positive fusional vergence demand is created by separating the target so that the target seen by the right eye is to the left of the target seen by the left eye. The common perception induced by a relative base-out demand is for the image to appear slightly smaller and closer in toward the observer; conversely, a relative base-in demand will produce the perception of the image becoming slightly larger and further out (away) from the observer. These spatial perception effects are referred to as SILO (smaller *in*, larger *out*). The SILO perception in the example described should cause the image to appear closer to the athlete than the screen and the image should seem slightly smaller. If the athlete can fuse the image without suppression, he or she is asked to report the

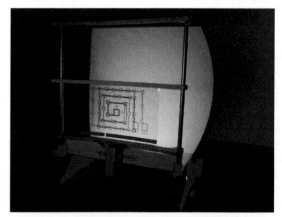

FIG. 8.12 A spirangle variable vectogram on a dynamic fusion slides holder (www.vteshop.com).

exact location of the target. The trainer can wave a hand or meter stick to help the athlete report the apparent plane of the target image; typically the trainer starts by waving his or her hand at the plane of the screen and slowly moves toward the athlete. This training enhances the sensitivity of extraocular muscle information for the discrimination of relative depth judgments.

Once the athlete becomes proficient at making depth localization judgments with the targets, the speed of stereopsis is enhanced. The athlete is first asked to localize a target with a moderate demand to positive fusional vergence and then turn and face away from the target. While the athlete is facing away, the positive fusional vergence demand is either increased or decreased a small amount. The athlete is then instructed to look again and quickly determine if the target is at the same relative location, slightly closer, or slightly further away. In this manner the athlete becomes more sensitive to small changes in spatial localization and receives feedback regarding rapid depth judgments.

Once the athlete can demonstrate consistently accurate precision and speed on this task, additional sensory integration burdens can be added. A balance board or mini-trampoline can be added to this procedure to add proprioceptive challenges for the athlete and help build performance automaticity. The mini-trampoline is used in a manner similar to that previously described for the balance board. The athlete is instructed to maintain steady balance while rhythmically jumping on the mini-trampoline and performing the vectogram or tranaglyph task. The athlete can also move from primary gaze position to other positions that simulate the task demands of the sport, such as viewing in baseball batting stance or golf putting stance.

Fixation disparity. Precise and stable eye alignment (measured as fixation disparity) has been suggested to be crucial in sports that require precise spatial localization.[1] Training targets that give the athlete visual feedback regarding eye alignment are readily available in many anaglyphic and polarized vision therapy activities used to improve vergence function, as previously described for simulated depth activities. For example, many vectograms have an "R" seen by the right eye directly above an "L" seen by the left eye. The vertical alignment of these letters indicates the status of fixation disparity. Other targets can be easily modified to provide alignment feedback, such as drawing nonius line markings inside the circles on the lifesaver card (Fig. 8.13). Sports Fixation Cards were developed by Bernell (www.bernell.com) for this purpose. These targets typically include a fusional

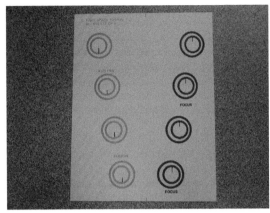

FIG. 8.13 Nonius line markings on a free space fusion card for feedback regarding fixation disparity.

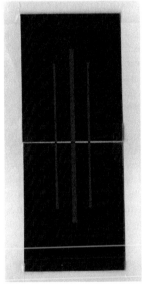

FIG. 8.14 Fixation disparity targets with no vergence demand using cross-polarizing filters and hand-drawn nonius lines; designed by Coffey.

vergence demand in addition to feedback regarding fixation disparity; however, it may not be necessary to enhance vergence ranges in some athletes. Dr. Bradley Coffey designed targets with no vergence demand (Fig. 8.14) by using cross-polarizing filters and hand-drawn nonius lines.

The initial goal of training is to refine the athlete's ability to maintain steady, stable alignment of the targets and develop the feeling of steady alignment. Once the athlete can easily achieve and maintain target alignment, the athlete is compelled to achieve alignment in progressively shorter periods, preferably attaining alignment instantaneously. The athlete should also move from primary gaze position to other positions that simulate the task demands of the sport, such as viewing in baseball batting stance or golf putting stance. Additional visual discrimination demands and sensory integration burdens can be added to further build automaticity of stable and precise eye alignment.

Spatial localization. Spatial localization tasks in "real" space may provide a useful bridge between simulated depth activities and the actual demands of sports performance. Additionally, mental imagery has been suggested to be a powerful tool for enhancing physical performance.[1] Studies have suggested that mental imagery may share the same types of neural processes as visual perception, which may have significant implications for depth judgments in sports.[41,42]

Coffey and Reichow[1] presented an SVT activity combining real space depth judgments with mental imagery calibrations. The athlete is positioned in front of an array of targets (varying sized papers, coffee cans, etc.) spaced at varying distances and visual directions. The athlete develops an internal calibration of distance estimation by tossing beanbags at the targets and noting error tendencies. The targets are then rearranged at different distances and directions, and the athlete is instructed to construct a mental image of each target location. Before tossing the beanbags to each new target location, the athlete is instructed to close his or her eyes, recall as vividly as possible the exact position of the target, and then toss the beanbag at the target with

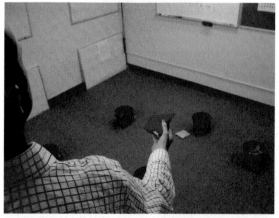

FIG. 8.15 A visual performance enhancement training activity combining real space depth judgments with mental imagery calibrations; created by Coffey and Reichow.

eyes still closed (Fig. 8.15). After each toss, feedback is provided to the athlete regarding performance accuracy. Once the athlete has achieved an appropriate level of performance accuracy, he or she is required to create a mental image of multiple targets and toss beanbags at all the targets before being allowed to access the visual feedback of performance accuracy. The practitioner may also wish to have the athlete perform this procedure monocularly to improve the use of monocular cues to depth. Although many variables can influence performance, this procedure may be particularly beneficial for sports in which the athlete's view of critical information is often interrupted by other participants or objects (e.g., basketball, soccer, hockey).

Peripheral vision

The processing of information from the peripheral visual fields is a practically universal element to successful sports performance, whether the task is to monitor teammates and opponents or maintain steady balance. Peripheral vision is critical to generate accurate saccadic eye movements and guide searching eye movements in most sports. The goal of SVT for peripheral vision is to enhance visual field awareness and responsiveness, often while simultaneously processing central visual information, and typically is not directed to extending the size of the visual fields.

Wayne peripheral awareness trainer. The Peripheral Awareness Trainer had a central circular module that contained a central fixation light and eight clear rods extending from it with red light-emitting diodes (LEDs) at each end (see Fig. 4.6). The athlete was instructed to hold a joystick, fixate centrally, and move the joystick in the direction of an LED when it was perceived by the peripheral visual field. This system was often discussed to enhance peripheral awareness in athletes; however, the product is no longer available, and there is currently no similar product available.

Spatial localization techniques. In sports such as trap or skeet shooting and gymnastics, precise peripheral localization is crucial to success. Some procedures have been developed that provide feedback regarding peripheral localization accuracy. Many of the devices discussed to enhance visual-motor reaction require peripheral visual processing to locate each stimulus as it is illuminated. These procedures can be modified to require precise peripheral localization by having the athlete fixate a central spot on the instrument panel. The athlete is instructed to rapidly point at the randomly illuminated button on the panel with a finger while maintaining central fixation and hold his or her finger on the spot where the finger touches the panel. The athlete is then allowed to look at his or her finger to see the accuracy of the localization. The process is repeated to build rapid accuracy of peripheral localization. Additional sensory integration burdens can be added to further build automaticity.

Coffey and Reichow[1] described a similar training procedure with a tachistoscope projector and a laser pointer. The athlete faces a screen with a central fixation spot and holds a laser pointer. A slide with a dot located in a random position is flashed tachistoscopically (e.g., 0.05 s), and the athlete is instructed to point the laser pointer at the position on the screen that the dot was seen. Feedback is provided by illuminating the slide so that the athlete can see the accuracy of his or her peripheral localization. As the athlete improves peripheral localization accuracy, the exposure time of the slide is reduced.

Split attention activities. Many sports demand that the athlete process central and peripheral information simultaneously, placing an almost insurmountable burden on the attention mechanism. When an athlete has developed superior visual performance skills, adding procedures that compel the athlete to split attention between central and peripheral information can be a powerful method of building automaticity. For example, the athlete is placed so that he or she centrally fixates a Hart chart and sees the Wayne Saccadic Fixator in the peripheral field of vision (Fig. 8.16). The athlete is instructed to call out the letters on the Hart chart in sequence while simultaneously hitting the buttons of the Wayne Saccadic Fixator as they are randomly lit in one of the visual-motor reaction programs. Additional sensory integration burdens can be added to further build automaticity.

Juggling. The act of juggling requires heightened peripheral awareness and excellent hand reaction and response speed. For athletes who cannot successfully juggle three objects (balls), learning the skill demands significant attention to improve peripheral awareness with hand coordination. Several websites have specific instructions for learning how to juggle (e.g., www.wikihow.com/Juggle-Three-Balls, www.instructables.com/id/how-to-juggle/), and these can be used to complement the instructions that the practitioner provides. Once the skill of three-ball juggling is mastered, additional sensory integration burdens can be added.

For team sports, the whole team can compete in daily juggling competitions in which everyone begins juggling simultaneously to determine who can continue the longest. As the athletes master the juggling technique, movement can be added to the competition. The team members are allowed to move around and bump into each other in an attempt to induce a teammate to drop a ball. This movement significantly increases the load on peripheral awareness while introducing split attention and foot reaction/response demands to the activity. To further challenge the anticipation skills of the athletes, the room can be darkened and a strobe light used to add a speed-of-recognition demand to the activity. Performance of this level of activity helps the athlete develop better control of visual attention during stressful motor performance, which should help transfer the improvements to the field of play.

Yardstick saccades. Yardstick saccades was described by Martin[156] to develop head control during saccadic eye movements. The procedure was explained with a yardstick; however, a meterstick is substituted in this description. The athlete is centered approximately 50 cm from the center of a meterstick (at the 50-cm mark) in primary gaze position. The task is for the athlete to fixate the 50-cm mark and locate the next higher mark (51 cm) by using peripheral awareness. The athlete completes an accurate saccade to that mark and makes a return saccade to the center point. This process is repeated for the next lower mark (49 cm). If performed smoothly and successfully, the athlete uses peripheral awareness to locate the mark two steps away (52 and 48 cm) and repeats the steps described earlier. This process continues until the

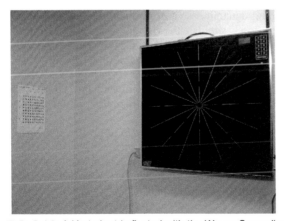

FIG. 8.16 A Hart chart is fixated with the Wayne Saccadic Fixator in the peripheral field of vision to split attention between central and peripheral information to build automaticity.

athlete can no longer locate the next centimeter mark with his or her peripheral vision. Further visual feedback can be provided with a visual afterimage, as previously described. This task initially is performed with the meterstick placed horizontally; however, the orientation can be adjusted to simulate the sport demands and enhance more superior and inferior aspects of peripheral vision. The goal is smooth, quick, and accurate saccadic eye movements with an expanded awareness of the peripheral visual fields (e.g., the athlete can see further out into the periphery on the meterstick). The drawback of using a meterstick is that the markings become a barrier to peripheral awareness, as the resolution capabilities are significantly reduced the further the image is from the macula. The Macdonald Form Field Recognition Cards and Peripheral Awareness Chart (available from www.bernell.com) use letters of increasing size from the center fixation point to address this.

Once the athlete can demonstrate consistently accurate precision and speed on this task, additional sensory integration burdens can be added. The use of a metronome is a particularly effective method for enhancing auditory-visual integration, and increasing the pace of the metronome can generate performance stress similar to athletic competition. When adding a metronome to this procedure, the athlete is challenged to saccade to each successive centimeter mark accurately with the beat from the metronome. The athlete must develop awareness of the attentional conditions that enhance peripheral awareness to apply this mental state to sport performance.

DECISION MECHANISM

Many SVT programs attempt to improve the speed and efficiency of the decision mechanism. This mechanism requires the athlete to know where crucial visual information exists, be able to direct attention to those crucial elements, select the best information from all that is available, organize and interpret the information in the most appropriate manner based on experience and memory of similar situations and information, and select the most accurate response with consideration of an anticipated action plan. A meta-analysis of 42 studies investigating perceptual-cognitive abilities in athletes found that sport experts were roughly 35% faster and 31% more accurate in their decision-making compared with lesser skilled athletes.[157] There exists a false dichotomy in the literature that suggests that training paradigms are either "sports vision training" or "perceptual-cognitive training" (PCT).[158] The notion is that SVT is an optometry-based program

that uses generic stimuli and responses to train elemental vision skills and that PCT uses sport-specific film or images to develop relevant perceptual-cognitive skills. This seems to be an academic dichotomy found mainly in the sports science literature because most sports vision practitioners employ elements of both approaches (and others) under the general label of SVT. Indeed, it is likely the combination of approaches that enhances the efficacy of SVT rather than one specific aspect of the training paradigms used.

Speed of Recognition

The ability to process visual information rapidly has been considered an essential element for success in fast-action sports. Athletes must analyze available temporal and spatial information during sports situations relatively quickly to make accurate decisions concerning performance responses. Most SVT programs that include activities designed to improve speed of recognition also attempt to increase the quantity of information that the athlete can process.

Tachistoscopic training

Tachistoscopes have been used for many years to enhance the ability to process visual information rapidly. Originally, slide projectors or similar instruments were used to present stimuli for short durations; more recently, computers provide a relatively easy platform for tachistoscopic training. Traditionally the athlete is instructed to recall a sequence of numbers that has been flashed for a very short period (e.g., 0.02 s). However, the use of numeric stimuli may confound the assessment and enhancement of speed of recognition in athletes. As previously discussed for training dynamic visual acuity, target parameters that more closely simulate the visual information processed in sport situations may provide a more effective approach to improve the visual information processing speed for athletes. Sport-specific images or stop-action video offers the athlete a more direct benefit to sports performance and should enhance transfer of skill development to the playing field.

The addition of a motor response to the presented stimuli is useful to approximate the completion of the motor reaction process. For example, the athlete may be instructed to move his or her feet (or racquet, hockey stick, glove) in the direction of an arrow stimulus placed in a random location on the training slide or computer monitor. This type of activity can also be performed with flash cards or computer programs at home by the athlete. If video footage is used, the athlete can complete the anticipated motor response to the video action that was stopped and feedback is provided concerning the accuracy of the predicted action. For example, video footage of a baseball pitch can be stopped at a designated time interval (e.g., 0.1 s) after release of the pitch and the batter responds with a swing (or no swing) corresponding to the anticipated trajectory of the pitch.

Brain-training games

Computer-based applications marketed as brain-training games have become popular, and some have targeted sports with tailored applications. There have been reviews and critiques about the use of commercial computer-based cognitive training programs and applications to improve aspects of visual perceptual performance for sports; however, many of the programs discussed were not specifically designed for sport application.[159–161] An example of a program designed for sport is HeadTrainer (www.headtrainer.com) with games designed to train five areas of mental function: focus and concentration, visual-spatial awareness, decision-making, processing speed, and memory. Brain HQ (www.brainhq.com) is another with a module that focuses on sports and games and targets four areas of cognition: reaction time, useful field of view, visual processing speed, and multiple object tracking (MOT). There are other computer-based applications, such as Lucid (www.getlucid.com), that target visualization and mindfulness attributes in athletes. These digital brain-training applications may be a useful adjunct to traditional SVT; however, there is no research currently that evaluates the effectiveness of these applications for enhancing sports performance.

Sports simulations and virtual reality platforms

Computerized simulations and virtual reality platforms have the potential to simulate game action without the physical and personnel demands of traditional sports practice. Simulation platforms provide training protocols that can mimic real game activities, allowing athletes to gain 'mental repetitions' that mimic actual plays being run in the first person with little-to-no risk of injury.[54] Research with customized virtual simulations has evaluated the capacity to utilize training with sport-specific simulations of table tennis,[162] baseball,[163–165] rugby,[166] and darts.[167] A study with high-school baseball players found that players who trained with an adaptive baseball batting virtual environment showed greater improvement in batting assessments as well as batting statistics in league play.[168] Similarly, training with simulated baseball pitch speeds has been shown to improve dynamic visual acuity and batting ability.[22] Many companies and products have emerged that target specific sports and many seem to

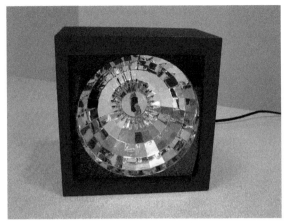

FIG. 8.17 A strobe light.

vanish quickly as well. Axon Sports (www.axonsports.com), StriVR (www.strivr.com), uHit by deCervo (www.decervo.com), the A.M.P. system (www.ampsystem.net), and Beyond Sports (www.beyondsports.nl) have developed digital training simulations for a variety of sports that are marketed toward athletes, coaches, officials, and trainers. While these applications are rapidly evolving to include new modules and technologies and show promise as an adjunct to traditional training, there are currently very few studies that have evaluated the capacity of simulations to improve sports performance.

Stroboscopic training

A strobe light (Fig. 8.17) or stroboscopic filters provide another method for the development of visual information processing speed.[51] A strobe light in a darkened room reduces the availability of visual information to the brief periods when the strobe light illuminates the room. The faster the flash rate of the strobe light, the greater the amount of information available to the athlete. Ultimately the athlete is encouraged to maintain performance of a sport-relevant activity with progressively less visual information as the flash rate on the strobe light is reduced. It is thought that performance under suboptimal stroboscopic conditions is similar to other forms of resistance training found in sports, such as altitude training for distance runners or a drag suit for swimmers.[54] Intermittent vision conditions have been shown to affect catching tasks[169,170] and reduce motion sickness in a variety of settings.[171] Studies have found more rapid improvements following strobe training in central visual field motion sensitivity and transient attention,[172] short-term visual memory,[173] accuracy and consistency in coincidence-anticipation timing with the Bassin Anticipation Timer,[174] and attention and acquisition of MOT and multiple object avoidance skills.[175] In sport application, strobe training (in addition to other training) has been shown to provide improvements in on-ice ice hockey skills,[176] visuomotor abilities in high-level badminton players,[177] as well as batting practice, batting averages, slugging percentage, and on-base percentage in collegiate baseball players.[13,23] Other sport-specific applications include effects on a one-handed ball catching task,[19] rehabilitation following anterior cruciate ligament injury,[178] and a reduction in the incidence of concussion in football.[17]

A typical example early in training has the athlete engaged in a motor performance task, such as the pitch-back activity previously described. The athlete throws a ball or beanbag into a pitchback net and attempts to catch it on the return flight. As the athlete's ability to catch improves, the ball or beanbag is thrown faster into the net, and more spin can be induced by the athlete during the throw. To add a level of unpredictability to the task, the ball can be thrown by another person, thereby requiring the athlete to rapidly judge the speed and trajectory of the ball during flight. The flash rate of the strobe light is gradually reduced so that the athlete must perform with less and less visual information.

The pitchback activity can be replaced with motor tasks that match the demands of the sport; for example, catching for baseball, softball, or football; service returns for tennis, racquetball, table tennis, or volleyball; or simulated game play for team sports such as basketball, softball, football, and volleyball. The practitioner must be careful to protect the athletes from injury when conducting strobe activities (e.g., use a batting cage with a machine rather than a real pitching/batting setup for stroboscopic batting). An original product called Strobespecs previously provided battery-powered liquid crystal strobe filters in an eyewear frame. Later similar products, such as the Nike Vapor Strobe, Senaptec Strobe (www.senaptec.com), PLATO Visual Occlusion Spectacles (www.translucent.ca), VIMA Rev Sport (www.vima.com), that also provide portable stroboscopic occlusion filters were developed. These devices are excellent for providing strobe demands during actual sports performance training because the athlete can wear the stroboscopic filters on the playing field during practice. The liquid crystal filtered lenses in these products alternate between transparent and opaque or semiopaque states that can be changed through various ranges of visual occlusion. The Senaptec Quad Strobe (Fig. 8.18) has segments of each lens that can be activated independently to customize the occlusion pattern during training.

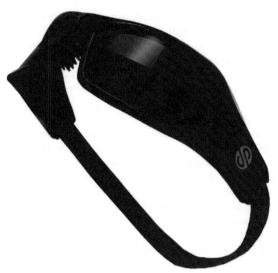

FIG. 8.18 Senaptec Quad Strobes (www.senaptec.com).

Multiple Object Tracking

Sports that require athletes to extract crucial visual information from a dynamically changing environment in order to make the best decision on how to respond appropriately use visual abilities that have been called multiple object tracking (MOT). Research has demonstrated that this form of visuospatial cognition is enhanced in expert athletes.[16,179-186] SVT programs have been developed that target MOT abilities, such as the CogniSens NeuroTracker (https://neurotracker.net), Neurotrainer (www.neurotrainer.com), and Senaptec Sensory Station (www.senaptec.com). This SVT platform provides an MOT paradigm (some also provide three-dimensional views) with added functions to increase the cognitive load. Athletes view a virtual or monitor-based space containing an initial set of identical balls/objects with a subset of balls/objects designated at the start of each trial to be tracked. Once the program is started, all the balls/objects move simultaneously throughout the volume of the space or cube for a period (usually 8–10 s) and then freeze in place for the athlete to identify where the designated balls/objects stopped. The speed and number of balls to be tracked are modified in an increasing staircase algorithm based on performance. The athlete can progress from sitting to standing or to carry out dual-task functions such as performing sport-specific movements while at the same time tracking targets.

Studies have found that NeuroTracker performance is correlated with actual game performance in professional basketball players[16] and that training with this program can selectively transfer to improved small-sided game performance in university-level soccer players.[186] However, a study of possible transfer effects from NeuroTracker training with elite athletes showed no significant transfer effects on tests of executive brain functioning.[187] Neurotrainer employs tasks in a virtual reality environment that are often presented in large fields of view. While Neurotrainer has been shown to be associated with peripheral vision improvements in visually impaired youth,[188] there are no studies of its efficacy at improving sport-specific visual abilities or performance. The Senaptec Sensory Station contains a training program for MOT; however, there are also currently no studies supporting the efficacy of this training platform.

EFFECTOR MECHANISM
Visual-Motor Reaction/Response (Eye-Hand, Eye-Foot, Eye-Body)
Many sport situations require the athlete to make a motor response to visual information, and the speed of visual and neuromuscular processing is often a valuable attribute for an athlete. The visual system is responsible for providing critical information regarding response characteristics of the athlete's hands, feet, and body position. Many programs designed to improve athletic performance in reactive sports include activities designed to enhance visual-motor reaction time, and it is a frequent element of SVT programs.

The enhancement of visual-motor reaction and response speed has two main goals. The primary goal is to reduce the time that elapses between the initiation of a visual stimulus and the commencement of an appropriate motor response to the stimulus. This part of the reaction time process involves the speed of visual information processing (perceptual mechanism) and the decision mechanism to instigate the effector mechanism accurately. In the parlance of the sports world, this ability is often referred to as quickness. An athlete with superior quickness is able to react earlier to visual information than other athletes. The second goal is to reduce the time required for the neuromuscular system to send the information to the muscles that need to be stimulated to make the appropriate motor response. This part of the reaction time process involves the speed of the effector mechanism and is often referred to as pure speed. An athlete with superior speed is faster at the required motor performance once the effector mechanism has been engaged. For example, a soccer goalkeeper with superior quickness will have a faster step toward a goal shot, and a goalkeeper with superior

speed will cover the distance to intercept the goal shot faster. The combination of exceptional quickness and speed offers the best potential for success.

Electronic devices
The Wayne Saccadic Fixator was the original instrument developed to evaluate and improve visual-motor reaction and response speed, and although it is no longer commercially available, there are many similar instruments. The Binovi Touch Saccadic Fixator, Dynavision D2, SVT (www.sportsvision.com.au), Vision Coach (www.visioncoachtrainer.com), BATAK Pro (www.batak.com), FitLight (www.fitlighttraining.com), Senaptec Sensory Station, Reflexion (www.reflexion.co), Sanet Vision Integrator (www.svivision.com), and the MOART system are commercially available devices. The instruments are similar in that they each consist of a two-dimensional panel or setup with an array of illuminated 'buttons'. The athlete is required to press a randomly lit button as rapidly as possible; then, another button is lit in a random position on the instrument, with this cycle repeated for an established period. FitLight is unique in that it employs wireless LED-powered lights that are controlled by a computer and can be flexibly placed at distances up to 50 yards from the controller, rather than embedded in a fixed board (see Fig. 4.7).

Typically, the athlete repeats a specific training program on the instrument in an attempt to improve his or her score. The instruments have programs in two primary modes: *proaction* refers to a self-paced mode for a set period in which each light stays lit until the button is pressed, while *reaction* refers to an instrument-paced stimulus presentation in which each light stays lit for a preset amount of time before automatically switching to another light, whether the button is pressed or not. As performance improves, the speed of the reaction training programs is increased to keep the athletes working at the threshold of their ability. Additional sensory integration burdens (e.g., balance board, stroboscopic eyewear) can be added to further build automaticity of visual-motor reaction and response speed.

Previous research with these instruments has varied considerably in scope and intent, with some devices utilized in several peer-reviewed studies, while others have very limited available research. Studies have shown that SVT using the Wayne Saccadic Fixator or Accuvision results in better performance on these instruments; however, these studies do not account for any practice effects in the research design.[18,189] A study with collegiate softball players found that a program of SVT improved performance on the Go/No Go assessment of the Senaptec Sensory Station.[21] Dynavision International has produced two primary visual-motor training devices, the Dynavision 2000 and the Dynavision D2, that have been used as part of SVT programs and concussion management protocols. Previous studies have utilized Dynavision instruments as part of multiweek training programs that included a number of additional training approaches. In a first study performed with collegiate baseball players, training sessions began 6 weeks prior to the season and occurred three times per week throughout the season. In conjunction with seven SVT studies that have included Dynavision, it was shown that batting averages, slugging percentage, and on-base percentage were all improved in collegiate baseball players as compared with the previous season when no vision training was performed[13] and that concussion incidence was reduced in collegiate football players.[17] In a study with youth field hockey players, performance on the Dynavision assessment task and a functional field of view assessment task both improved compared to a control group; however, there was no difference in the MOT assessment (a transfer task).[14] This study shows evidence of specific learning but does not provide support for transfer of this learning to other tasks or generalization to on-field performance. While these studies collectively provide evidence that programs utilizing the Dynavision instruments produce some benefits, it is important to note that all these studies also involved training with other activities, so the precise contribution of the Dynavision training has yet to be clearly determined.

The instruments discussed in this section are most often used to train eye-hand reaction, but there are some instruments that provide a method to train eye-foot response. The HD Sensor Board developed by the Quick Board (www.thequickboard.com/) consists of a rubber mat positioned on the ground with sensor pads in five locations (see Fig. 4.8). The mat is connected to a control device that provides visual stimulus and feedback information about the movement responses. Galpin et al.[190] found that 4 weeks of training with the Quick Board produced significant improvements in foot speed, choice reaction, and change of direction in moderately active adults. The FitLight units can be configured similar to the Quick Board for this type of training as well as a host of other arrangements that can be tailored for certain movement skill development.

Visual-Motor Reaction/Response Games

Many games require rapid motor responses to visual stimuli for success. For example, table tennis compels the athlete to perform extremely quick eye-hand responses, which should have a salutary effect on eye-hand responses in other sports applications. Even some video games can provide an environment for the development of eye-hand response speed, although the nature of the motor response (e.g., thumbs) may not engage the gross motor neuromuscular system required in most sports. The pitchback stroboscopic activities described earlier also provide an excellent environment for increasing visual-motor reaction and response speed.

Coincidence-anticipation timing

Many fast-action sports involve reaction and responses to visual information approaching the athlete. For example, a tennis player must determine when and where an opponent's serve will arrive on his or her side of the court and anticipate this location early enough to initiate the proper motor response. Predictive visual information concerning the space-time behavior of critical factors in fast-action sports can provide a significant advantage in determining and executing the most appropriate motor responses.[191–201] Therefore many visual performance enhancement training programs include activities designed to heighten coincidence anticipation skills. The goals for this area of enhancement are to improve the accuracy and consistency of visual-motor anticipation timing.

Bassin Anticipation Timer or Senaptec Synchrony. The Bassin Anticipation Timer (www.lafayetteinstrument.com) is an instrument most often used to assess coincidence anticipation. As described in Chapter 4, the instrument consists of a track of LED lights that make a "runway" of various lengths (see Fig. 4.8). The LEDs are illuminated sequentially down the runway in rapid succession to simulate the apparent motion of the stimulus lights traveling at velocities of 1–500 mph. The task requires the athlete to anticipate when the target light will be illuminated as the LEDs are sequentially illuminated along the z-axis approaching the athlete and to make a motor response that coincides with the illumination of the target light. The velocity of the stimulus lights can be calibrated to simulate the action speeds encountered in the athlete's sport, in effect simulating the stimulus parameters experienced by the athlete (e.g., the pitch speeds in baseball batting). Similar to the Bassin Anticipation Timer, the Senaptec Synchrony (see Fig. 8.19) is a more portable option for coincidence-anticipation training. Visual and verbal feedback is provided to the athlete concerning each performance so that the athlete can begin to

(A) **(B)**

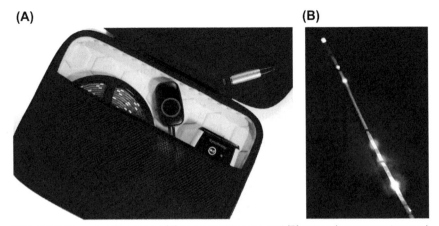

FIG. 8.19 Senaptec Synchrony **(A)** in a portable case and **(B)** set up (www.senaptec.com).

internally calibrate coincidence-anticipation accuracy. Many athletes report improved visual concentration during sport performance after training with these instruments. In sport application, Bassin anticipation timing training (in addition to other training) has been shown to enhance batting practice performance in collegiate baseball players.[23]

Stroboscopic training. A strobe light or stroboscopic filters provide another method for the development of coincidence-anticipation skills, in addition to improving visual information processing speed. The emphasis is placed on motor responses to approaching objects, such as that described in the pitchback activity.

The development of visual performance enhancement procedures is limited only by individual or collective creativity. The sports vision practitioner should perform a visual task analysis for each sports team or athlete for whom these services are designed. The relevant and critical visual skills initially should be isolated for performance enhancement. Visual skill integration and sensory integration demands are gradually introduced to challenge the athlete and build automaticity of performance. The practitioner, athlete, and the athlete's support network should develop strategies to assist in the transfer of enhanced visual performance to the playing field by incorporating vision performance aspects into sport skill practice and mental preparations for competition. A home-based program of visual skill procedures should be prescribed at the conclusion of visual performance enhancement therapy to provide the athlete a structure for maintaining skill development and for continuing performance improvements. Although many of the reports in the literature supporting SVT are anecdotal or significant flaws in the research

designs preclude a definitive conclusion, a logical relation exists between visual performance and sports performance. Ample evidence exists that visual skill performance can be enhanced with well-designed procedures; therefore enhancement of visual skill performance should provide the athlete an additional advantage when preparing for competition.

NUTRITION AND VISUAL PERFORMANCE
In addition to SVT approaches, supplementation of nutrients that contribute to optimal visual performance should be considered. There has been a significant amount of research in the recent years into the effects of nutrients on visual performance, not only in the aging population but also in young, healthy individuals. Lutein (L) and zeaxanthin (Z) are plant-derived carotenoids that are found to be concentrated in the eye and brain. L and Z are concentrated within the inner layers of the fovea, specifically at Henle fiber layer, and act as a filter for light.[202,203] The macular pigments have peak absorbance for short-wavelength light (400–500 nm) and filter light before it reaches the cone photoreceptors. The peak energy of both blue haze and sky light is 460 nm, which coincides with the peak absorbance of the macular pigments (similar to yellow-tinted filters).[204]

Visual Effects of Lutein and Zeaxanthin
There is mounting evidence from placebo-controlled, double-blind trials that the density of the macular pigment has an effect on glare disability and discomfort, photostress recovery, and contrast enhancement. Less discomfort is reported from short-wavelength light in those with a higher concentration of macular

pigment, as well as less glare disability.[205,206] Supplementation with L and Z has shown an improvement in glare disability that was proportional to the level of macular pigment increase.[206–208] The same trend can be seen with photostress recovery following exposure to bright light, and visual discomfort.[207,208] The ability to perform optimally under intense glare conditions may be improved by increasing macular pigment density.

Recent research has demonstrated a linear relationship between macular pigment density and contrast enhancement,[209] and supplementation with L and Z has been shown to improve contrast sensitivity at 6 and 12 cycles/degree.[210] As the macular pigments selectively filter short-wavelength light, it has been proposed that those with a higher density of macular pigments have an expanded visible range (approximately 30%) due to the preponderance of short-wavelength light in the atmosphere.[211] Therefore the ability to detect a target such as a baseball or tennis ball against a blue sky is enhanced with increasing macular pigment.

Neural Effects of Lutein and Zeaxanthin

Although the presence of L and Z in the macula is well recognized, these carotenoids are also concentrated in the brain. Randomized, double-masked, placebo-controlled trials of young healthy subjects have shown that macular pigment density is linked to L and Z levels in the brain,[212] and the level present is related to functions such as cognition, reaction time, and temporal visual processing.[213–215] Neuroimaging to measure the relation of L and Z to brain structure in vivo has confirmed that L and Z influences white matter integrity, particularly in regions vulnerable to age-related decline.[216] L and Z are incorporated in cell membranes and axonal projections, which serve to enhance interneuronal and neural-glial communication.[217] Recently, supplementation with carotenoids has been shown to increase critical flicker frequency thresholds, visual motor reaction time, and temporal contrast sensitivity function compared with a placebo control group, improving processing speed by an average of 10%–20%.[214,215] In dynamic, reactive situations, this may enhance the ability to evaluate critical visual information faster. For example, more rapid visual processing allows a baseball batter to process more visual information regarding the judgment of the speed and trajectory of a pitched ball.

Nutrition Recommendations for Athletes

To help athletes achieve optimal visual performance, recommendations should include modifications to diet to increase intake of carotenoids and supplementation with purified forms of L and Z. Placebo-controlled studies have found that macular pigment density can be increased by an average of about 20% with supplementation.[205,206] Recent studies have used 20 mg of dietary Z in the supplements for those who are young and healthy, compared to lower concentrations for the aging population (the AREDS 2 formula has only 2 mg of Z).[207,214,215] For competitive athletes, care should be taken to recommend supplements that have been certified by the National Science Foundation (NSF) for content, including for substances banned in sports. In addition to the visual performance improvements found with supplementation, evidence exists that L and Z have protective effects for the retina from photooxidative damage.

For those athletes who experience difficulties with glare, photostress, and contrast judgment, increasing macular pigment density offers a potential method to improve these functions by enriching natural physiology. Some athletes do not see a benefit from filter recommendations to help with glare disability, and filters can be cumbersome to change when moving between bright light and shadow. It may be that improvement in L and Z concentrations in the macula can provide enhanced visual function without the reduction in overall luminance that occurs with external filter use. In addition, supplementation with L and Z may help reduce photosensitivity symptoms following sport-related concussion.

ACKNOWLEDGMENT

The author recognizes and acknowledges the influence of Drs. Bradley Coffey and Alan W. Reichow for much of the information contained in this chapter.

REFERENCES

1. Coffey B, Reichow AW. Visual performance enhancement in sports optometry. In: Loran DFC, MacEwen CJ, eds. *Sports Vision*. Oxford: Butterworth-Heinemann; 1995: 158–177.
2. Coffey B, Reichow AW. Optometric evaluation of the elite athlete. *Probl Optom*. 1990;2:32.
3. Cohen AH. The efficacy of optometric vision therapy. *J Am Optom Assoc*. 1988;59:95.
4. Ciuffreda KJ. The scientific basis for and efficacy of optometric vision therapy in nonstrabismic accommodative and vergence disorders. *Optometry*. 2002;73:735.
5. Ciuffreda KJ, Wang B. Vision training and sports. In: Hung GK, Pallis JM, eds. *Biomedical Engineering Principles in Sports*. New York: Kluwer Academic/Plenum; 2004: 407–433.

6. West KL, Bressan ES. The effect of a general versus specific visual skills training program on accuracy in judging length-of-ball in cricket. *Int J Sport Vis.* 1996;3:41.

7. Quevedo-i-Junyent L, Sole-i-Forto J. Visual training program applied to precision shooting. *Ophthalmic Physiol Optic.* 1995;15:519.

8. McLeod B. Effects of eyerobics visual skills training on selected performance measures of female varsity soccer players. *Percept Mot Skills.* 1991;72:863.

9. Kofsky M. Sports vision visual training and experimental program with Australian Institute of Sport basketball players. *Aust J Optom.* 1988;6:15.

10. Bressan ES. Effects of visual skills training, vision coaching and sports vision dynamics on the performance of a sport skill. *Afr J Phys Health Educ Recreat Dance.* 2003; 9:20−31.

11. Balasaheb T, Maman P, Sandhu JS. The impact of visual skills training on batting performance in cricketers. *Serbian J Sports Sci.* 2008;2:17−23.

12. Hopwood MJ, Mann DL, Farrow D, Nielsen T. Does visual-perceptual training augment the fielding performance of skilled cricketers? *Int J Sports Sci Coach.* 2011; 6:523−535.

13. Clark JF, Ellis JK, Bench J, et al. High-performance vision training improves batting statistics for University of Cincinnati baseball players. *PLoS One.* 2012;7:e29109.

14. Schwab S, Memmert D. The impact of a sports vision training program in youth field hockey players. *J Sports Sci Med.* 2012:624−631.

15. Deveau J, Ozer DJ, Seitz AR. Improved vision and on-field performance in baseball through perceptual learning. *Curr Biol.* 2014;24(4):R146−R147.

16. Mangine GT, Hoffman JR, Wells AJ, et al. Visual tracking speed is related to basketball-specific measures of performance in NBA players. *J Strength Condit Res.* 2014;28: 2406−2414.

17. Clark JF, Graman P, Ellis JK, et al. An exploratory study of the potential effects of vision training on concussion incidence in football. *Optom Vis Perf.* 2015;3:116−125.

18. Jenerou A, Morgan B, Buckingham RS. A vision training program's impact on ice hockey performance. *Optom Vis Perf.* 2015;3:139−148.

19. Wilkins L, Gray R. Effects of stroboscopic visual training on visual attention, motion perception, and catching performance. *Percept Mot Skills.* 2015;121:57−79.

20. Zwierko T, Puchalska-Niedbal L, Krzepota J, et al. The effects of sports vision training on binocular vision function in female university athletes. *J Hum Kinet.* 2015;49:287−296.

21. Appelbaum LG, Lu Y, Khanna R, Detwiler K. The effects of sports vision training on sensorimotor abilities in collegiate softball athletes. *Athl Train Sports Health Care.* 2016;8(4):154−163.

22. Kohmura Y, Nakata M, Kubota A, et al. Effects of batting practice and visual training focused on pitch type and speed on batting ability and visual function. *J Hum Kinet.* 2019;70:5−13.

23. Liu S, Ferris LM, Hilbig S, et al. Dynamic vision training transfers positively to batting performance among collegiate baseball players. *Psychol Sport Exerc.* 2020. https://doi.org/10.1016/j.psychsport.2020.101759.

24. Abernethy B, Wood JM. Do generalized visual training programmes for sport really work? An experimental investigation. *J Sports Sci.* 2001;19:203.

25. Quevedo L, Sole J, Palmi J, et al. Experimental study of visual training effects in shooting initiation. *Clin Exp Optom.* 1999;82:23.

26. Wood JM, Abernethy B. An assessment of the efficacy of sports vision training programs. *Optom Vis Sci.* 1997;74: 646.

27. Allard F, Starkes JL. Perception in sport: volleyball. *J Sport Psychol.* 1980;2:22.

28. Allard F, Graham S, Paarsalu ME. Perception in sport: basketball. *J Sport Psychol.* 1980;2:14.

29. Starkes JL, Deakin J. Perception in sport: a cognitive approach to skilled performance. In: Straub WF, Williams JM, eds. *Cognitive Sport Psychology.* Lansing, NY: Sport Science; 1984:115−128.

30. Allard F, Burnett N. Skill in sport. *Can J Psychol.* 1985;39: 294.

31. Helsen W, Pauwels JM. The use of a simulator in the evaluation and training of tactical skills in football. In: Reilly T, Lees A, Davids K, et al., eds. *Science and Football.* London: E&FN Spon; 1987:493−497.

32. Starkes JL. Skill in field hockey: the nature of the cognitive advantage. *J Sport Psychol.* 1987;9:146.

33. Garland DJ, Barry JR. Sports expertise: the cognitive advantage. *Percept Mot Skills.* 1990;70:1299.

34. Lisberger SG. The neural basis for learning of simple motor skills. *Science.* 1988;242:728.

35. Gottlieb GL, Corcos DM, Jaric S, et al. Practice improves even the simplest movements. *Exp Brain Res.* 1988;73:436.

36. Bjurwell C. Perceptual-motor behavior in sport: the double reaction. *Percept Mot Skills.* 1991;72:137.

37. Mahoney M, Avener J. Psychology of the elite athlete: an exploratory study. *Cognit Ther Res.* 1977;1:135.

38. Meyers AW, Cooke CJ, Cullen J, et al. Psychological aspects of athletic competitors: a replication across sports. *Cognit Ther Res.* 1979;3:361.

39. Greenspan MJ, Feltz DL. Psychological interventions with athletes in competitive situations: a review. *Sport Psychol.* 1989;3:219.

40. Davis H. Cognitive style and nonsport imagery in elite ice hockey performance. *Percept Mot Skills.* 1990;71:795.

41. Schuster C, Hilfiker R, Amft O, et al. Best practice for motor imagery: a systematic literature review on motor imagery training elements in five different disciplines. *BMC Med.* 2011;9:75.

42. Finke RA. Mental imagery and the visual system. *Sci Am.* 1986;254:88.

43. Harris DV, Harris BL. *The Athlete's Guide to Sports Psychology: Mental Skills for Physical People.* New York: Leisure Press; 1984.

44. Heil J. Imagery for sport: theory, research, and practice. In: Straub WF, Williams JM, eds. *Cognitive Sport Psychology.* Lansing, NY: Sport Science Associates; 1984: 245−252.

45. Suinn RN. Imagery and sports. In: Straub WF, Williams JM, eds. *Cognitive Sport Psychology.* Lansing, NY: Sport Science Associates; 1984:253–271.

46. Ahissar M, Hochstein S. Task difficulty and the specificity of perceptual learning. *Nature.* 1997;387:401–406.

47. Seitz AR, Watanabe T. The phenomenon of task-irrelevant perceptual learning. *Vis Res.* 2009;49:2604–2610.

48. Shibata K, Yamagishi N, Ishii S, Kawato M. Boosting perceptual learning by fake feedback. *Vis Res.* 2009;49:2574–2585.

49. Birnbaum MH. Automaticity in fusional vergence therapy. *J Am Optom Assoc.* 1995;66:471.

50. Groffman S. Consideration of individual characteristics and learning theory in vision therapy. In: Press LJ, ed. *Applied Concepts in Vision Therapy.* St Louis: Mosby; 1997:51–52.

51. Leslie S. Sports vision therapy in motion. In: Press LJ, ed. *Applied Concepts in Vision Therapy.* St Louis: Mosby; 1997.

52. Shams L, Seitz AR. Benefits of multisensory learning. *Trends Cognit Sci.* 2008;12(11):411–417.

53. Xiao LQ, Zhang JY, Wang R, et al. Complete transfer of perceptual learning across retinal locations enabled by double training. *Curr Biol.* 2008;18:1922–1926.

54. Appelbaum LG, Erickson G. Sports vision training: a review of the state-of-the-art in digital training techniques. *Int Rev Sport Exerc Psychol.* 2016;11:160–189.

55. Crist RE, Li W, Gilbert CD. Learning to see: experience and attention in primary visual cortex. *Nat Neurosci.* 2001;4:519–525.

56. Bavelier D, Green CS, Pouget A, Schrater P. Brain plasticity through the life span: learning to learn and action video games. *Annu Rev Neurosci.* 2012;35:391–416.

57. Deveau J, Seitz AR. Applying perceptual learning to achieve practical changes in vision. *Front Psychol.* 2014;5:1166.

58. Dahlin E, Neely AS, Larsson A, et al. Transfer of learning after updating training mediated by the striatum. *Science.* 2008;320(5882):1510–1512.

59. Broadbent DP, Causer J, Williams AM, Ford PR. Perceptual-cognitive skill training and its transfer to expert performance in the field: future research directions. *Eur J Sport Sci.* 2015;4:322–331.

60. Woods AC. Report from the Wilmer Institute on the results obtained in the treatment of myopia by visual training. *Trans Am Acad Ophthalmol Otolaryngol.* 1945;49:37.

61. Ewalt HW. The Baltimore myopia control project. *J Am Optom Assoc.* 1946;17:167.

62. Rowe AJ. Orthoptic training to improve the visual acuity of a myope. *J Am Optom Assoc.* 1947;18:494.

63. Epstein LH, Greenwald DJ, Hennon D, et al. Monocular fading and feedback training. *Behav Modif.* 1981;5:171.

64. Gil KM, Collins FL. Behavioral training for myopia: generalization of effects. *Behav Res Ther.* 1983;21:269.

65. Collins FL, Pbert LA, Gil KM. The effects of behavioral training for improving visual acuity in emmetropic and myopic volunteers. *Behav Med Abst.* 1984;5:142.

66. Gil KM, Collins FL, Odom JV. The effects of behavioral vision training on multiple aspects of visual functioning in myopic adults. *J Behav Med.* 1986;9:373.

67. De Valois KK. Spatial frequency adaptation can enhance contrast sensitivity. *Vis Res.* 1977;17:1057.

68. Adini Y, Sagi D, Tsodyks M. Context-enabled learning in the human visual system. *Nature.* 2002;415:790.

69. Ricci JA, Collins FL. Visual acuity improvement following fading and feedback training. III: effects on acuity for stimuli in the natural environment. *Behav Res Ther.* 1988;26:475.

70. Bailliet R, Clay A, Blood K. The training of visual acuity in myopia. *J Am Optom Assoc.* 1982;53:719.

71. Low FN. The peripheral visual acuity of 100 subjects. *Am J Physiol.* 1943;140:83.

72. Low FN. Some characteristics of peripheral visual performance. *Am J Physiol.* 1946;146:573.

73. Low FN. Peripheral visual acuity. *Arch Ophthalmol.* 1951;45:80.

74. Saugstad L, Lie I. Training of peripheral visual acuity. *Scand J Psychol.* 1964;5:218.

75. Johnson CA, Leibowitz HW. Practice effects for visual resolution in the periphery. *Percept Psychophys.* 1979;25:439.

76. Collins FL, Epstein LH, Hannay HJ. A component analysis of an operant training program for improving visual acuity in myopic students. *Behav Ther.* 1981;12:692.

77. Beard BL, Levi DM, Reich LN. Perceptual learning in parafoveal vision. *Vis Res.* 1995;35:1679.

78. Hildreth HR, Meinberg WH, Milder B, et al. The effect of visual training on existing myopia. *Am J Ophthalmol.* 1947;30:1563.

79. Marg E. Flashes of clear vision and negative accommodation with reference to the Bates method of visual training. *Am J Optom Arch Am Acad Optom.* 1952;24:167.

80. Gallaway M, Pearl SM, Winkelstein AM, et al. Biofeedback training of visual acuity and myopia: a pilot study. *Am J Optom Physiol Optic.* 1987;64:62.

81. McKee SP, Westheimer G. Improvement in vernier acuity with practice. *Percept Psychophys.* 1978;24:258.

82. Fahle M, Edelman S. Long-term learning in vernier acuity: effects of stimulus orientation, range and of feedback. *Vis Res.* 1993;33:397.

83. Regan D, Beverly KI, Cyander M. The visual perception of motion in depth. *Sci Am.* 1979;241:136.

84. Regan D, Beverley KI. Illusory motion in depth: aftereffect of adaptation to changing size. *Vis Res.* 1978;18:209.

85. Beverley KI, Regan D. Separable aftereffects of changing-size and motion-in-depth: different neural mechanisms? *Vis Res.* 1979;19:727.

86. Regan D, Beverley KI. Looming detectors in the human visual pathway. *Vis Res.* 1978;18:415.

87. Regan D, Cyander M. Neurons in area 18 cat visual cortex selectively sensitive to changing size: non-linear interactions between responses to two edges. *Vis Res.* 1979;19:699.

88. Regan D, Gray R. Binocular processing of motion: some unresolved questions. *Spatial Vis.* 2009;22:1–43.

89. McLeod P, McLaughlin C, Nimmo-Smith I. Information encapsulation and automaticity: evidence from the visual

control of finely timed actions. In: *Attention and Performance XI*. Hillsdale, NJ: Erlbaum; 1985:391−400.

90. Judge SJ, Bradford CM. Adaptation to telestereoscopic viewing measured by one-handed ball-catching performance. *Perception*. 1988;17:783.

91. von Hofsten C, Rosengren K, Pick HL, et al. The role of binocular information in ball catching. *J Mot Behav*. 1992;24:329.

92. GJP S, Whiting HTA. The acquisition of catching under monocular and binocular conditions. *J Mot Behav*. 1992;24:320.

93. Ogle KN. *Researches in Binocular Vision*. New York: Hafner; 1964.

94. Cline D, Hoffstetter HW, Griffin JR. In: Radnor PA, ed. *Dictionary of Visual Science*. 3rd ed. 1980:641. Chilton.

95. Griffin JR, Borsting EJ. *Binocular Anomalies: Theory, Testing and Therapy*. 5th ed. Santa Ana, CA: Optometric Extension Program Foundation; 2010:116−117.

96. Hart WM. Entoptic imagery. In: Moses RA, Hart WM, eds. *Adler's Physiology of the Eye*. St Louis: Mosby−Year Book; 1987:383−384.

97. Di Russo F, Pitzalis S, Spinelli D. Fixation stability and saccadic latency in elite shooters. *Vis Res*. 2003;43:1837.

98. Deveau J, Lovcik G, Seitz AR. Broad-based visual benefits from training with an integrated perceptual-learning video game. *Vis Res*. 2014;99:134−140.

99. Blackburn RH. Perception of movement. *Am J Optom*. 1937;14:365.

100. Graham CH, Cook C. Visual acuity as a function of intensity and exposure time. *Am J Psychol*. 1937;49:654.

101. Ludvigh EJ. The gradient of retinal illumination and its practical significance. *Am J Ophthalmol*. 1937;20:260.

102. Langmuir I. The speed of the deer fly. *Science*. 1938;87:233.

103. Ludvigh E. Extrafoveal visual acuity as measured with Snellen test-letters. *Am J Ophthalmol*. 1941;24:303.

104. Ludvigh E. Visibility of the deer fly in flight. *Science*. 1947;105:176.

105. Ludvigh E. The visibility of moving objects. *Science*. 1948;108:63.

106. Ludvigh EJ. Visual acuity while one of viewing a moving object. *Arch Ophthalmol*. 1949;42:14.

107. Westheimer G. Eye movement responses to a horizontally moving visual stimulus. *AMA Arch Ophthalmol*. 1954;52:932.

108. Hulbert SF, Burg A, Knoll HA, et al. A preliminary study of dynamic visual acuity and its effects in motorist's vision. *J Am Optom Assoc*. 1958;29:359.

109. Ludvigh EJ, Miller JW. Study of visual acuity during the ocular pursuit of moving test objects. I. Introduction. *J Opt Soc Am*. 1958;48:799.

110. Miller JW. Study of visual acuity during the ocular pursuit of moving test objects. II. Effects of direction of movement, relative movement, and illumination. *J Opt Soc Am*. 1958;48:803.

111. Burg A, Hulbert SF. Dynamic visual acuity and other measures of vision. *Percept Mot Skills*. 1959;9:334.

112. Burg A, Hulbert S. Dynamic visual acuity as related to age, sex and static acuity. *J Appl Psychol*. 1961;45:111.

113. Miller JW, Ludvigh E. The effect of relative motion on visual acuity. *Service Ophthalmol*. 1962;7:83.

114. Weissman S, Freeburne CM. Relationship between static and dynamic visual acuity. *J Exp Psychol*. 1965;69:141.

115. Burg A. Visual acuity as measured by dynamic and static tests: a comparative evaluation. *J Appl Psychol*. 1966;50:460.

116. Kirshner AJ. Dynamic acuity a quantitative measure of eye movements. *J Am Optom Assoc*. 1967;38:460.

117. Barmack NH. Dynamic visual acuity as an index of eye movement control. *Vis Res*. 1970;10:1377.

118. Brown B. Resolution thresholds for moving targets at the fovea and in the peripheral retina. *Vis Res*. 1972;12:293.

119. Brown B. Dynamic visual acuity, eye movements and peripheral acuity for moving targets. *Vis Res*. 1972;12:305.

120. Brown B. The effect of target contrast variation on dynamic visual acuity and eye movement. *Vis Res*. 1972;12:1213.

121. Hoffman LG, Rouse M, Ryan JB. Dynamic visual acuity: a review. *J Am Optom Assoc*. 1981;52:883.

122. Jendrusch G, Wenzel V, Heck H. The significance of dynamic visual acuity as a performance-influencing parameter in tennis. *Int J Sports Med*. 1998;19.

123. Long GM, Rourke DA. Training effects on the resolution of moving targets-dynamic visual acuity. *Hum Factors*. 1989;31:443.

124. Long GM, Riggs CA. Training effects on dynamic visual acuity with free head viewing. *Perception*. 1991;20:363.

125. Seiderman A, Schneider S. *The Athletic Eye: Improved Sports Performance through Visual Training*. New York: Hearst Books; 1983.

126. Reichow AW, Stern NS. Athlete and optometrist: performance oriented. *OEP Curriculum II*. 1986;59:35.

127. Revien L. Eyerobics *[videotape]*. Great Neck, NY: Visual Skills; 1987.

128. Gregg JR. *Vision and Sports: An Introduction*. Stoneham, MA: Butterworth Publishers; 1987.

129. Sherman A. Sports vision testing and enhancement: implications for winter sports. In: Casey M, Foster C, Hixson E, eds. *Winter Sports Medicine*. Philadelphia: F.A. Davis; 1990:78−84.

130. Wilson TA, Falkel J. *Sports Vision Training for Better Performance*. Champaign, IL: Human Kinetics; 2004.

131. Griffin JR, Borsting EJ. *Binocular Anomalies: Theory, Testing and Therapy*. 5th ed. Santa Ana, CA: Optometric Extension Program Foundation; 2010:33−37.

132. Scheiman M, Wick B. *Clinical Management of Binocular Vision: Heterophoric, Accommodative, and Eye Movement Disorders*. Philadelphia: Wolters Kluwer Health; 2020:20−22.

133. Leslie S. Sports vision: therapy in motion. In: Press LJ, ed. *Applied Concepts in Vision Therapy*. St Louis: Mosby; 1997:109−110.

134. Hebb DO. *The Organization of Behavior: A Neurophysiological Theory*. New York: John Wiley & Sons; 1949.

135. Piaget J. Development and learning. In: Ripple R, Rockcastle V, eds. *Piaget Rediscovered*. Ithaca, NY: Cornell University; 1964.

136. Case R. *The Mind's Staircase: Exploring the Conceptual Underpinnings of Children's Thought and Knowledge*. Hillsdale, NJ: Erlbaum; 1991.

137. Peachey GT. Minimum attention model for understanding the development of efficient visual function. *J Behav Optom*. 1991;2:199.

138. Land MF. Vision, eye movements, and natural behavior. *Vis Neurosci*. 2009;26:51–62.

139. Wilson M, Causer J, Vickers J. Aiming for excellence: the quiet eye as a characteristic of expertise. In: Baker J, Farrow D, eds. *Handbook of Sport Expertise*. London: Routledge/Taylor and Francis; 2015:22–37.

140. Gegenfurtner A, Lehtinen E, Saljo R. Expertise differences in the comprehension of visualizations: a meta-analysis of eye-tracking research in professional domains. *Educ Psychol Rev*. 2011;23:523–552.

141. Vickers JN. Origins and current issues in quiet eye research. *Curr Issues Sport Sci*. 2016;1:1–11.

142. Wilson MR, Richards H. Putting it together: skills for pressure performance. In: Collins D, Button A, Richards H, eds. *Performance Psychology*. Edinburgh, UK: Elsevier; 2011:337–360.

143. Vickers JN. *Perception, Cognition, and Decision Training: The Quiet Eye in Action*. Champaign, IL: Human Kinetics; 2007.

144. Vine SJ, Wilson MR. Quiet eye training: effects on learning and performance under pressure. *J Appl Sport Psychol*. 2010;22:361–376.

145. Vine SJ, Moore LJ, Wilson MR. Quiet eye training facilitates competitive putting performance in elite golfers'. *Front Psychol*. 2011;2:8.

146. Moore BC, Vine SJ, Cooke A, et al. Quiet eye training expedites motor learning and aids performance under pressure: the roles of response programming and external attention. *Psychophysiology*. 2012;49: 1005–1015.

147. Harle S, Vickers JN. Training quiet eye improves accuracy in the basketball free throw. *Sport Psychol*. 2001;15: 289–305.

148. Oudejans RRD, Koedijker JM, Bleijendaal I, Bakker FC. The education of attention in aiming at a far target: training visual control in basketball jump shooting. *Int J Sport Exerc Psychol*. 2005;3:197–221.

149. Vine SJ, Wilson MR. The influence of quiet eye training and pressure on attention and visuomotor control. *Acta Psychol*. 2011;136:340–346.

150. Wood G, Wilson MR. Quiet-eye training, perceived control and performing under pressure. *Psychol Sport Exerc*. 2012;13:721–728.

151. Causer J, Holmes PS, Williams AM. Quiet eye training in a visuomotor control task. *Med Sci Sports Exerc*. 2011;43: 1042–1049.

152. Miles CAL, Vine SJ, Wood G, et al. Quiet eye training improves throw and catch performance in children. *Psychol Sport Exerc*. 2014;15:511–515.

153. Hughes PK, Blundell NL, Walters JM. Visual and psychomotor performance of elite, intermediate and novice table tennis competitors. *Clin Exp Optom*. 1993;76:51.

154. Omar R, Kuan YM, Zuhairi NA, et al. Visual efficiency among teenaged athletes and non-athletes. *Int J Ophthalmol*. 2017;10:1460–1464.

155. Clark JF, Graman P, Ellis JK. Depth perception improvement in collegiate baseball players with vision training. *Optom Vis Perf*. 2015;3:106–115.

156. Martin WF. *An Insight to Sports Featuring Trapshooting and Golf*. Seattle: SportsVision; 1984:155–159.

157. Mann DTY, Williams AM, Ward P, Janelle CM. Perceptual-cognitive expertise in sport: a meta-analysis. *J Sport Exerc Psychol*. 2007;29:457–478.

158. Hadlow SM, Panchuk D, Mann DL, et al. Modified perceptual training in sport: a new classification framework. *J Sci Med Sport*. 2018;21:950–958.

159. Harris DJ, Wilson MR, Vine SJ. A systematic review of commercial cognitive training devices: implications for use in sport. *Front Psychol*. 2018;9:709.

160. Walton CC, Keegan RJ, Martin M, Hallock H. The potential role for cognitive training in sport: more research needed. *Front Psychol*. 2018;9:1121.

161. Renshaw I, Davids K, Araujo D, et al. Evaluating weaknesses of "perceptual-cognitive training" and "brain training" methods in sport: an ecological dynamics critique. *Front Psychol*. 2019;9:2468.

162. Todorov E, Shadmehr R, Bizzi E. Augmented feedback presented in a virtual environment accelerates learning of a difficult motor task. *J Mot Behav*. 1997;29: 147–158.

163. Gray R. Behavior of college baseball players in a virtual batting task. *J Exp Psychol Hum Percept Perform*. 2002;28: 1131–1148.

164. Fink PW, Foo PS, Warren WH. Catching fly balls in virtual reality: a critical test of the outfielder problem. *J Vis*. 2009; 9(13), 14.1–8.

165. Zaal FTJM, Bootsma RJ. Virtual reality as a tool for the study of perception–action: the case of running to catch fly balls. *Presence*. 2011;20:93–103.

166. Miles HC, Pop SR, Watt SJ, et al. A review of virtual environments for training in ball sports. *Comput Graph*. 2012; 36:714–726.

167. Tirp J, Steingrover C, Wattie N, et al. Virtual realities as optimal learning environments in sport – a transfer study of virtual and real dart throwing. *Psychol Test Assess Model*. 2015;57:57–69.

168. Gray R. Transfer of training from virtual to real baseball batting. *Front Psychol*. 2017;8:2183.

169. Lyons J, Fontaine R, Elliott D. I lost it in the lights: the effects of predictable and variable intermittent vision on unilateral catching. *J Mot Behav*. 1997;29:113–118.

170. Bennett S, Ashford D, Rioja N, Elliott D. Intermittent vision and one-handed catching: the effect of general and specific task experience. *J Mot Behav*. 2004;36:442–449.

171. Reschke MF, Somers JT, Ford G. Stroboscopic vision as a treatment for motion sickness: strobe lighting vs. shutter glasses. *Aviat Space Environ Med*. 2006;77:2–7.

172. Appelbaum LG, Schroeder JE, Cain MS, Mitroff SR. Improved visual cognition through stroboscopic training. *Front Psychol.* 2011;2:276.

173. Appelbaum LG, Cain MS, Schroeder JE, et al. Stroboscopic visual training improves information encoding in short-term memory. *Atten Percept Psychophys.* 2012; 74:1681–1691.

174. Smith TQ, Mitroff SR. Stroboscopic training enhances anticipatory timing. *Int J Exerc Sci.* 2012;5:344–353.

175. Bennett SJ, Hayes SJ, Makoto U. Stroboscopic vision when interacting with multiple moving objects: perturbation is not the same as elimination. *Front Psychol.* 2018;9: 1290.

176. Mitroff SR, Friesen P, Bennett D, et al. Enhancing ice hockey skills through stroboscopic visual training. *Athl Train Sports Health Care.* 2013;5:261–264.

177. Hulsdunker T, Rentz C, Ruhnow D, et al. The effect of 4-week stroboscopic training on visual function and sport-specific visuomotor performance in top-level badminton players. *Int J Sports Physiol Perform.* 2018;14:343–350.

178. Grooms D, Appelbaum LG, Onate J. Neuroplasticity following anterior cruciate ligament injury: a framework for visual-motor training approaches in rehabilitation. *J Orthop Sports Phys Ther.* 2015;45:381–393.

179. Cavanagh P, Alvarez GA. Tracking multiple targets with multifocal attention. *Trends Cognit Sci.* 2005;9(7): 349–354.

180. Memmert D. Pay attention! A review of visual attentional expertise in sport. *Int Rev Sport Exerc Psychol.* 2009;2(2): 119–138.

181. Memmert D, Simons DJ, Grimme T. The relationship between visual attention and expertise in sports. *Psychol Sport Exerc.* 2009;10:146–151.

182. Zhang X, Yan M, Yangang L. Differential performance of Chinese volleyball athletes and nonathletes on a multiple-object tracking task. *Percept Mot Skills.* 2009; 109:747–756.

183. Faubert J, Sidebottom L. Perceptual-cognitive training of athletes. *J Clin Sport Psychol.* 2012;6:85–102.

184. Faubert J. Professional athletes have extraordinary skills for rapidly learning complex and neutral dynamic visual scenes. *Sci Rep.* 2013;3:1154.

185. Romeas T, Faubert J. Soccer athletes are superior to non-athletes at perceiving soccer-specific and non-sport specific human biological motion. *Front Psychol.* 2015;6: 1343.

186. Romeas T, Guldner A, Faubert J. 3D-multiple object tracking task performance improves passing decision-making accuracy in soccer players. *Psychol Sport Exerc.* 2016;22:1–9.

187. Moen F, Hrozanova M, Stiles T. The effects of perceptual-cognitive training with neurotracker on executive brain functions among elite athletes. *Cogent Psychol.* 2018;5: 1544105.

188. Nyquist JB, Lappin JS, Zhang R, Tadin D. Perceptual training yields rapid improvements in visually impaired youth. *Sci Rep.* 2016;6:37431.

189. Zupan MF, Arata AW, Wile A, et al. Visual adaptations to sports vision enhancement training. *Optom Today.* 2006; 43(May 19):43–48.

190. Galpin AJ, Li Y, Lohnes CA, Schilling BK. A 4-week choice foot speed and choice reaction training program improves agility in previously non-agility trained, but active men and women. *J Strength Condit Res.* 2008;22: 1901–1907.

191. Sharp RH, Whiting HTA. Information processing and eye-movement behavior in a ball catching skill. *J Hum Mov Stud.* 1975;1:124.

192. Franks IM, Weicker D, Robertson DGE. The kinematics, movement phasing and timing of a skilled action in response to varying conditions of uncertainty. *Hum Mov Sci.* 1985;4:91.

193. Bootsma RJ, van Wieringen PCW. Visual control of an attacking forehand drive. In: Meijer OG, Roth K, eds. *Complex Movement Behavior: The Motor-Action Controversy.* Amsterdam: North-Holland; 1988:189–199.

194. Bootsma RJ. *The Timing of Rapid Interceptive Actions: Perception-Action Coupling in the Control and Acquisition of Skill.* Amsterdam: Free University Press; 1988.

195. Bootsma RJ. Accuracy of perceptual processes subserving different perception-action systems. *Q J Exp Psychol.* 1989; 41A:489.

196. Bootsma RJ, van Wieringen PCW. Timing an attacking forehand drive in table tennis. *J Exp Psychol Hum Percept Perform.* 1990;16:21.

197. Bootsma RJ. Predictive information and the control of action. *Int J Sport Psychol.* 1991;22:271.

198. Savelsbergh GJP, Whiting HTA, Bootsma RJ. "Grasping" tau. *J Exp Psychol Hum Percept Perform.* 1991;17:315.

199. Bootsma RJ, Peper CE. Predictive visual information sources for the regulation of action with special emphasis on catching and hitting. In: Proteau L, Elliott D, eds. *Vision and Motor Control.* Amsterdam: North-Holland; 1992:285–314.

200. Bootsma RJ, Oudejans RRD. Visual information about time-to-collision between two objects. *J Exp Psychol Hum Percept Perform.* 1993;19:1041.

201. Siegel D. Response velocity, range of movement, and timing accuracy. *Percept Mot Skills.* 1994;79:216.

202. Krinsky NI, Landrum JT, Bone RA. Biologic mechanisms of the protective role of lutein and zeaxanthin in the eye. *Annu Rev Nutr.* 2003;23:171–201.

203. Landrum JT, Bone RA. Lutein, zeaxanthin, and the macular pigment. *Arch Biochem Biophys.* 2001;385: 28–40.

204. Bone RA, Landrum JT, Cains A. Optical density spectra of the macular pigment in vivo and in vitro. *Vis Res.* 1992; 32:105–110.

205. Stringham JM, Hammond BR. The glare hypothesis for macular pigment function. *Optom Vis Sci.* 2007;84: 859–864.

206. Stringham JM, Hammond BR. Macular pigment and visual performance under glare conditions. *Optom Vis Sci.* 2008;85:82–88.

207. Hammond BR, Fletcher LM, Roos F, et al. A double-blind, placebo-controlled study on the effects of lutein and zeaxanthin on photostress recovery, glare disability, and chromatic contrast. *Invest Ophthalmol Vis Sci.* 2014;55: 8583–8589.

208. Stringham JN, Garcia PV, Smith PA, et al. Macular pigment and visual performance in glare: benefits for photostress recovery, disability glare, and visual discomfort. *Invest Ophthalmol Vis Sci.* 2011;52: 7406–7415.

209. Renzi LM, Hammond BR. The effect of macular pigment on heterochromic luminance contrast. *Exp Eye Res.* 2010; 91:896–900.

210. Nolan JM, Power R, Stringham J, et al. Enrichment of macular pigment enhances contrast sensitivity in subjects free of retinal disease: central retinal enrichment supplementation trials – report 1. *Invest Ophthalmol Vis Sci.* 2016;57:3429–3439.

211. Wooten BR, Hammond BR. Macular pigment: influences on visual acuity and visibility. *Prog Retin Eye Res.* 2002;21: 225–240.

212. Vishwanathan R, Neuringer M, Snodderly DM, et al. Macular lutein and zeaxanthin are related to brain lutein and zeaxanthin in primates. *Nutr Neurosci.* 2013;16:21–29.

213. Renzi-Hammond LM, Bovier ER, Fletcher LM, et al. Effects of a lutein and zeaxanthin intervention on cognitive function: a randomized, double-masked, placebo-controlled trial of younger healthy adults. *Nutrients.* 2017;9: 1246–1259. https://doi.org/10.3390/nu9111246.

214. Bovier ER, Renzi LM, Hammond BR. A double-blind, placebo-controlled study on the effects of lutein and zeaxanthin on neural processing speed and efficiency. *PLoS One.* 2014;9(9):e108178.

215. Bovier ER, Hammond BR. A randomized placebo-controlled study on the effects of lutein and zeaxanthin on visual processing speed in young healthy subjects. *Arch Biochem Biophys.* 2015;15(572):54–57.

216. Mewborn CM, Terry DP, Renzi-Hammond LM, et al. Relation of retinal and serum lutein and zeaxanthin to white matter integrity in older adults: a diffusion tensor imaging study. *Arch Clin Neuropsychol.* 2017;17:1–14. https:// doi.org/10.1093/acn/acx109 [Epub ahead of print].

217. Stahl W, Sies H. Effects of carotenoids and retinoids on gap junctional communication. *Biofactors.* 2001;15: 95–98.

CHAPTER 9

Sports Vision Practice Development

Successful practices that provide sports vision services share some common approaches and experiences. First, the eye care professionals have a passion for helping athletes to see their sport better. Second, the initial services offered were typically modest and did not require significant expenditure for instrumentation at the beginning. Many practices begin by informing existing patients in the practice about the types of services available. Third, connections were developed with members of the athletic community that fostered growth of this area of practice. At this stage of development, decisions must be made about acquiring additional instrumentation to provide more opportunities to help athletes and also to distinguish the expertise provided in this area. Ultimately, the key to sports vision practice development is getting the message out that you have something unique to offer. It is important to keep in mind that your practice in this area should be well developed before any aggressive advertising of services, as this can be a very costly mistake.

For most practices, the internal marketing of services should be in place before external marketing. External marketing brings new patients to the practice. If patients do not receive what was promised in the external marketing message, your practice will go downhill faster than if you did not market at all. Look at all the communication opportunities within the practice experience and make them consistent with your message. Marketing a sports vision practice is similar to marketing any vision practice, with the exception that you are promoting a particular niche in eye care. This chapter discusses developing a marketing plan to promote sports vision.

Table 9.1 shows a self-assessment exercise listing several communication opportunities available to a practice. Complete the exercise and use your responses to determine what to change within your practice to make it more sports vision friendly. The following paragraphs contain some suggestions relative to many marketing techniques.

INTERNAL MARKETING

Brand Identity and Image

When positioning your practice consider what image to project. One way to look at image is that it represents your brand. What is your brand? What is special about you that will motivate patients (athletes) to choose you over the competition? This question is especially important to ask in highly competitive areas.

Patients have much more to do than think about eye care and eyewear. The eye care provider is responsible for educating the public about what the practice has to offer. What do you have to offer?

The book *Eyecare Business: Marketing and Strategy* provides exercises to help develop your practice brand and image, which tell a story about you.[1] This story is what your patients will use when speaking about you. Their words are "word of mouth" marketing, which has always been the leading marketing technique for the healthcare industry. Trust and competence are so important in healthcare that most patients choose a provider on the basis of what trusted individuals say. What do you want your patients to say about you? What story should they tell?

Following is an example story: "We provide many eye care services and products to help athletes perform at the highest level, whatever age or sport. Our practice will take special care to ensure that you have the best vision, eye protection, and program options to improve visual performance skills, which will give you an advantage over the competition. Whether you are a weekend warrior or a professional athlete, new technology is available to help you to see your sport better. We are dedicated to providing you the tools to perform at your highest ability."

Before you decide on marketing techniques, think about your practice brand and practice story. Begin with this and develop a practice message. All communications should be consistent with this image and brand, or conflict will occur in the minds of your patients and prospective patients regarding who you are. Communication occurs during every interaction a consumer has with you and your practice. Orchestrating what occurs during these interactions results in your ideal image and brand. This image and brand should be expressed throughout the patient visit.

Theme

One of the best ways to communicate your brand and story is through a practice theme. The theme, or slogan,

TABLE 9.1
Marketing Technique Self-Evaluation Form.

Marketing Technique	Successful	Needs Improvement	Not Using but Want to	Not Appropriate
Marketing plan				
Survey				
Brand identity/image				
Name				
Theme				
Niche				
Logo				
Quality				
Pricing				
Selection				
Direct mail				
Demographics research				
Newspaper inserts				
Refrigerator magnets				
Newspaper advertisements				
Courses and lectures				
School educational programs				
Seminars				
Trunk shows				
Medical practitioner referrals				
Contests				
Scholarships and awards				
Community activities				
Public relations				
Clubs and associations				
Outside signs				
Reputation				
Word of mouth				
Availability of financing				
Hours of operation				
Days of operation				
Free consultations				
Speed				
Service				
Phone hold messages				
Smiles				
Welcome to the office				
Office brochure				
Biographic sketch				
Information packet				

TABLE 9.1 Marketing Technique Self-Evaluation Form.—cont'd				
Marketing Technique	**Successful**	**Needs Improvement**	**Not Using but Want to**	**Not Appropriate**
Practice location				
Building appearance				
Parking lot				
Window displays				
Website				
Office appearance				
Reception area design				
Color				
Decor				
Furniture				
Staff greeting				
Staff appearance				
Attire				
Attitude				
Attention				
Library				
Electronic bulletin board				
Videos				
Counter cards				
Product brochures				
Samples				
Demonstrators				
Business cards				
Advertising and publicity reprints				
Refreshments				
Treats				
Television				
Reading materials				
Miscellaneous				
Bathrooms				
Music				
History form				
History questions				
Posters				
Testimonials				
Diplomas, awards				
News articles				
Photos of celebrity patients				
Equipment				
Explanations of benefits				

Continued

TABLE 9.1				
Marketing Technique Self-Evaluation Form.—cont'd				
Marketing Technique	**Successful**	**Needs Improvement**	**Not Using but Want to**	**Not Appropriate**
Scripts for assistants				
Dispensing mats				
Examination room appearance				
Neatness				
Saying hello				
Explaining test procedures				
Human bonding				
Models				
Pictures				
Lenses				
Written materials				
Articles				
Books				
Prescription pad				
Saying goodbye				
Referral cards				
Examination summaries				
Dispensary design				
Sales training				
Lens packages				
Frame displays				
Merchandise displays				
Gift packages				
Fee slips/receipts				
Follow-up				
Phone calls				
Cards and letters				
Stationery				
Newsletters				
Special invitations				
Gifts				
Recall				
Tie-in with other professionals				
Team sponsorships				
Cooperative funding				
Radio advertisements/shows				
Television advertisements/shows				
Magazine advertisements/articles				
Billboards				
E-mail bulletins				

is a phrase that describes what you stand for. This should be used on all your communications to give patients the message you want them to remember. The reader should be able to tell what your office emphasis is based on reading your theme. What do you think is emphasized in the following themes?

Correction, protection, and enhancement for athletes
Sports Vision: correction, protection, and enhancement
Sports Vision: A winning advantage
Seeing your way to championships
The athlete's edge: sports vision
SuperVision, SuperCaring
See better, play better
Vision for sports
Specializing in sports vision for all athletes
See like a pro athlete

If someone saw those words associated with you, would they perceive what you want them to perceive about you? If so, that is a theme for you.

Niche

Consider whether you are interested in a particular aspect of sports vision. Sports vision is already a niche within vision care, but you may want to emphasize refractive surgery, contact lenses, or sports vision training. You may only want to work with athletes at the college or professional level, or perhaps you prefer those younger than 18 years. In a highly competitive area, you may want to carve out a certain part of sports vision that is being underserved. Decide on your niche and make it part of your story.

Practice Logo

Your logo is a symbol representing what you stand for. Every time someone sees your logo, you want them to think about what you have to offer. Potential patients may not read your direct mail, but they will see your logo. If the logo is properly chosen, they will think "sports vision" when they see it. The logo can be used several ways to promote your practice. Besides having it on all your office communications, you can write a paragraph on why the logo was chosen and what it represents. This can be included in "welcome to the office" materials or your website. You can send an e-mail or letter explaining the new logo to existing patients. Many companies in the ophthalmic industry send out such a letter when changing their logos. Additionally, the sign for the practice can communicate the emphasis of sports vision (see Fig. 9.1).

Quality

Although you may not think of quality of products and services as a marketing tactic, the quality of what you

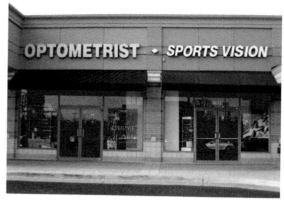

FIG. 9.1 External sign highlighting sports vision at the Northern Virginia Doctors of Optometry. (Courtesy of Keith Smithson, O.D.)

offer communicates something to your patients. Educate your patients about the benefits of high-quality products and services so they can make an educated decision on how to spend their hard-earned money.

Pricing

Pricing goes along with quality. You can provide high-quality service and high-quality products at a high cost, but not at a low cost. If you do provide high-quality services and products at a low cost, you will not be in business long. An early strategy could be to provide the services and products at a reduced cost until you build a demand. You may even choose to give away services and products to opinion shapers within the community in the hope they will spread the word and generate new patients. A common approach is to assist a local school or team with a vision screening as part of the annual preparticipation health assessment. While the screening will not directly generate revenue, it will likely generate referrals to your practice for comprehensive vision exams, eyewear needs, and other sport-related services. In addition, your participation in the event will help develop important relationships within the sports community while providing a platform for educating the community about the importance of vision and eye care for optimal sports performance.

Each practitioner must establish fees for sports vision services that reflect the local health and fitness economy. The practice should determine appropriate fees for a comprehensive sports vision evaluation, sports vision training sessions, and consultation services. For individual athletes, the practitioner can use a fee-per-session approach or charge a global fee for a package of services.

When establishing a relationship with a team or club, the agreement can entail per-session fees or a retainer fee for needed services. The team or club management and doctor must agree on which method better suits the relationship. One advantage of a retainer for the team and doctor is that the doctor does not need to justify the fee for each office visit or training session; this way the team has no concerns about the doctor making recommendations for care that are unnecessary simply to increase income from the team. The doctor should ascertain an appropriate retainer fee for the range and frequency of services that are likely to be provided and negotiate effectively with the team management.

Selection
Product selection is an area in which you can outperform the competition. Few general practices have a good choice of protective eyewear, lenses for athletes, and sports vision training services. Unfortunately, the patient population does not know this unless you tell them. Provide the best selection of services and products for the athlete and communicate this every chance you get. If the competition does not provide what you provide, they are not really competing. A good example of this is special spectacle designs for hunters and shooters.

Choose your practice brand identity, name, theme, niche, logo, quality, pricing, and selection and you will be ready to develop the internal marketing opportunities to send a consistent message to anyone coming to the practice setting. Remember to be consistent in all your communications and keep the practice brand promise you make to the patient.

MARKETING OPPORTUNITIES BEFORE THE PATIENT ENTERS THE OFFICE
Consumers form perceptions about businesses during every contact. Many perceptions are formed before the consumer has even entered the business premises. Your patients form opinions about you when they call for an appointment; visit your website; note the practice location, building appearance, and parking lot; and see the window displays. Use each of these opportunities to enhance the chance they perceive you in the manner you desire.

Telephone Hold Messages
No one likes being put on hold, but it is expected with busy practices. Use this opportunity to educate the caller about what you have to offer in the area of sports vision. Remember, consumers have more to worry about than eye care. For example, few know much about corneal refractive therapy (also known as ortho-keratology), nutrition and vision, or sports vision training to improve visual skills. State in your on-hold message that you can potentially improve their ability to perform in sports.

Making the Appointment by Telephone
While making the appointment the receptionist can note the age of the caller and perhaps ask whether he or she plays sports and alert him or her to services that may be of benefit. An example of new technology is the availability of computerized evaluation and training programs, such as the Senaptec Sensory Station or RightEye. Nearly all athletes could potentially benefit from this technology. After making the appointment, the receptionist could say, "Dr _____ is using new technology that can assess visual performance and compare your skills to a database of athletes at any competition level. With this information, recommendations for methods to improve vision can be individualized in order to help you achieve optimal performance in your sport." This scripted information can generate enthusiasm for the upcoming visit, lessening the chance of a no-show and positioning your practice as current with new technologies. This is also a good time to ask the patient to download a sports-specific history form from the practice website to complete in advance of the appointment.

Website
More consumers are evaluating service providers by visiting their websites, and many use websites to make appointments. Use your website to convey your message to prospective patients. You should refer to it in your external marketing for those who want more information. Provide links to companies whose products you sell, and be sure to include your theme and logo. You may want to provide a sports vision history form to be completed before patients come to the office. Sport-specific history questions can effectively communicate your expertise and educate the prospective patient about the range of services provided by your practice. You and your staff must follow up with the patient responses to sport-specific questions, however, to attain the potential practice benefits of this tool. Your website can generate enthusiasm, reducing the number of no-show patients and resulting in patients generating referrals.

"Welcome to the Office" Mailing
You can also mail information about your practice to new patients. This can take the form of an office brochure or an information packet consisting of a

presentation folder with a "welcome to the office" letter, biographic sketches of staff and doctors, and product and service brochures. Although costly, professional mailings separate you from the competition. To be more successful than others, you must do what others do not, or will not, do. This welcome packet is a good example of providing more than the competition. You can also give the patient the option of receiving the same information by e-mail, which reduces the cost to the practice to just the time it takes to send it.

Practice Location

Where does the average consumer expect a sports vision practice to be located? Answer this question for your community and you will send the correct message to potential patients. Good locations are sports training facilities, physical therapy and orthopedic surgery buildings, and facilities in proximity to athletic fields, stadiums, or gyms. All have the advantage of a location where athletes typically frequent. You may also be able to demonstrate the benefits of the products easier if you are near an athletic field where you can demonstrate the difference or instruct patients on proper use of what you prescribed.

Often the patients of a physical therapist or sports physician become a sports vision patient when the two practices share a reception room or are in the same building. Choose a location where others work with athletes. You can often share the cost of external marketing pieces with these other professionals.

Parking Lot

Sometimes the first perception a patient builds about an office is the parking, or lack thereof. The appearance of your parking lot sends a message to your patients. Ask yourself how you can make the parking lot consistent with your image as a sports vision specialist. Perhaps you can include a basketball hoop, with the basketball key painted on the lot; banners of local sports teams; or even a scoreboard giving scores of games.

Window Displays

Many practices have large windows near the entrance to the office. Patients and prospective patients walk by these windows before entering the practice or may wait for a ride near them. In either case use them to communicate that you are an expert on sports vision and have benefits to offer the athlete.

MARKETING IN THE RECEPTION ROOM

Your office space is one of the primary ways to communicate with your patients. Patients may not be able to

tell if you have the most up-to-date equipment and instruments, but they can tell if your color scheme, carpeting, draperies, and decor are modern. Examine your office from the point of view of the consumer and consider what it says. Is the message consistent with your desired image and brand? A good way to ascertain if you have modern colors and decor is to observe fashions in trendy restaurants. They typically redecorate frequently in order to keep a fresh, modern appearance. Eyewear display vendors may offer expertise in office decor for free or at a reduced price. Their expertise often can result in a greater return on your investment in office design.

While waiting, patients look at everything in the reception area. They see every cobweb and outdated magazine. They notice how staff dress, how they move, and how they treat others. They hear every word said and how it is said. Therefore consider offering an experience that is enjoyable and educational. Use the reception area as a classroom and provide opportunities to learn about what you offer and how it can benefit them. Brainstorm everything you can include that fits your image and brand and is practical based on your office design.

Office Design and Decor

As a sports vision specialist, you may want to use the colors of the local professional or collegiate teams in your area. Fans will appreciate the fact that you support the local teams (Of course, this can lead to interesting banter from those who root for opposing teams). You may want to decorate it like a sports store or sports bar. You can include pennants, sports memorabilia, and photographs, especially from thankful patients who are known in the community. Decor that includes photos of athletes or teams you have sponsored or worked with are consistent with a sport-oriented practice (see Fig. 9.2); however, you must be careful about getting appropriate permissions for the public display of patient information.

Staff Appearance

Staff appearance communicates a message to your patients. What clothes convey that they work with sports vision? Surgical greens may imply work with eye injury or surgery, whereas sport shirts with your logo and theme may convey an athletic focus. Staff members who are fit and passionate about sports send the message that your practice is focused on helping patients to succeed in athletic endeavors.

Patient Education

Properly designed, the reception area can offer information on services and products for patients. Use every

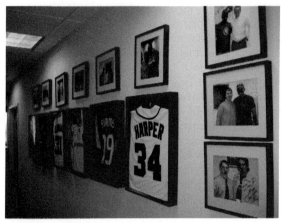

FIG. 9.2 Internal decor at the Northern Virginia Doctors of Optometry highlighting work with athletes and sports teams. (Courtesy of Keith Smithson, O.D.)

opportunity to educate them regarding the services provided and benefits derived from treatments. If you have not already sent a "welcome to the office" packet, then hand them one when they arrive. This packet can be customized to the sport or age of the patient and can include information about the practice and the products and services that may be of a benefit to the patient. Use libraries to impress them with what you know. Stock a bookcase with books on vision and sports, including textbooks. Develop a system for loaning the books to patients if they ask to borrow them. Seeing the complexity of the textbooks will impress them with your knowledge. Electronic bulletin boards and media monitors can display game scores and highlight new technology and how it can benefit them. Have counter cards, brochures, posters, demonstrators, and advertisement and publicity reprints readily available to waiting patients so they can learn more about the various aspects of eye care.

Patient-Centered Office

An experience that is enjoyable helps ensure that patients are more apt to return, especially families. If no distraction is available for children, they will resist coming to the office—either as a patient or brought by a parent who is a patient. Make a sports vision practice athlete-centered. Provide video games for the young and maybe a separate glassed-in area for the children. Allow them to be seen by their parents playing with video games, plastic kitchens and workshops, or blocks. With the proper environment, children may be excited about coming to your practice.

How do you treat friends who come to your home? Typically you offer them a refreshment and snack. Providing the same in your office positions you as a friend to your patients, and people generally like doing business with friends. Make your patients comfortable and enhance your sports vision brand by providing sporting events on monitors, magazines with a sports theme such as *Sports Illustrated,* and the sports section from the newspaper.

Bathrooms

A bathroom typically is not thought of as a marketing technique, but the office's bathroom communicates something to your patients, which is what marketing is all about. A bathroom that is meticulously clean and patient friendly says something about your service. It says you pay attention to small details and understand the consumer's needs. If staff are careful about the bathroom, the staff likely are careful about vision care. Include makeup mirrors, hairspray, hand lotion, and tissues to anticipate the needs of your patients. Many patients will visit the bathroom to check their appearance after an eye examination. The room can be made more appealing by posting the sports page and having decorations on the wall that include information about sports vision, sport-tinted contact lenses, etc. Remind them that you can relate to their needs. Provide information about sports vision to read.

Music

Music is always a difficult choice in any office because it is impossible to address the preferences of every patient. As a sports vision expert, you may be able to avoid this by broadcasting sports talk show stations or game commentaries, which would convey the message that you are all about sports, effectively separating you from other eye care professionals.

COMMUNICATION DURING PATIENT HISTORY AND PRETESTING

The next opportunity to communicate with your patient is during completion of the patient history form. The patient history form can be used to make patients aware of needs they may not have realized when making the appointment. The history form can be used to gather information that you would otherwise not garner. For example, history may reveal risk factors requiring someone active in outdoor sports to protect the eyes from sunlight. A patient may mention a type of recreation that puts him or her at risk for eye injury, such as basketball. A sports vision practice should ask specific questions regarding sports activities (see Chapter 4 and Appendix A). Does the patient play tennis, golf, baseball, racquetball, basketball, or other sports? How often? Do patients use any eye protection during the sport? Do they wish they could see better when playing the sport? A checklist of all sports activities is useful for a sports vision history form. As previously mentioned, follow-up regarding the information the patient provides is crucial. For example, for a patient who indicates skeet shooting as a recreational pursuit, the examination and dispensing services should provide evaluation and recommendations specifically suited for this sport.

Many medications can cause mydriasis, which may decrease the depth of focus and increase the effect of higher order aberrations on vision. A good history lets you give the proper counseling on the effect these medications may cause on vision during sports.

Pretesting Room

Often patients are seated in a pretesting room before tests are conducted by a technician. While in the room, they will look around, as they do in the reception area. Posters, testimonials, diplomas, awards, news articles, and Health Insurance Portability and Accountability Act (HIPAA)-compliant photos of special patients can be placed on the walls in this room and can be a strong support for your recommendations.

Counter cards, brochures, dispensing mats, and copies of office marketing materials can also be displayed. Use the pretesting room to educate patients about the services you offer.

Technician Review of History Form

A well-trained technician can review the history form and recognize treatment possibilities for the athlete. The technician can discuss opportunities with the athlete by saying, "I see from the history that you play racquetball. There are new protective goggles that are lightweight and look cool while still providing necessary protection for your eyes. Here is a brochure about the new protective frames made for racquetball players." Or the technician may say, "I see from your history form that you are taking allergy medications that may affect the way your pupils respond to sunlight. Combined with the time you spend playing golf outside, you should protect your eyes from the sun. Here is a brochure about sun eyewear specially designed for golf to give you better vision and protect your eyes from developing cataracts and macular degeneration. The doctor can discuss whether these lenses are appropriate for you."

Staff training is a key element to a successful practice. Regular, weekly staff meetings can be an important opportunity to provide ongoing training and update staff, ultimately facilitating staff to feel empowered to help each patient get the most benefits from the office visit. Train your assistants how to look at the history form and match the history with probable treatment options. Give your staff materials to educate the patient on what you offer. These steps will help not only your patients and practice but also the staff to have a rewarding work experience.

Pretesting Scripts for the Technician

The technician can further educate the patient about the value of examination procedures by explaining their value in relation to the patient's particular needs. For example, the technician may say, "I am now going to test your peripheral vision, which you use to detect the ball out of the corner of your eye when playing basketball" or "I am going to test your depth perception to make sure you can judge distances as well as possible as when you are playing baseball."

A well-trained technician can relate binocular vision, visual field, and color vision tests to sports and convey the message that you provide an excellent examination experience. "The doctor will use these test results and history information to deliver an eye examination designed to your specific needs."

THE DOCTOR'S EXAMINATION

After pretesting examination, the patient typically is led to a doctor's examination room. The patient may review the brochures and educational materials obtained from the technician while waiting for the doctor. The examination room should be decorated with diplomas, awards, recognitions, photos of eye conditions, or other materials that convey the image of a sports vision specialist.

The Human Bond Before the Business Bond

Marketing experts say the doctor must form the human bond before the business bond, and the human bond can be on any subject other than the business at hand. Sports vision is an excellent topic for the athletic patient who never considered speaking to the doctor about improved performance through better vision. A discussion about similar sports interests can assist in developing a relationship with the patient, enhancing the chances he or she will adhere to the prescribed treatment after the examination. When the patient returns for another visit, a mention of "How's your golf game?" can immediately bond the patient to the doctor. Casual discussion about your experiences with sports can enhance your image as someone who understands the needs of the athlete patient.

Creating the human bond goes a long way in building trust between the doctor and patient. The human bond results in more loyalty, enthusiasm, and referrals. This is also important when working with sports teams. Developing relationships with the team personnel is an important element for gaining the trust of the organization. For many teams, the athletic training staff is a critical connection to foster. Athletic trainers are allied healthcare professionals who, under the direction of the team physician, manage the overall care of the athletes. Athletic trainers are the center of the sports medicine team that can include a network of physicians in a variety of specialties (including eye care), nutritionists, psychologists, coaching staff, strength and conditioning trainers, and administrators. In the athletic trainer's capacity to facilitate everything from injury prevention to comprehensive rehabilitation, they are an excellent ally in helping develop and implement a program to address the visual needs of the athletes on the team. Athletic trainers can also be your advocate with all the important stakeholders and translate program goals into practical messages that will resonate with the team.

Explaining the Value of the Examination Procedures

Eye care practitioners often incorrectly assume that patients know what is going on during the examination. Unless the procedure is explained, patients have no idea of the benefit. For example, retinoscopy has been performed for hundreds of years, yet few patients know the value of the procedure. A simple description such as, "I am shining a light off the back of your eye and focusing it up close where I am looking, so it will get blurry for you. This tells me what your eye needs without asking you any questions. Half the tests I do today don't require you to say anything, that way you do not have to worry about giving the right answers." This explanation dispels the worry of many patients that they will give the wrong response and get the wrong lenses.

Link examination procedures to patients' particular sports needs whenever possible. When assessing visual performance, it is essential that patients put forth their best effort in order to have a meaningful result. Understanding why the assessment is important for their sport can help provide the necessary motivation to perform optimally. Assessment explanations may also be used

to prepare the patient for prescribed treatments such as contact lenses, polarized sun lenses, sports vision training, and sports protective eyewear. By talking throughout the examination, the time will be no longer and the patient will be much more engaged in the process. Explained properly, the patient will not be surprised at the recommended treatment and may be eager to proceed with the recommendations.

Sports Vision Instrumentation

A significant challenge when developing a sports vision practice is determining what instrumentation to invest in. There are some natural limitations based on the space available in the practice (see Fig. 9.3 for a sample sports vision training area) and also how much capital expenditure is reasonable before there is a revenue stream. As described early in this chapter, it is often wise to start by offering a modest level of services without a significant investment in instrumentation. As expertise is developed and opportunities are created, investment in advanced technologies strongly communicates your practice's dedication to providing high-level care to athletes. The practice needs to determine what visual performance skills are important to assess and prioritize a list of instruments that meet those needs. The same approach can be used with sports vision training instrumentation. In many practices, it is wise to concentrate on equipment that is portable and easy to implement.

The practice should develop a budget for acquiring instruments that are based on revenue generation from this aspect of the practice. As more athletes seek

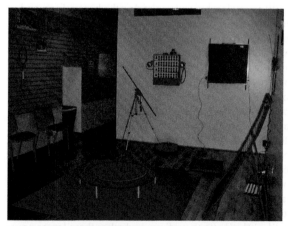

FIG. 9.3 Example of the sports vision testing and training room at the XTREMESIGHT Performance Clinic. (Courtesy of Fred Edmunds, O.D.)

sports vision services, the instrumentation and services can be expanded to meet the growing demand. It is also vitally important that, prior to making a purchase, the practitioner understands what the instrumentation is capable of and how it can be incorporated into the practice. You can gather this important information from colleagues who use the instrumentation, from company sales representatives, and from conferences with an exhibit hall where you can have a hands-on demonstration. A significant element of the return on investment is how useful the instrumentation is for your practice needs, so decisions regarding these purchases are very important.

The Case Presentation

The case presentation is the doctor's chance to put everything together for the patient to understand. Studies show that a patient remembers 60% more if a visual aid is used during an explanation.[2] Models, pictures, lenses, videos, written materials, samples, and demonstrations may be used to explain the patient's needs (based on history and examination) and the solutions to these needs. Often doctors are so caught up in data gathering that they do not spend enough time communicating what they can offer the patient. This is the most important part of the examination process for the patient, and this is how patients judge how "good" the doctor is. Patients want good explanations from their doctors, so spend extra time on this part of the eye examination.

An examination summary form can be used to summarize the findings and prescribed treatments (see Appendix B). This form can make the patient aware of everything involved in the examination and the complexity of vision care. Handing an examination summary form to a patient is a good example of doing something that other doctors do not, or will not, do. This act can help you stand out as special to your patients. There are computer-based assessment programs that provide a visual performance profile at the completion of the assessments, as described in Chapter 4, and these are excellent visual aids for describing the athlete's visual strengths and "opportunities." With athletes, it is better not to describe "weaknesses," but to rather adopt a more positive message of discussing opportunities to improve performance.

With athletes, it is recommended that you discuss actions or interventions that the athlete can adopt immediately. It is important that the athlete recognizes a tangible benefit to the vision care services provided. Determining what the athlete's greatest needs are and offering quick and effective options to improve are essential steps for gaining the trust and confidence of the athlete. Like most patients, athletes do not have extensive knowledge about vision and intervention options, so it is important to provide a tangible benefit immediately. The athlete is more likely to return for follow-up care recommendations if there is a perceived benefit.

Recommendations by the doctor are often referred to as the "power of the white coat." Patients are more apt to spend money on products and services if the doctor discusses them with the patient and makes a strong recommendation or prescription. Offices that leave the explaining of lens features to the opticians have less compliance with the prescription. Use the power of your "white coat" to improve the lives of your patients, but be careful not to cross the line into coaching. One of the biggest mistakes an eager doctor can make is to recommend changes to an athlete's sports performance that is beyond the scope of his or her expertise. If there are some potential changes in the biomechanics of the sport that the practitioner thinks will benefit the athlete, it is much better to communicate those recommendations directly with the coaches or trainers. If the coaches and trainers see a potential benefit to the recommendations, it will be much more effective for them to implement those changes than for the doctor to. Your deference to their expertise in the sport will demonstrate your team-focused approach to vision care.

After the examination, you may want to hand the patient a few referral cards. A referral card is a business card that says on the back, "The greatest compliment our patients can give is the referral of their friends and loved ones. Thank you for your trust." If you feel as if you bonded well with the patient, then hand them a few cards and say, "If you know of family or friends who could benefit from my services, I'll be glad to see them." Some doctors say this is the single most important tool they have used to generate new patients.

When working with sports teams, access to the doctor is paramount. Provide the athletic training staff with your mobile phone number so that they can contact you at any time, and provide a backup contact in case you are not available. With elite-level teams, when a problem arises, it often needs to be attended to quickly and effectively. Your availability communicates your dedication to the team.

Communicating the Benefits in the Dispensary

The patient typically is next escorted to the dispensary, where the recommendations are restated and demonstrated by the optician. Sales training is a benefit to the person in this position because he or she is required to "close the sale" and explain the fees. Sometimes objections must be overcome and the value of the prescribed product or service restated. Have your staff develop scripts to explain the benefits and overcome common concerns.

Demonstrators, Displays, and Written Materials

Demonstrators, displays, and written materials can be used to show the patient what to expect from the prescribed product or service. Lens packages are an excellent way to present fees and options without going through every lens option. Think of the "value meal" offered by fast-food restaurants. This concept is a simple way to bundle all the options and present them to the consumer. The computer and auto industries have used bundling for many years. Presenting lens options as best, better, and good can help the optician explain what is ideal for the patient. Bundling may also be used to join products together with services such as contact lenses. What sports vision services and products can you bundle together and offer patients?

Fee Slips and Receipts

When presenting the bill, a fee slip or receipt should act as a marketing technique by including your logo, theme, and a list of available services and products. Show patients what you stand for and what you offer on the fee slip. Patients often do not realize the wide variety of services and products offered by eye care professionals. Their exposure to vision care may consist only of a general eye examination and a limited choice of lenses. Listing many of the services and product choices on your receipt can help educate patients that there is more to eye care than simply a basic examination and glasses.

With sports teams or student athletes, you may choose to provide some services as a gift in-kind or in exchange for advertising. The value of the services provided can be used as a business tax credit, or advertising for the practice can be placed in game programs, signage in the stadium, or on the team's website.

Dispensary Decor

The decor of the dispensing area should be consistent with the sports vision theme of the practice. Team memorabilia, colors, and sports themes can be reinforced. Modern decor is consistent in conveying that your practice is consistent with the latest technology. Merchandise displays can make the observer aware of what is available to them.

EXTERNAL MARKETING

Once all the internal marketing strategies are implemented and aligned with your practice brand and image, you are ready to develop external marketing to attract new patients. If the internal marketing is not in place, you will not keep the promise made by your theme and story and thus lose patient trust sooner, leading to the demise of your business faster than if you did no marketing at all. A survey of top practices in Southern California showed that external marketing was not necessary once word of mouth and reputation were strong.[3] To get to that point, however, external marketing is required to get the "mouths" in and give them the message to spread. Box 9.1 shows several marketing techniques that can be used to bring in new patients.

External marketing techniques should depend on what has been most effective in the past; be most fun, easiest to do, and free or inexpensive; fill a present need; and be something of interest to someone on staff.

Direct Mail

Although no one seems to want to receive "junk" mail, direct mail is still an effective method by which people learn about products and services. Many eye care practitioners attempt direct mailings at some point, while many professionals scoff at using direct mail, citing the irritation of junk mail. Often the strength of direct mail is simply reminding recipients that they can benefit from certain services or products. In a hectic

> **BOX 9.1**
> **Marketing to Established and New Patients**
>
> Direct mail
> Research demographics
> E-mail
> Newspaper inserts
> Refrigerator magnets
> Newspaper advertisements
> Courses and lectures
> School educational programs
> Seminars
> Trunk shows
> Referrals from medical practitioners
> Contests
> Scholarships and awards
> Community activities
> Public relations
> Club and association memberships
> Outside signs
> Reputation
> Word of mouth

world, direct mail can remind them that eye care is important. Your name, logo, and theme on a direct mail piece can suggest they receive that care from you.

Many professionals send out direct mail pieces only once and lament how the effort did not result in any additional sales. Common mistakes such as omission of a phone number or address, misspellings, and postal errors regarding bulk rates can defeat even the best direct mail intentions.

A successful direct mail campaign includes at least four direct mailings a year. Each should result in an increased response. Ideally, the fourth mailing will provide the greatest success. Marketing experts state that people must hear a message at least three times before they respond to it. For example, it takes 27 opportunities to notice a sign 9 times and it takes 9 times to pay attention to the message 3 times. Direct mailings work better than signs because recipients must look at the piece to make the decision to throw it away. Eye care practitioners can expect a gross return on investment of 10 times from four direct mailings a year.

The success of direct mail also increases by targeting the proper population. As a sports vision specialist target athletic trainers, physical therapists, orthopedists, sports medicine physicians, sports psychologists, coaches, gyms, and any group associated with sports, such as little league baseball. Sending letters, newsletters, or postcards to targeted groups about what you offer costs little and can result in big returns for your practice.

E-mail Bulletins

If you have the e-mail addresses of important referral sources, you may want to communicate with them in that medium. Remember, a message can be deleted with the press of a button but the reader will still be reminded you exist. You could ask recipients how they prefer to learn about new technologies that may help their athletes. Sending e-mails to former patients and those who inquire about the practice can also result in building the sports vision portion of your office.

Newspaper Inserts

Inserts are full-page advertisements in newspapers that are an inexpensive way to deliver information to the general community. The cost can be as low as $45 per 1000 papers, but prices vary depending on the size of the newspaper's circulation. Although the consumer may not read the entire flyer, again, he or she must look at it long enough to throw it away. It will remind them you exist and may be timed perfectly to someone who has recognized the need for eye care services and products.

Another advantage of inserts is that the medium is separate from other newspaper information. An insert is much more noticeable than an advertisement tucked away on a page with several columns of news articles or other advertisements. The insert can also be reused in other forms of marketing, such as direct mail, posted flyers, or office information presented in the reception area or that of another healthcare provider.

Refrigerator Magnets

If you enjoy working with young people, refrigerator magnets are a must. No parent has enough refrigerator magnets to post all their children's school work and notices. An advantage of a refrigerator magnet is that it can put your name in front of prospective patients every day for a year or more. Design it like a mini brochure, including your logo, theme, and contact information. Many offices send a calendar refrigerator magnet to encourage use.

Newspaper Advertisements

Some people like to learn about services available to them through their local newspaper. Local papers often do not have the technology to include newspaper inserts. In those cases, a well-placed advertisement, run on a regular basis, may convey to the community what you offer. Make sure your advertisements include all the benefits of your products and services. Often a combination of several small benefits, rather than one particular benefit, inspires a potential patient to choose you. Think of every possible benefit you can offer the athlete and list it in the advertisement along with your logo, theme, and contact information. Placing advertisements in the newspaper can also position you for free public relations exposure.

Newspaper Columns

If you prove to be adept at writing and enjoy it, then offer to write a column for your local newspaper. Include samples of topics that may be useful to the paper to use when they have space to fill. Relationships with newspaper decision-makers can offer many opportunities to get your name into print.

Public Relations

Ask the salesperson who handles your newspaper advertisements and inserts to introduce you to the sports or science editor of your newspaper. You can establish your credibility as an authority in eye care by providing information to him or her in the form of press releases and articles you have written supporting the releases. Follow the release with a phone call from your office manager and offer to be interviewed on pertinent topics.

Although eye care practitioners may be well versed on new eye care technologies, the sports or science editor may not. Be a resource that journalists can trust to clarify information they may have heard elsewhere. Offering complimentary eye examinations and sports vision evaluations to opinion shapers such as newspaper editors can demonstrate your ability to improve their standard of living. Stories involving vision in sports can be distinctive and compelling, which is attractive to newspaper editors.

Consider local radio stations, cable television stations, and magazines and other periodicals as an audience for public relations announcements.

Courses, Lectures, and Workshops

Personal contact is the second most powerful marketing tool according to surveys concerning optometry. Courses and lectures establish you as an authority in the field. Send out a letter from your office manager each year offering to give a specific lecture or workshop to service organizations and community associations. Athletic trainers are often very receptive to an in-service on the triage and management of sports eye injuries, presenting an excellent opportunity to build a relationship. Creating an eye injury triage kit can be an excellent marketing tool because it is useful for the athletic trainers, and it can be branded with your practice information. The contents of the kit and triage card are described in Chapter 7 (see Table 7.3). Another good workshop opportunity is teaching contact lens insertion and removal because athletic trainers are often called on during practices or competitions to help athletes with contact lens challenges. By seeing you in person, the prospective patient or referral source will be more comfortable choosing you as a practitioner or member of the team's medical staff.

You can also hold lectures and workshops in your office. This can be an excellent opportunity to demonstrate what services your practice is dedicated to providing. Even if few participants show up, the ones that do attend could be key referral sources. Advertising the lecture also provides opportunities for exposure.

Referrals From Medical Practitioners

Saying you have something to offer is simple, but getting trusted medical practitioners to say you have something to offer can be more effective in convincing a prospective patient to come to you. Market to prospective professional referral sources by sending them letters, brochures, and referral pads. Offer complimentary examinations and refer to them in return. Developing relationships with key medical practitioners can develop into strong referral sources. Often their staff can be even more effective in busy medical offices. Have your staff take them out to lunch and encourage referrals.

Contests

If your brand identity is someone who is fun, a lottery-style drawing could be effective. You can advertise the contest and receive free exposure from your local newspaper or radio station. Add those entering the contest to your mailing list. The prizes for a sports vision practice should be related to sports, such as sports sunglasses or goggles.

For elementary schools a poster contest can be appropriate. For higher grades an essay on the importance of vision in sports could be effective.

Community Activities

People like to buy from friends. The more involved you are with the community, the more friends you will make. Make sure they learn of your qualifications through patient education pieces. Offer to contribute time and money to their causes and build loyalty for supporting the community.

One important fact to remember, however, is to act like a professional. Some eye care practitioners build their practice through community activities and others are unsuccessful. If you want the public to come to you as a doctor, you must fit their image of a doctor. Often this means certain expected behaviors. If you cannot act like a doctor (whatever that means for your community), then do not try to build your practice through community involvement. You may be the life of the party, but that person may not be a doctor to whom others are willing to trust their eyes.

Consider building your practice by joining service clubs, youth sports organizations, booster clubs, alumni organizations, or other sport-related associations and clubs.

Other marketing techniques that may build your practice include billboards, team sponsorships, radio advertisements, radio shows, television advertisements, television shows, magazine advertisements, and magazine articles. Sponsoring a local youth team puts your logo and name on their uniforms, reminding everyone that vision is an important part of sports and that you are there to help athletes. Advertising on a stadium or arena billboard or in a team media guide associates you with high-achieving athletes and bonds you with the fans. If you are the eye care provider for high-achieving athletes, you may be perceived as better than other eye doctors. Some offices pay professional teams large sums of money to advertise that they are the eye doctors for the team. If you have a large practice, this level of sponsorship may be beneficial.

Special Invitations

Your marketing plan should include as many opportunities as possible to give prospective patients an excuse to come to the office and learn about you and what you offer. Invitations can take the form of an open house, patient appreciation day, community service day, or sports vision screening day. You can send out invitations to learn more about new frame releases, new sports vision contact lenses, sport-tinted contact lenses, disposable bifocal contact lenses, refractive surgeries, and other new procedures and services. Invite athletic trainers, strength and conditioning coaches, physical therapists, sports medicine practitioners, orthopedists, sports psychologists, and coaches to your practice for a special open house. In addition, you may want to consider invitations for members of the local law enforcement or military who require excellent visual performance in their occupations.

Often you can partner with an optical or pharmaceutical company to provide cooperative funds to pay for the special event. They may send sales representatives to help with contact lens application and removal or frame experts.

Reputation

The ultimate goal of all external marketing is to build a desired reputation. Once the community learns to associate you and your office with desired characteristics, the patients will want to go nowhere else. Reputation is built by getting patients to your practice with a promise to provide what they want and then fulfill this promise through the practice experience and internal marketing. Once a good reputation is achieved, the strongest marketing tool of all is available to you—word of mouth.

Word of Mouth

Consumers are better educated than ever before. They have grown skeptical through advertisements that promise one thing and provide another. Now consumers have a greater number of products and services to spend their money on than at any other time in history. Trusting a friend or colleague to confirm what the prospective patient has learned through a website or marketing pieces is critical in choosing an eye care provider. For this reason, word of mouth continues to be the primary marketing technique to bring in patients. Always remember when designing patient communications that satisfied patients have the mouths; you are responsible for putting the words into them.

Use every communication opportunity available to place positive words in your patients' mouths. Restate what you stand for and retell your story. Once you have others telling your story and building your reputation, you have arrived. You are the sports vision expert! The core principle is to deliver high-quality vision care by being prepared to meet the needs of your athlete patients. Remember, vision is a key aspect of human performance, but it is only one aspect of the complex equation. When you make misleading or grandiose claims, the door of opportunity may be closed. It is more difficult to get opportunities a second time when you have failed to deliver the first time. Be careful about making false claims about what you can deliver—it is much better to have the athlete tell your story.

REFERENCES

1. Moss GL, Shaw-McMinn PG. *Eyecare Business Marketing and Strategy.* Boston, MA: Butterworth-Heinemann; 2001, 98−106, 115.
2. Levinson JC. *Guerilla Marketing Attack.* Boston, MA: Houghton Mifflin; 1989:8.
3. Katzaroff J, Hopkins J, Shaw-McMinn PG. *A Survey of Marketing Methods by Private Practitioners in Southern California* [thesis], Southern California College of Optometry Student Research Papers, 97−28 to 97−39. California: Fullerton; 1997.

2006
American Optometric Association
Sports Vision Screening Protocols

July 2006
STEPHEN BECKERMAN, O.D., F.A.A.O.
STEVEN HITZEMAN, O.D., F.A.A.O

CONTENTS

<u>CONSENT</u>

For the consent to participate in a vision screening and research study

Read the following to the Athlete:

> I, the undersigned, give my permission for a Sports Vision Screening to be performed on me by the members of the AOA Sports Vision Section Screening Team (AOA SVSST). In granting this permission, I release agents and representatives of the Junior Olympics and the AOA SVSST from any and all liability, which may arise from the screening examinations or tests. I realize that a screening should not be considered a complete examination and that responsibility for any recommended follow-up care is mine alone.
>
> Having come to the AOA SVSST for this screening, I voluntarily consent to allow the information in my record (including test results, photographs and other pertinent information) to be inspected (reviewed) and/or used for the purpose of research, student education, scientific studies or other professional purposes. During my examination, the clinician or optometrist assigned to me will explain the benefits and risks of specific testing procedures to me. I understand that my name will remain confidential (will not be used) if the information in my record is reviewed.
>
> Furthermore, I am aware that I may refuse to allow the use of my record, but that such refusal would in no way affect the level of care to which I am entitled.

Present the above information to the Athlete and allow for questions to be asked.

> If the Athlete agrees to the vision screening have him/her to sign in the appropriate location on the recording form. If the athlete is a minor, have their legal guardian sign the form.

HISTORY

It is important to get an accurate ocular and medical history in order to fully utilize the screening information. Ask the Athlete the following questions about their ocular and medical health and sport's involvement. Allow the Athlete to ask questions and offer additional information and record the answers in the appropriate area on the recording form.

Demographic info:

Patient initials:

Age (at time of screening):

Sport: record primary competitive sport

1. baseball	12. softball
2. basketball	13. sailing
3. hockey	14. gymnastics
4. football	15. karate/martial arts
5. volleyball	16. surfing
6. soccer	17. field hockey
7. track	18. power lifting
8. tennis	19. jump aerobics
9. swimming	20. water polo
10. wrestling	21. other
11. golf	

Male/ Female:

Competition level: record highest level achieved
1. grade school
2. jr. high
3. high school
4. jr. college
5. college NCAA division 2/3
6. college NCAA division 1
7. professional (minor league)
8. professional (major league)
9. recreational
10. control

Rx History

What was the date of your last eye Exam in an Eye Doctor's office?
What is your Eye Doctor's name?

Do you wear corrective lenses?
If yes, do you wear them for sports?

Ask which of the following describe the Athlete's current spectacles.
- None
- ASTM f803 approved Eyewear (Prescriptive)
- Plano Polycarbonate Shield
- Standard Spectacle

If the Athlete uses contact lenses ask which of the following applies.
- Soft Sphere Daily Wear
- Soft Sphere Extended Wear
- Soft Disposables
- Soft Toric
- Rigid Gas Permeable

Ocular Symptoms

Ask the Athlete if they ever experience or have been told they have any of the following symptoms:

-Difficulty seeing	*-Reduced Peripheral Vision*
-Sensitivity to lights	*-Reduced Performance as Stress Builds*
-Lack of Consistency of Play	
-Easily Distracted from Visual Target	*-Headaches*
	-Poor Depth Perception
-Difficulty following moving objects	*-Blurred Vision After Close Work*

Ask the Athlete if they have any reason to believe they have an eye or vision problem.

Medical History

Ask the Athlete to describe their current medical health and to list any medications they are currently taking.

LENSOMETRY

Evaluates: The sphere, cylinder, and axis of the Athlete's current optical prescription. Perform lensometry on the prescription that the Athlete most often uses for sport's activities.

Basic Components of a Lensometer

All lensometers have the same basic parts and features although the designs vary. These components are:

1. Viewing Telescope

     This allows the image of the target mire formed by the unknown lens to be viewed. The telescope is focused for optical infinity therefore the mire image will appear clear only if light emerging form the unknown lens into the telescope is parallel.

2. Eyepiece   The eyepiece is where the observer looks into the lensometer. This must be focused to make the internal reticule clear. The reticule is a black crosshair that in some models has a series of concentric circles and/or hashmarks used to measure prism. The reticule must be in focus in order to obtain an accurate neutralization of unknown lenses.

3. Target (Mires)

     These are object lines inside the body of the lensometer, which are focused by turning the power wheel. They are two perpendicular sets of either 2 or 3 lines. The lines of one set are spaced closely together and the lines of the other set are spaced more widely apart.

4. Power Wheel

     This is an external wheel, which is rotated until the internal mire targets are clear. The sphere and cylinder components of the prescription are read off a scale on power wheel when the mires are in focus.

5. Cylinder (axis) Wheel

     This is an external wheel that rotates the mires. It is calibrated in degrees in order to indicate the orientation of the minus cylinder axis of the lens when the mires are properly positioned.

6. Lens Stage (Table)

This is a horizontal platform that supports the lower edge of the glasses. It can be moved up or down in order to accommodate different frames.

7. Lens Stop

The lens to be measured is placed against the lens stop. The area of the lens centered on the lens stop is the area measured.

8. Lens Holder

This is a spring-loaded arm that holds the lens firmly against the lens stop when it is released.

9. Lens marker

This is a three dot marking system used to mark a horizontal line across a lens. It is used to mark the optical center of the lens when the mire pattern is centered on the reticule.

10. Prism compensator

This device is used to compensate for the displacement of the mires from the center of the reticule. A scale on the compensator allows the prism magnitude and direction to be determined. The compensator is set on zero unless prism is being measured.

Preparing the Lensometer:

1. Focus the eyepiece

First, set the power wheel to zero. Next rotate the eyepiece completely out, counterclockwise, until the reticule is blurred. Then rotate the eyepiece slowly inward until the reticule is clear and distinct. *See figure 1*

2. Re-set the prism compensator

If the lensometer has a prism compensator, it must be re-set to zero. When you look into the lensometer if the mire patterns are not centered on the reticule then the prism compensator is not set at zero.

Neutralizing the lenses

1. Always measure the right lens first.

2. Place the pair of glasses in the lensometer with the concave surface away from you. *See figure 2*

3. Center the lens by aligning the target in the center of the eyepiece reticule by moving the lens up, down, to the right, or to the left. Once the lens is centered move the stage so that it supports the bottom of the frame. Carefully release the lens holder so that the lens is held firmly in place.

4. Turn the power wheel to very high plus. Then slowly turn the power wheel towards the minus direction and rotate the axis wheel until the sphere mires (small narrow lines) come into sharp focus. If the cylinder mires (wider lines) come into focus first rotate the axis wheel 90 degrees so that the sphere mires are in focus. If the sphere and cylinder mires come into focus at the same time the lens is spherical.

5. Now find the cylinder power. Do not move the axis wheel. The axis has already been determined. Continue turning the power wheel in the minus direction until the cylinder mires are clear. The difference between the new power reading shown on the power wheel and the original sphere power is the amount of minus cylinder power in the lens. Read the axis of the cylinder from the axis wheel. *See figure 3.*

Examples

1. Power wheel reading when the sphere mires are in focus = -1.00 D
   Axis wheel reading when the sphere mires are in focus = 175 degrees
   Power wheel reading when the cylinder mires are in focus = -3.00 D

   Rx = -1.00 -2.00 x 175

2. Power wheel reading when the sphere mires are in focus = +2.00 D
   Axis wheel reading when the sphere mires are in focus = 45 degrees
   Power wheel reading when the cylinder mires are in focus = +0.50 D

   Rx = +2.00 -1.50 x 045

Recording

1. Always record the sphere and cylinder power and the axis location as three digits. For example:

Correct	Incorrect
+1.00 -0.50 x 045	+1.00 - .50 x 45

2. If the lens is spherical record "sph" or "DS". For example:

-3.00 DS

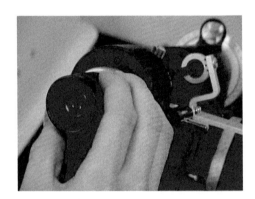

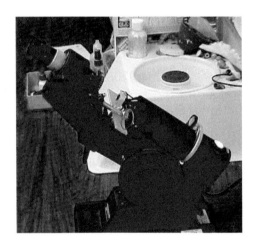

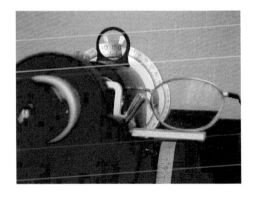

VISUAL ACUITY (SNELLEN)

Evaluates: The Snellen chart uses minimum separable angle techniques to determine visual acuity. The fraction result that is obtained is the reciprocal of minimum angle of resolution (this is based on one minute of arc).

Test Distance: 20 feet

Illumination: Standard illumination

Position: Standing relaxed

Critical Factors:
Sequence for testing is OD followed by OS

Criterion: Crisp 20/20 (1 minute of arc) OD, OS

Instructional Set:
"Please cover your left eye and read the row of letters above the red line. Then the smallest line below the red line you can with out squinting. Guess if you have too." Repeat this with the right eye covered.

Record: Record BVA (best visual acuity) as the smallest line where the patient gave >50% correct.

STANDARD CHART ANSWERS

200:E
100:F,P
70:T,O,Z
50:L,P,E,D
40:P,E,C,F,D
30:E,D,F,C,Z,P
25:F,E,L,O,P,Z,D
20:D,E,F,P,O,T,E,C
15:L,E,F,O,D,P,C,T
13:F,D,P,L,T,C,E,O
10:P,E,Z,O,L,C,F,T,D

<u>COVER TEST</u>

Evaluates: This test assesses the presence and magnitude of a phoria or a tropia (strabismus). If motor fusion is present (there is no strabismus) the cover test measures the demand put on the Athlete's fusional vergence system.

Equipment: Occluder, Snellen chart, near point target, and a prism bar.

Set-up: This test is done at both distance (20 feet) and near (16 inches). The Athlete should wear his/her habitual Rx for the distance being tested. The room illumination should be full. For distance testing the target should be a isolated Snellen letter 2 lines above best visual acuity for the patient's poorer seeing eye. *See figure 1*. For near testing the target should be an isolated near target letter. *See figure 2*.

Instructions: Inform the athlete that this test measures the ability of his/her eyes to work as a team. Instruct the athlete to look at a particular detail of the target letter ("look at the tip of the A"). Tell the athlete to keep that detail clear throughout the entire test. It is very important that the athlete does not look around during this test.

Procedure: 1. First perform the unilateral cover test (UCT). This portion of the test determines if a strabismus (tropia) is present. Begin the UCT with the occluder in the midline position (over the patient's nose). Cover the patient's right eye while observing the left eye. Repeat this several times noting any movement of the left eye only. Then cover the patient's left eye while observing the right eye. Again, repeat this several times noting any movement of the right eye only. Be sure to hold the occluder over the eye for 2-4 seconds to allow the deviating eye (if present) to regain fixation. Note the direction and magnitude of any movement. If no movement is present on this test the athlete does not have a strabismus. Perform the above procedure at both distance and near. *See figure 3*.

2. Now perform the alternating cover test (ACT). This allows the determination of the presence of a phoria if a tropia has already been ruled out by performing the unilateral cover test. Alternately occlude the right and left eye for at least 5 cycles. Watch the eye that is uncovered as you move the occluder to the other eye. It is important to make sure the athlete is not binocular at any time. The occluder is in place over the eye for 2-4 seconds but it should be moved quickly between the eyes in order to avoid binocularity. Note the direction of the movement of the eye as it is uncovered in order to determine the type of deviation present.

1. If the eye moves in when uncovered = exo deviation (the eye was out)
2. If the eye moves out when uncovered = eso deviation (the eye was in)
3. If the eye moves down when uncovered = hyper deviation (eye was up)
4. If the eye moves up when uncovered = hypo deviation (eye was down)

Also perform the ACT at both distance and near. *See figure 4*

3. In order to determine the magnitude of the deviation hold the appropriate base prism over 1 eye and perform the alternating cover test.
BO prism for eso
BI prism for exo
BD prism for hyper
BU prism for hypo
Begin with low amounts of prism and increase the amount of prism and repeat alternate occlusion until no motion is seen. The magnitude of the deviation is determined when no motion is noted. *See figure 5.*

Recording: Phorias: record the magnitude and direction of the deviation.
Tropias: Record the type of deviation, laterality (unilateral or alternating), magnitude of the deviation (in prism diopters), frequency of the deviation (constant or intermittent), and the direction. The prime sign (') indicates a near deviation.
P = phoria

T= tropia = strabismus
E= eso deviation
X = exo deviation

Examples: 2 XP = 2 prism diopters of exophoria at distance
10 EP′ = 10 prism diopters of esophoria at near
5 CLET = 5 prism diopter constant left esotropia at distance
30 IAXT′ = 30 prism diopter intermittent alternating exotropia at near

Referral Criteria: Any strabismus that is present.
A phoria greater than 2 exo or 2 eso at distance.
A phoria greater than 6 exo or 2 eso at near.

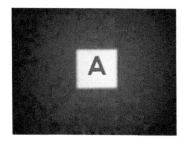 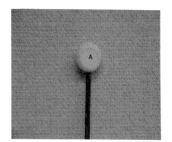

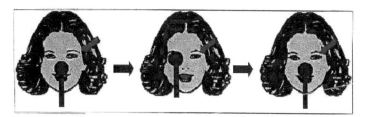

Figure 3: Unilateral cover test.

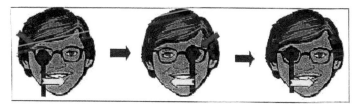

Figure 4: Alternating cover test. Be sure to watch the eye being uncovered. Movement is in the direction of the yellow arrow.

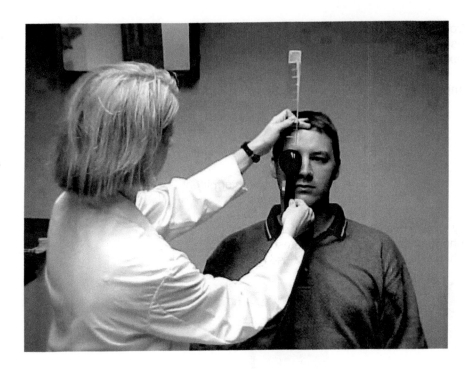

<u>NEAR POINT OF CONVERGENCE (NPC)</u>

Evaluates: The ability of the eyes to converge while maintaining fusion.

Equipment: Near point target, PD ruler

Set-up: The athlete can either sit or stand and should be wearing his/her habitual Rx. The near target should be fully illuminated. Hold the PD ruler with the zero mark at the eye's center of rotation. *See figure 1.*

Instructions: Instruct the athlete to look at the near target. Tell the athlete that you are going to be bringing the target in towards his/her nose. Instruct the athlete to report if the target becomes blurry or splits into two targets. Tell the athlete to maintain fixation on the target at all times.

Procedure: Start with the fixation target slightly below the athlete's eye level at 50cm.

Bring the target slowly up the midline towards the nose. If the patient reports two targets or if the examiner notices an eye turn, note the distance from the eye. This is the break point.

Now bring the target back towards yourself until the patients reports that the target is now one or until you witness the eyes regaining bifixation. This is the recovery point.

Recording: Record the break point and recovery point in centimeters. Also note if diplopia was reported or if the examiner saw an eye deviation. If the athlete maintains bifixation all the way to his/her nose record TN (to nose).
Examples: 5/8 (broke at 5cm and recovered at 8cm)

Referral Criteria:
Any break or recovery greater than 12/15cm.

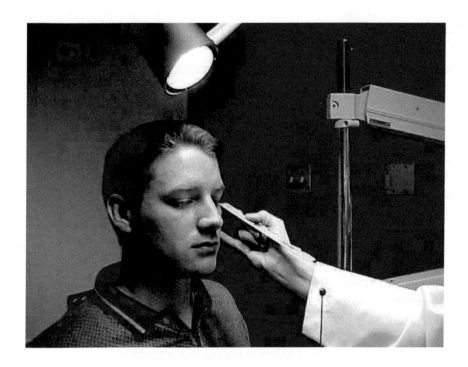

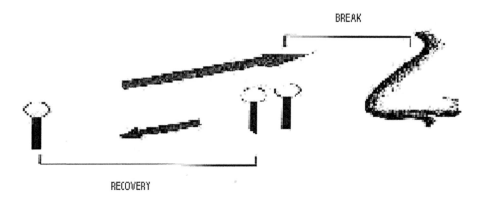

BREAK

RECOVERY

<u>COLOR VISION</u>
(Color Vision Testing Made Easy)

Evaluates: To detect the presence of any red-green color deficits.

Test Distance: 75 cm (30 inches)

Illumination: True Daylight Illuminant (TDI), Standard Illumination "C"

Position: Sitting or standing

Critical Factors:

Binocular testing

Criterion: If the athlete was able to identify 8 out of 9 plates, the test is complete.   If the athlete identified the sample plate but scored less than 8, present all of the 9 plates a second time.

Instructional Set:

Part 1: "Please tell me if you see a circle (or ball) on these cards."   Present the first card to the binocular athlete and allow 3 seconds per plate. If they fail the first attempt, repeat the test.

Part 2: "Please tell me what object you see on each of these cards. Do you see a dog, boat, balloon, or nothing?"

Recording: Record the number of correct responses attempted out of nine (X/9) by the trial number. Don't include the demonstration card in this number. Classify any color deficiency.

STANDARD CHART ANSWERS:

Part 1

Card No.	Normal Color	Deficient Color Vision	Normal Color	Deficient Color Vision
1	☐	☐	☐	☐
2	☐	Nothing	☐	Nothing
3	☐	☐	☐	☐
4	☐	Nothing	☐	Nothing
5	☐	☐	☐	☐
6	☐	Nothing	☐	Nothing
7	☐	Nothing	☐	Nothing
8	☐	Nothing	☐	Nothing
9	☐	Nothing	☐	Nothing

Part 2

	Normal Color Vision	Deficient Color Vision
☐A☐	Boat	Nothing
☐B☐	Balloon	Nothing
☐C☐	Dog	Nothing

If patient responds ☐car☐, then diagnose as malingering.

COLOR VISION
(Ishihara Color Plates)

Evaluates: Presence of any deficits in sensitivity to various wavelengths of light

Test Distance: 50 cm

Illumination: True Daylight Illuminant (TDI), or Standard illuminant type "C"

Position: Sitting or standing

Critical Factors:
Binocular testing

Criterion: The athlete is not allowed to miss any plates binocularly. If any plates are missed, retest monocularly. The first plate is for demonstration and should not be missed by anyone, or the athlete may be malingering. For plates 1-15, only show every other plate (1, 3, 5, etc...), then show plates 16 and 17.

Instructional Set:
"Look at the plates and tell me what the dots form."

Recording: Record the number of correct responses (X/10) per response attempted. Classify person as Red-Green deficiency, Protan, Deutan, or Total Color deficiency.

Example of Color Plate

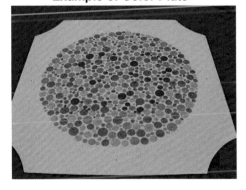

Example of proper testing position

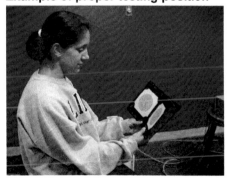

Answers for Ishihara Color Plates (Normative and Color Deficient responses):

Plate	Normal Person	Person with Red-Green Deficiencies				Person with Total Color Blindness
1	12	12				12
2	8	3				X
3	29	70				X
4	5	2				X
5	3	5				X
6	15	17				X
7	74	21				X
8	6	X				X
9	45	X				X
10	5	X				X
11	7	X				X
12	16	X				X
13	73	X				X
14	X	5				X
15	X	45				X
		Protan		Deutan		
		Strong	Mild	Strong	Mild	
16	26	6	(2) 6	2	2 (6)	
17	42	2	(4) 2	4	4 (2)	

RANDOT STEREOPSIS

Evaluates: Near sensitivity to binocular disparity depth information presented vectographically.

Test Distance: Exactly 40cm

Illumination: Normal room lighting

Position: Sitting or standing.

Critical Factors:

Must test the forms located in the six boxes on the right side of book first. All six boxes must be correctly identified before the test is continued. Then test the circles, there must be no head tilting, or turning of the book. Time limit of 5 seconds per line for response. Test at **exactly** 40 cm. **Note:** Many patients have difficulty at #6, please encourage guessing until #10.

Criterion: 6/6 on forms and 7/10 dots without hesitation
Norms: 8.71 $\pm$ 1.94

Instructional Set:

Have the athlete wear vectographic spectacles over habitual Rx. Present the example figures shown below and on the cover of the book to the athlete and have them identify those figures in the six boxes on the right side of the book by asking, "What shapes do you see hidden in each of these panels?" If all figures are seen, present the rows of circles on the left. "Tell me which of the circles, left, middle, or right appears to be floating slightly above the other circles." Have the judgement made on all ten rows of stimuli.

Record: Record the number of figures identified correctly. The first incorrect response on the circles will be considered the limit of disparity except when the patient identifies two consecutive finer stimuli correctly.

ANSWER KEY

Scoring Key:		Sec of Arc at 16 in:	Scoring Key:		Sec of Arc at 16 in:
1 $\Rightarrow$	L	400	6 $\Rightarrow$	M	50
2 $\Rightarrow$	R	200	7 $\Rightarrow$	L	40
3 $\Rightarrow$	L	140	8 $\Rightarrow$	R	30
4 $\Rightarrow$	M	100	9 $\Rightarrow$	M	25
5 $\Rightarrow$	R	70	10 $\Rightarrow$	R	20

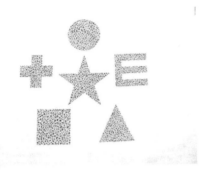

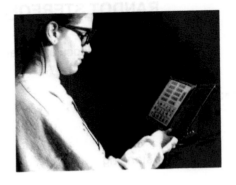

Example of Stereo forms

Example of proper testing position

PUPILS

Evaluates: The direct, consensual, and afferent pupillary responses.

Equipment: Fixation target with low accommodative demand, transilluminator.

Set-up: The athlete is standing with his/her eyes directed at a fixation target 20 feet across the room.

Instructions: Explain to the athlete that you are assessing how well his/her eyes react to light. Instruct the athlete to keep fixation on the distant target while you shine the transilluminator in his/her eyes.

Procedure: Shine the light into the right eye, without interfering with the athlete's visual axis, and observe the size of the pupil and the speed of the constriction in the right eye for three cycles. This is the direct response of the right eye.

Continue to shine the light in the right eye, while observing the pupil of the left eye for 3 cycles. This is the consensual response of the left eye.

Shine the light into the left eye and observe the direct response of the left eye for three cycles and the consensual response of the right eye for three cycles.

Check the athlete's pupils for an afferent pupillary defect (APD) by moving the light alternately between both eyes rapidly, while sustaining a period of 4 seconds per eye. Observe the responses of the eyes as the light moves to each of them. Be sure to indicate for each eye whether or not constriction occurs (normal) or if an initial dilation occurs (abnormal) as the light shines on the eye.

Recording: Record the relative appearance of the pupils (pupils equal round: PER), if the pupils were responsive to light (RL), and if a APD is present or not (- or + APD). Be sure to record any difference in size or shape between the two pupils.

Referral Criteria:

Any abnormal response including diminished light response, presence of an APD, or differences between size and shape.

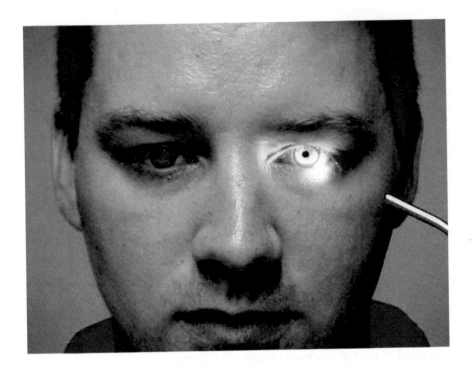

OCULAR MOTILITIES

Evaluates: This test assesses the athlete's ability to perform conjugate eye movements.

Equipment: Transilluminator

Set-up: The athlete should stand facing the examiner 50cm away. The room illumination should be full and the athlete should remove his/her habitual Rx.

Instructions: Tell the athlete that you are testing the ability of his/her eyes to move in different directions. The athlete should be instructed to keep their head still and to follow the light with their eyes. *See figure 1.* Instruct the athlete to report if he/she feels pain or has double vision at any time during the test.

Procedure: Beginning in primary gaze move the penlight into the cardinal positions indicated in the physiological "H" pattern. *See figure 2.* Be sure to move the penlight to the athlete's extreme limits of gaze. Throughout the procedure observe the smoothness of movement, the accuracy of following the penlight, and the extent of eye movement. At the extreme limits of a healthy person's gaze it is normal to observe a low amplitude nystagmus, termed end-point nystagmus.

Recording: If the athlete follows the penlight smoothly and accurately in all positions record FROM (full range of motion). Record the presence of any pain, diplopia, or restriction in the position that it occurred.

Referral Criteria:
     The presence of any oculomotor restriction.

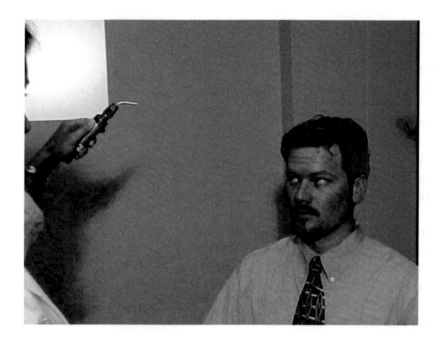

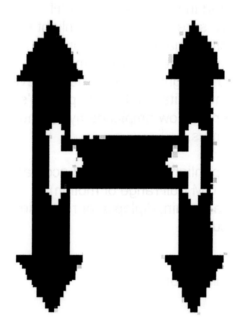

Figure 2: Physiological H pattern

<u>PURSUITS/SACCADES</u>

Evaluates: The quality of the athlete's pursuits and saccades.

Equipment: Two near targets of different colors.

Set-up: The athlete should stand facing the examiner 50cm away. Room illumination should be full and the athlete should wear his/her habitual sport's Rx.

Instructions: - Pursuits: Tell the athlete that you are testing his/her ability to follow a moving near target. Instruct the athlete to look at the target and follow it wherever it goes only using his/her eyes and without moving his/her head.

- Saccades: Tell the athlete that you are assessing his/her ability to change fixation from one target to another. Instruct the athlete to look at one near target and to look at the other target as quickly and accurately as possible when you call the color of the second target.

If any head movement occurs during either test instruct the athlete to try to hold their head still and only move their eyes. If the athlete is unable to resist head movement grade them as a 1 on that section.

Procedure: - Pursuits: Use one near target and move it left to right, right to left, up and down, down and up, and then in a circular pattern. Be sure to maintain the 50cm working distance and not to exceed a pattern greater than the circumference of the athlete's face.   *See figure 1.*

- Saccades: Use both near targets held at a distance of 10cm apart. Direct fixation from one target to the other for a total of 5 cycles. Be careful not to get into a predictable rhythm.   *See figure 2.*

Recording: Record according to the following scales.

Pursuits: 4+   smooth and accurate
3+   one fixation loss
2+   two fixation losses (fail)
1+   more than two fixation losses or any head movements (fail)

Saccades: 4+   smooth and accurate
                   3+   some slight undershooting
                   2+   gross undershooting or overshooting
                            or increasedlatency (fail)
                   1+   inability to do task or greatly
                            increased latency, any head
                            movements

Referral criteria: A score of 2+ or 1+ on either test.

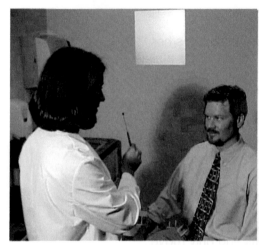

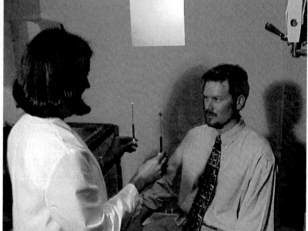

DOMINANT EYE/HAND

(WISCONSIN SPORTS VISION PROJECT [WSVP] DOMINANCE WAND)

Evaluates: To determine the dominant eye and hand.

Test Distance: The examiner is 10 feet from the athlete.

Illumination: Standard illumination

Position: Standing relaxed

Critical Factors:

The athlete is to hold the handle of the WSVP dominance wand with both hands and arms extended, in the midline of the body a few feet below primary gaze. The examiner points to their dominant eye and instructs the athlete to slowly raise their arms in the midline and capture the eye within the circle.

Instructional Set:

"Hold the wand between both hands at the center of your body. Look at the eye I'm pointing to with both eyes open. Bring the wand up and look at my eye through the hole."

Record: Record whether the patient is left or right handed. Circle the dominant eye, and record strong, mild/moderate preference, or central or cyclopean tendency, or alternate/undetermined preference. Refer to diagram at station.

STRONG   **MILD/MODERATE**   **CYCLOPEAN**

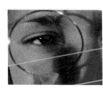   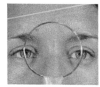

note: Alternating non-established athletes will appear as mild/moderate with both eyes (eye dominance may switch from one to the other)

DOMINANT EYE/HAND

Evaluates: To determine the dominant eye

Test Distance: An isolated 20/40 letter is placed 6 to 15 feet from the athlete.

Illumination: Standard room

Position: Standard relaxed

Critical Factors:

Insure the athlete is looking through the circle aperture and not moving it once the task is understood. The athlete's body needs to be centered with the target.

Instructional Set:

"Look at the target across the room with both eyes open. While holding the circle aperture, bring it up and center the distant object in the circle." The examiner is to cover up the right eye and ask "Can you still see the object through the circle?" Cover the left eye and ask if the object is still seen.

Recording: The dominant eye sees the object while the other eye is covered. Record <u>OD dominant</u> or <u>OS dominant</u>. Record whether patient is right or left handed.

AUTOREFRACTION

Evaluates: The refractive error objectively with the use of an automated instrument. Either a desk top or a hand held autorefractor can be used.

DESK TOP

Set-up: Use standard room illumination. The athlete should be seated with his/her chin in the chin rest and forehead against the forehead rest. The athlete should remove his/her habitual Rx.

Procedure: -Turn the instrument on.

-Adjust the chin rest and the instrument for the Athlete. Position the instrument to allow for measuring the right eye first. *See figure 1.*

-Instruct the Athlete to fixate on a specified target.

-Look at the monitor to ensure proper alignment and fixation. Use the instruments landmarks designated for proper alignment. *See figure 2.*

-Push the button that will begin the objective evaluation.

-The instrument may voluntarily move to the left eye once it is finished testing the right eye. If not, manually adjust the instrument to test the left eye.

-Press the print button in order to receive a readout of the indices found. *See figure 3.*

HAND HELD: Nikon Retinomax

Set-up: Use standard room illumination. The athlete should be seated comfortably with his/her eyes in primary gaze and his/her habitual Rx removed. Focus the eyepiece for the examiner by rotating it until the text inside is clear. Release the forehead by pushing in gently. The rest will then release. The angle of the eyepiece can be adjusted according to both the examiner's and the athlete's height. The adjustments should allow that the instrument is held perpendicular to the athlete's line of sight.

Procedure: -Direct the athlete to look into the Retinomax. They should see a character riding a rocket to the moon. Ask them to keep looking at this target throughout the testing.

-Begin by testing the right eye. The instrument will assume the right eye is being tested first if it is set on automatic. Hold the instrument so that the line on the left side of the Retinomax lines up with the lateral canthus and the line on the top of the instrument is at midpupil. If the instrument is lined up correctly, the pupil should be centered when you look into the eyepiece.

-The examiner should move in and out until the circle of dots in the center of the eyepiece are focused clearly. Once this is accomplished, press the trigger on the handle and the instrument will automatically begin taking readings.

-Before you start taking readings you will see "R0/L0" on the right in the eyepiece in the lower portion of the screen. This represents the number of readings taken on the right and left eyes. The instrument needs at least eight readings to accurately average the information. As the Retinomax takes reliable readings the number on the right side will increase up to eight. Once you reach "R8/L0" you are ready to test the left eye. The "R0/L0" on the top of the screen takes Keratometry readings. Don't be concerned with this information at this station.

-The Retinomax will automatically respond to shift to the left eye. Just be sure that you are centered in the middle of the pupil with the circle of dots focused clearly. You do not need to touch the trigger again. Continue to take readings until the screen reads "R8/L8".

-Aim the Retinomax toward the front of the printer at a distance of no more than 50 centimeters. Press the button located on the top of the Retinomax for 2 to 3 seconds until you hear a beep from the Retinomax and a responsive beep from the printer. The tones are slightly different so that you can distinguish them.

- The printer will begin immediately after the beep. The reading with the asterisk is the averaged reading. Record this value as the autorefraction information on the screening form.

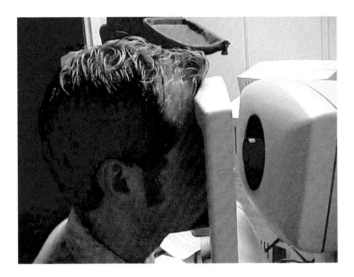

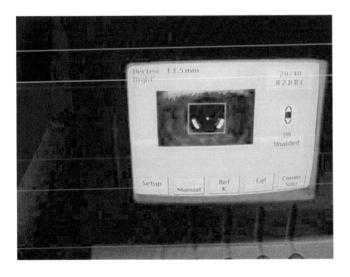

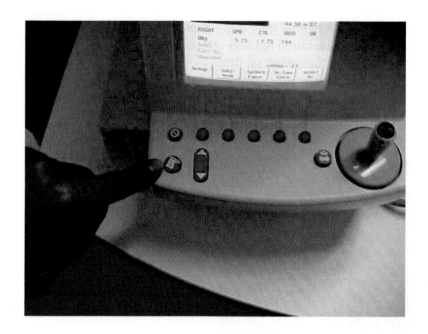

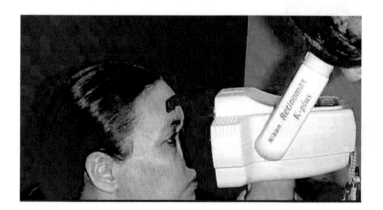

EXTERNAL EVALUATION

Evaluates: External and anterior segment health of the eye.

Illumination: Dim

Position: Athlete seated. If biomicroscope is available, have athlete put their chin in the chin rest and have their forehead touching the upper bar.

Critical Factors:
Steady fixation to a target point as directed by the examiner.

Criterion: **LIDS**- Look at the edges of the eyelids. Observe for signs of inflammation, discharge, and crusting or debris on the eyelids. If crusting debris is found, the athlete may have blepharitis.

CONJUNCTIVA- The peripheral conjunctiva should appear smooth. Note the presence of papillae (a vessel is located in the center) or follicles (a raised bump with out a central vessel). If the papillae are very large, GPC may be present. Common disorders of the bulbar conjunctiva include Pinguecula and Pterygia, these should be noted if the athlete has either or both conditions. Also note if the athlete has any injection (this is graded on a 1+ to 4+ scale).

CORNEA- Scan the cornea for any scarring, note location and level within the cornea layer if a scar is found. Infiltrates (made up of Polymorphonuclear leukocytes) should also be noted.

ANTERIOR CHAMBER- Look for signs of cell and flare (both are graded on a 1+ to 4+ scale with 1+ being trace and 4+ dense). The depth of the chamber angle is measured by comparing the depth of the anterior chamber with the corneal thickness at the limbus.

LENS- Look for any opacifications and note location: anterior of posterior subcapsular, cortex, or nucleus.

Instructional Set: "This procedure evaluates the health of the front of the eye. Place your chin on the rest and forehead against the bar. Try to keep your head still and hold your eyes on whatever target I direct you to."

Record: Record status of lids, conjunctiva, cornea, anterior chamber, and lens.

<u>**SLIT LAMP**</u> *(fig. 1)*

Head Rest   Beam Width Adjustment Knob   Magnification Adjustment

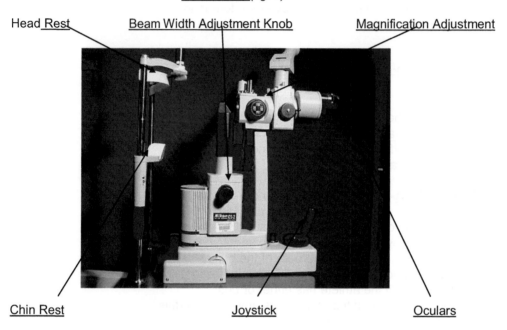

Chin Rest   Joystick   Oculars

EXTERNAL EYE *(fig. 2)*

Lids   Conjunctiva   Cornea

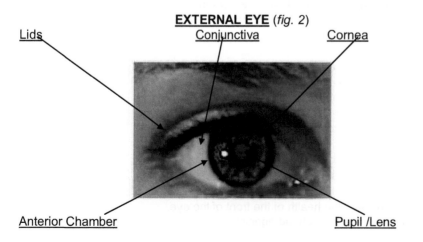

Anterior Chamber   Pupil /Lens

INTERNAL EVALUATION

Evaluates: The health of the internal structures of the eyes.

Equipment: A direct ophthalmoscope, a distant target

Set-up: The athlete should be seated and the target should be set up at 20 feet. The room illumination should be dim in order to encourage dilation of the pupils.

Instructions: Tell the athlete that you are evaluating the health of the back of his/her eye. Instruct him/her to look at the distance target and continue to look in the direction of the target if you get in the way.

Procedure: Hold the ophthalmoscope with your right hand, placing it over your right eye in order to examine the athlete's right eye. Position yourself at about 15 degrees off the axis of the athlete's eye in order to allow the athlete to continue to fixate on the distance target. *See figure 1.*

Dial in +8.00D to +10.00D in the ophthalmoscope in order to investigate the iris of the athlete.

Slowly reduce the power in the ophthalmoscope (less plus/more minus) in order to focus on the vitreous. Monitor the vitreous for clarity.

Continue to reduce plus in order to focus on the fundus. Look for the red reflex.

Evaluate the optic nerve head including the disc margin, rim tissue (contour and color), and the cup/disc size and depth.

Evaluate the adjacent posterior pole including the macular area and the surrounding vasculature. Note the following: color and clarity of the macular area, presence of a foveal reflex, and the artery/vein (A/V) ratio.

Recording: Record the cup/disc ratio, the A/V ratio, and the macular status.

Referral Criteria:
Refer if any abnormal findings are found.

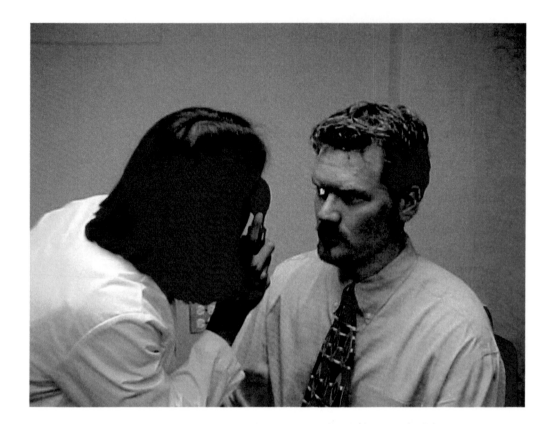

EYE MOVEMENTS-OBER II

Evaluates: This series of tests assesses fixation status, saccadic speed and accuracy, and the quality of pursuits at distance. Test I evaluates the ability to point the eyes accurately. Test II measures how quickly the eyes move from point to point and Test III evaluates the ability to track a moving object.

Set-up: Turn on the computer and click on the "Visa 4.3" icon. Click on the first icon on the Visa home page tool bar. Go to "Input Subject & Test Data". Enter the name, class (enter 'JO'), test (enter 'v'), sex, and date of birth of the athlete. Click on "measure" and prepare to do "Fixation Maintenance".

The athlete should be standing at a 5 feet test distance and the room illumination should be standard. It is important that the athlete be eye level with the targets. The goggles must be properly adjusted and calibrated to the athlete's pupillary distance.

Instructions and Procedure:

Test I - Fixation maintenance. Instruct the athlete to look at the center 'O' target without moving his/her eyes or head until you tell them to. Allow *at least* 25 seconds (4 screens) to pass before telling the athlete to stop or move his/her eyes. Press the 'enter' key (or click on OK) to begin the test. Click on "stop" to end the test. The software will take you to the next test.

Test II - Motilities - Lateral Saccades. Tell the athlete to move his/her eyes back and forth between the two 'X's' as fast as he/she can. The two 'X's' should be separated by 50 cm. Stress accuracy and speed during this procedure, avoiding head movements. Test this for *at least* 25 seconds, beginning and ending the procedure the same as for Test I.

Test III - Tracking. Instruct the athlete to again alternate fixations between each 'X' for 5-10 seconds. Begin and end this procedure as before.

At the end of these 3 procedures you will be asked if the measurement is OK or you need a retest. Click on OK and you will have a Visual Skills Profile containing the data. If data is not available (only '0's) you will need to repeat the procedure, but you should expect to see 0's in the tracking portion of the results.

Record "fixations" (under Fixation Maintenance) as **"Fixation Loss/10 sec."** Record "excursions" (under Motilities) as the **"Saccadic Speed/15 sec."** Select the eye (right or left) with the best test results (the lower the number, the better the result). The "Tracking" data is not used.

Note: After every 5 subjects exit the extra subject windows by clicking on the X on the superior right side of the subject windows. Failure to limit the number of open windows will significantly slow down the computer

Pursuits: Note: The Pursuit section is not routinely done at Junior Olympics

Return to the Visagraph 4.3 toolbar and click on 'new' (File menu.) Enter the same data as before in the "Input Subject & Test Data" box (it may already be entered from the initial tests II, III, and I) except enter the word 'Pursuits' in the comment section. Click on 'measure' to begin the next test.

Test I - Fixation Maintenance (this test is used for 'Pursuit Fixation Loss'). The athlete views the swinging ball from a distance of 4 feet. Instruct the athlete to fixate on one letter or the black line (switch to another letter if the ball rotates) during the horizontal ball swing, a total lateral swing of ~50-55 cm. The athlete should view the ball for ~ 25 seconds. Begin and end the test as before.

Test II - Motility This part of the procedure is only necessary for calculation purposes. Instruct the patient to alternate fixation between each 'X.' for ~ 5-10 seconds before ending the test.

Test III - Tracking This part of the procedure is only necessary for calculation purposes. Follow the identical instructions as for the previous Test II.

At the end of these 3 procedures you will be asked if the measurement is OK or you need a retest. Click on OK and you will have a Visual Skills Profile containing the data. If only '0's are presented, you will need to repeat the procedure.

Record "Pursuit Fixation Losses / 10 sec" as the 'fixation' data under the Fixation Maintenance section (lowest for either right or left eye.) The other data is ignored for this test. Close this page when completed and return to Visagraph 4.3 toolbar.

	Age< 7	Age 7-11	Age 12-15	Age 16-25	Age> 25
Fixation loss 10 sec	10±7	8±6	7±5	6±4	4±3
Saccadic Speed 15 sec	17±8	20±7	24±8	28±8	29±6
Pursuit Fixation Loss 10 sec	26±7	24±6	21±6	17±6	15±6

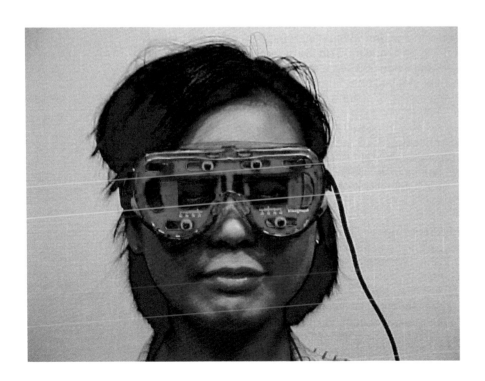

Threshold Dynamic Visual Acuity

Evaluates: This test assesses the subject's ability to resolve a 20/40 Snellen letter while it is in motion.

Testing distance: 10 feet.

Illumination: Standard room illumination.

Positioning: The athlete should be standing with feet comfortably apart. Testing is done binocularly with the athlete's habitual distance prescription.

Standard Parameters:

Track size 980 pixels X 40 pixels
Stimulus (letter) size 9mm (30pixels, or 20/40 equivalent)
Stimulus color Black
Target color White
Speed 10
Stimulus exposure time 200 msec

Instructions and Procedure:

Instructions to athlete:

"Watch the center of the screen. When I start the test, you will see a white ball going back and forth on the screen. Follow the ball with your eyes and when you see a letter flashed on the ball, call out the letter that you see. The target may speed up or slow down during testing. Continue to follow the target until I tell you to stop."

From the computer desktop, click on the "DynamicAcuity" icon. Click on "run session" Program defaults to standard test parameters. Give patient instructions and press any key to begin test. Test ends automatically and record scores on screen.

Responses and Recording.
When the athlete calls out a letter, press the space bar on the keyboard. Enter the letter that the athlete called out. Press enter to run next trial.

The software will stop automatically when a threshold is reached; Record the Mean, Median, and Standard Deviation Dynamic Acuity Scores that are displayed on the screen.
To abort a trial press F2

ACUVISION 1000 EYE HAND COORDINATION

Evaluates: The ability to visually direct the hand to a target in an efficient manner.

Test Distance: The athlete is 30 inches from the front of the instrument. The center green target light of the instrument should be at eye level.

Illumination: Medium room illumination. Faceplate illumination ranges between 0.65ft candles at the center to 2.50ft candles at the peripheral portions of the faceplate.

Positioning: The athlete should be standing, centered equidistant from right to left edge of the instrument. The athlete should wear appropriate athletic footwear.

Testing Sessions:

> **Speed = 7/Mode = FF120/Fixation = Off/Brita = 9/Map = Ne/Sound 9**

For ages less than 7, use the following parameters:

> **Speed = 7/Mode = rF60/Fixation = Off/Brite = 9/Map = Ne/Sound 9**

Instructional Set:

"This device assesses your ability to use your eyes to guide hand movements in space. While you are watching the board, red lights will appear in your peripheral vision. Using the fingertips of either hand, attempt to press the red lights as they appear. There will be a total of 120 test lights (ages <7 have 60 lights). The light will move to the next location after about 1 second if you don't press it. If you correctly press a light, it will immediately appear at another location. Try to find the lights with yours eyes as fast as you can, but try not to move your head.

Criterion: During each trial monitor the presence or absence of head movement and body movement. Rate this on a scale of 0 to 4 with 4 being excessive movement of the head or body.

Junior Olympics 1997

	Grade schl.	Jr. High	High Schl.	Cntrl./coach	Entire pop.
Acu#	30+17	52+12	67+13	55+28	53+22
Acu-Late	29+12	35+8	25+11	34+24	27+12
Acu-Time	95+12	88+5	82+7	80+2	87+11

For each trial, record the # of correct hits, the number of late responses, and the time used to complete the trial. Print out a hard copy of the distribution of points after the trial.

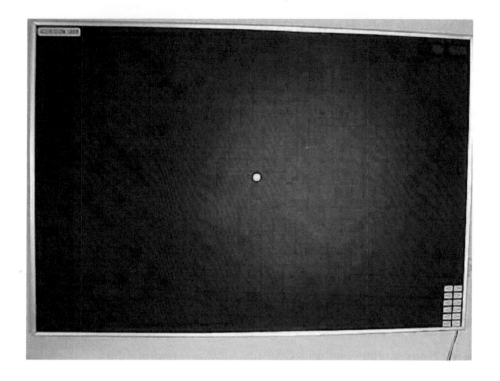

Speed/Mode/Fixation/Brite/Map/Sound buttons

WAYNE FOOTSPEED

Evaluates: Perceptual reaction time and motor footspeed.

Test Distance: 7 feet.

Illumination: Standard room (Approx. 7ft candles)

Position: Athlete stands with left foot on the center footplate, knees bent in a ready position.

Critical Factors:

Do not allow athlete to put pressure on left footplate until instructional set is completed. Footplates are secured horizontally separated by 7 feet on a hard surface. Push Enter-9-99-Enter to program the test.

Criterion: Junior Olympics 1997

	Grade Shcl.	Jr. High	High Shcl.	Cntrl./coaches	Entire pop.
Footspeed	.66+.6	.49+.18	.48+.19	.55+.39	.54+.29
Release Footspeed	1.5+.6	1.2+.6	1.2+.3	1.6+.9	1.3+.5

Instructional Set:

"This test evaluates reaction time and footspeed. When you place your weight on the center footplate a green light will illuminate on the board in front of you. After about 3 seconds a beep will sound and a red light will appear on the board at the 12:00, 3:00, 6:00, or 9:00 position. If a light appears at 12:00 move to the front footplate as fast as you can. 3:00 to the right, 6:00 behind you, 9:00 to the left. As soon as you hear the beep and see the light change, move as fast as you can and touch the other footplate with your right foot. We will do this three times."

Record: Record the release time first followed by footspeed. Two numbers will flash, the footspeed number is followed by a period. Record the direction of movement by checking a box on the score sheet for each of the trials. Enter the trials for each position in the computer.

Reprogram Codes: 1 => 13
2 => 0
3 => 0
4 => 3
5 => 4
6 => 0

WAYNE SACCADIC FIXATOR

Test Distance: 30 inches

Evaluates: Visual motor response to visual stimuli based on a precise, visually guided motor response (finger pressing a lighted target). Measures eye-hand coordination.

Illumination: 20 foot candles incident on the instrument in a dimly lit room.

Position: Center of instrument at eye level. Subject should be able to reach top and bottom of instrument without changing the test distance.

Critical Factors:

Illumination and the test distance are critical. Testing is conducted using one finger of the dominant hand. Both sub-tests one and two run for 30 seconds. Allow a demonstration of the task by allowing the athlete to correctly press 5 lights then restart the test by touching the green light.

Sub-test 1 (Proaction): Enter; 9,1,<enter>
Sub-test 2 (Reaction): Enter; 9,21,<enter>

Criterion: Proaction: Mean= 42   Std. Dev.=5
Reaction: Mean= 27   Std. Dev.=4
Speed: Mean= 94   Std. Dev.=13

Instructional Set:

"This instrument measures eye-hand coordination and hand speed. For the first test, using either hand, I want you to touch the lighted circles. As soon as you touch another circle will light up in another random position. Touch as many circles as you can in 30 seconds."

"The second test is similar to the first except the light may not wait for you. If you don't get it in time the light is going to move to a new location so keep on trying to touch it. The faster you start going the faster the lights will start moving. Try to get as many as you can in 30 seconds."

Recording: Sub-test 1: Record # of buttons touched (from display)
Sub-test 2: Record # of buttons touched and presentation speed. Hit #3 to access presentation speed.

Program Codes:

Proaction	Reaction
1 ⇒ 1	1 ⇒ 14
2 ⇒ 30	2 ⇒ 30
3 ⇒ 0	3 ⇒ 57
4 ⇒ 3	4 ⇒ 3
5 ⇒ 1	5 ⇒ 1
6 ⇒ 0	6 ⇒ 0
7 ⇒ 0	7 ⇒ 0
8 ⇒ 0	8 ⇒ 0
9 ⇒ 0	9 ⇒ 0

WAYNE SACCADIC FIXATOR (HAND SPEED)

Evaluates: Visual motor response to visual stimuli based on a precise, visually guided motor response (finger pressing a lighted target). Also measures eye-hand coordination and hand speed.

Test Distance: At comfort of the subject

Illumination: Critical at 40-70 cd/M^2 incident on the instrument in a dim room.

Position: Center of instrument at eye level. Subject should be able to reach 3:00 and 9:00 position of instrument without changing the test distance.

Critical Factors:

Illumination and the test distance are critical. The subjects gaze their eyes at one point or follow the stimulus and the subject may only use one hand but any finger.

Sub-test 3 (Hand-Speed): Enter; 9,18,<enter>

Criterion: Hand-Speed: O.28 $\pm$ 0.07

Instructional Set:

"This instrument measures eye   -hand coordination and hand speed. You can use all your fingertips of any one hand. I want you to touch this button (9:00), then touch this button (3:00). Do this only on time." Record speed. " Do it again." Record sp   eed. "One last time. Now, try to do it faster" Record again.

Recording: Record all three trials. Circle the best one and enter it into the computer.

Program Codes: 1 $\Rightarrow$ 11   6 $\Rightarrow$ 0
2 $\Rightarrow$ 0   7 $\Rightarrow$ 0
3 $\Rightarrow$ 3600   8 $\Rightarrow$ 0
4 $\Rightarrow$ 4   9 $\Rightarrow$ 0
5 $\Rightarrow$ 1

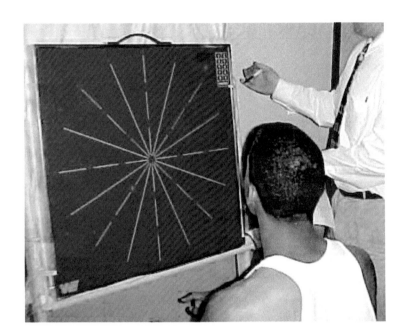

WAYNE SACCADIC FIXATOR (BALANCE BOARD)

Evaluates: Visually directed balance

Test Distance: 7 feet

Illumination: Standard room

Position: Standing on balance board facing the Wayne Saccadic Fixator

Critical Factors:

Good balance to start procedures. Stable position. Allow the athlete to move the board in the various directions to get a feel of the balance shifts required.

Enter; 9,26,<enter>

Criterion: To be determined

Instructional Set:

"This instrument measures visually dire   cted balance. While you balance on the board, a light will appear at the 12:00, 3:00, 6:00, or 9:00 positions. If it appears at the 12:00 position, tilt the board forward, if 3:00, tilt right, if 6:00, tilt back, and if 9:00 tilt left. Be very careful not to go in the wrong direction, since any wrong move will lose all your points. The task will continue for 30 seconds."

Record: Record the number attained after 30 seconds.

Program Codes: $1 \Rightarrow 11$
$2 \Rightarrow 0$
$3 \Rightarrow 0$
$4 \Rightarrow 3$
$5 \Rightarrow 1$
$6 \Rightarrow 121$
$7 \Rightarrow 0$
$8 \Rightarrow 0$
$9 \Rightarrow 0$

WAYNE PERIPHERAL AWARENESS TESTER (P.A.T.)

Evaluates: Visual motor response time (via lever press) to peripheral stimuli in eight visual field locations.

Test Distance: 30 inches

Illumination: 3-5 foot candles

Position: Standing relaxed with center of Wayne Saccadic Fixator at the subjects eye level. Alignment is especially critical with those athletes whose spectacle Rx might restrict their visual field.

Critical Factors:

All PAT screening should be performed in accordance with PAT diagnostic testing protocols: Instrument should be mounted against a neutral light-colored background. It is critical that the patient fixates on the red center light of the unit continuously during the testing procedure.

Enter; 9,125,<enter>

Criterion: Criteria < 0.6 sec per location.

Instructional Set:

"This instrument measures peripheral vision. I'd like you to always keep your eyes on this center yellow light. When you see a light at any one of the edges, move the joystick quickly in the direction of that light and release it. One of the lights will turn on every 2-4 seconds."

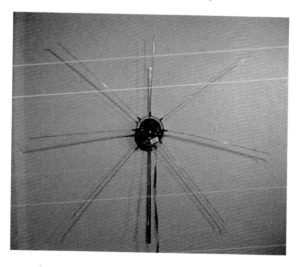

TACHISTOSCOPE

Evaluates: Speed and span or recognition

Test Distance: Athlete is 10 feet form the screen

Illumination: 35 foot/candles

Position: Standing comfortable

Critical Factors:

Numbers must be 3.5 cm high (20/80 acuity). There will
be 6 numbers per set and each set is shown at 0.05sec.

Criterion:

Junior Olympics 1997

Grade school	Jr. High	High School	Cntrl./coaches	entire pop.
9+4	12+3	13+3	13+2	12+4

Instructional Set:

"On the wall between the 2 stickers there will appear a set of
numbers such as these." Push the external shutter to show 6
numbers. "They will appear this fast." Push shutter initiate to
show how fast they will appear. "Look between the 2 stickers,
remember the numbers in order and recite them back to me."
Each athlete has 3 trials (18 total numbers).

Record: Number correct out of 18 (three trials).

Scoring: Subject allowed one transposition per slide, example: numbers
as they appear (123456) they recite (1234<u>65</u>) number correct
equals 5 out of 6 because 4 were correct plus 1 point for
transposition.

Answers:

	<u>Set 1:</u>	<u>Set 2:</u>	<u>Set 3:</u>	<u>Set 4:</u>	<u>Set 5:</u>
<u>Demo:</u>	360842	842907	728053	264073	739201
<u>1:</u>	254698	302658	394625	628149	583902
<u>2:</u>	628407	620174	873142	802476	831927
<u>3:</u>	602391	905281	984527	219684	730159

TACHISTOSCOPE CONTROL PANEL

Shutter Initiate   Shutter Time   Interval Timer   External Shutter

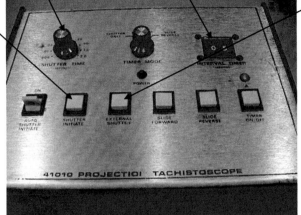

VECTORVISION CONTRAST SENSITIVITY

Evaluates: Visual contrast sensitivity; visual discrimination ability.

Test Distance: 12.5 feet

Illumination: Test is backlit with an internal light source.

Position: Standing relaxed

Critical Factors: Test only OD, OS

SPATIAL FREQUENCY EXAMPLES FOR VARIOUS TESTING DISTANCES IN CYCLES/DEGREE

	ROW A	ROW B	ROW C	ROW D
8 Feet	3	6	12	18
10 Feet	3.75	7.5	15	22.5
12.5 Feet	4.7	9.4	18.75	28.1

Criterion:

Junior Olympics 1997

	Grade School	Jr. High	High School	control/coaches	entire pop
CSFOD1	6+2	6+1	6+1	6+2	6+2
CSFOD2	6+2	6+2	6+2	6+2	6+2
CSFOD3	6+2	6+2	6+2	5+6	6+2
CSFOD4	6+2	6+2	6+2		6+2

Instructional Set:
"On each panel there are two rows of circles, for each pair one of the circles will contain some lines. Tell me for each pair whether the top or bottom contains the lines. Some of the lines will be faint, try to guess if you're unsure."

Record: Record the number or grids called correctly in each of the four plates on the Vectorvision chart.

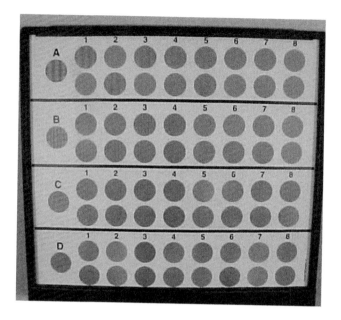

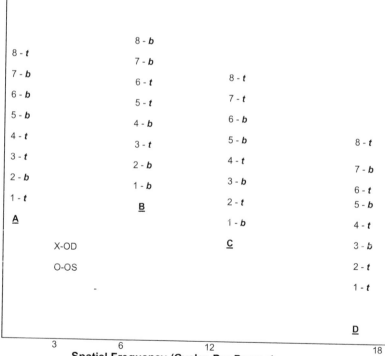

8 - *t*

7 - *b*

6 - *b*

5 - *b*

4 - *t*

3 - *t*

2 - *b*

1 - *t*

<u>A</u>

8 - *b*

7 - *b*

6 - *t*

5 - *t*

4 - *b*

3 - *t*

2 - *b*

1 - *b*

<u>B</u>

8 - *t*

7 - *t*

6 - *b*

5 - *b*

4 - *t*

3 - *b*

2 - *t*

1 - *b*

<u>C</u>

8 - *t*

7 - *b*

6 - *t*

5 - *b*

4 - *t*

3 - *b*

2 - *t*

1 - *t*

<u>D</u>

X-OD

O-OS

-

3   6   12   18

Spatial Frequency-(Cycles Per Degree)

HOWARD DOLMAN STEREOACUITY TEST

Evaluates: Stereoacuity or depth perception at distance.

Test Distance: The athlete is 6 meters from the zero point of the scale on top of the apparatus to the athlete's eye.

Illumination: Normal Room Illumination

Positioning: Athlete should be seated in front and level with the apparatus. The athlete should be wearing appropriate sports vision correction. Be sure the athlete cannot see the guide tracks on top and bottom on the inside of the box. Adjust chair accordingly.

Testing Sessions:

Four trials should be done for each rod separation in front and behind. Trials are done at 9, 6, 4, 2 and 1 cm separation. Four trials are performed at each separation distance, two trials with the right rod in front and two trials with the left rod in front. Start with the largest separation first. Only move to the next shorter separation if the athlete correctly identifies the movable rod in front or behind the stationary rod 3 out of the 4 trials. When moving the rod in front or behind, stand in front of the box. Stereoacuity is recorded as the last trial that was correctly identified 3 out of 4 times. The athlete should only be given approximately three to five seconds for each response, and he/she shouldn't move their head during the test. After three seconds, urge the patient to answer. If they do not answer, then consider that a fail for that trial. Do not inform the patient of the number of trials or the number of times the left or right rod is in front. Do not pause between testing of different separations. Do not test strabismics or amblyopes.

Instructional Sets:

"This device helps to measure your distance depth perception. There are two rods in the box in front of you. When you see the rods, immediately tell me which one is in front; either left or right."

Test Results:

Separation Distance	Stereoacuity
9cm	30.94"
6cm	20.63"
4cm	13.75"
2cm	6.88"
1cm	~3.44"

Record:

Separation Distance	Presentation: Rod in Front
9cm	R, L, L, R
6cm	L, R, L, R
4cm	L, L, R, R
2cm	R, L, R, L
1cm	R, L, L, R

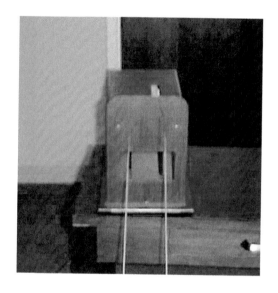

BASSIN ANTICIPATION TIMER

Evaluates: Visual anticipation skills; the ability to anticipate the arrival of the lights at the end of the track.

Test Distance: 3 feet away from the end of the track.

Illumination: 6-7 L (dim room)

Protocol: The patient demonstration is conducted with the speed at 10 mph. Do 1 trial at this speed. When the patient understands the task, increase the speed to 50 mph. Record the results of the next three trials.

Record: When the light is reacted to before it arrives, it is recorded with a plus sign. If reacted to late, it is recorded with a minus.

Position: Standing relaxed with track perpendicular to shoulders

Critical Factors: Athlete understands to stop the light on at the last position

Criterion: Computer average + sign for early / - sign for late

Instructional Set:

The patient is instructed that the row of lights represent a target that is approaching you. The athletes task is to stop the light exactly at the end of the track by pushing the hand held trigger. "I will let you practice on the slow balls, so you will learn how it works, then we will speed it up".

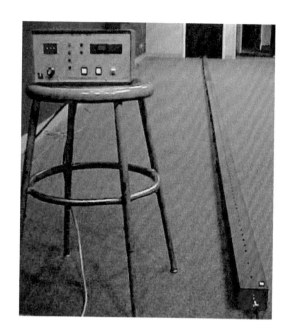

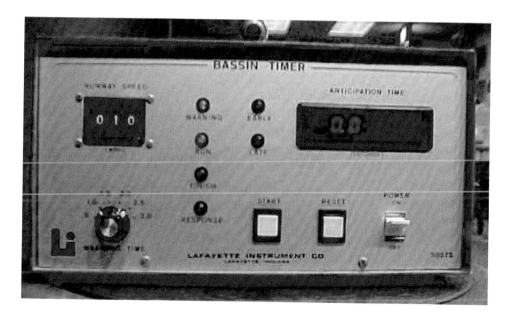

WESSON - FIXATION DISPARITY CARD

Evaluates: This test is used to evaluate phoric posture

Set - up: The athlete should be standing with his/her head straight. The test should be performed at a near distance of 16 inches and a far distance of 10 feet. Standard room illumination should be used and the athlete should wear **vectograph** glasses.

Procedure: Turn on the mallot box and instruct the athlete to look at the box. Ask the athlete to watch the bottom arrow and notice if the top arrow is to the right, left, or directly above the bottom arrow. Next, have the athlete look at one of the horizontal arrows and notice if the other horizontal arrow is above, below, or horizontally aligned with the arrow of fixation.

Recording: Record the associated phoria. Note that with standard vectograph glasses the top arrow to the right indicates eso posture and the top arrow to the left indicates exo posture. In addition, the right arrow higher indicates left hyperphoria.

Referral criterion:
Eso or exo greater than one or any vertical deviation.

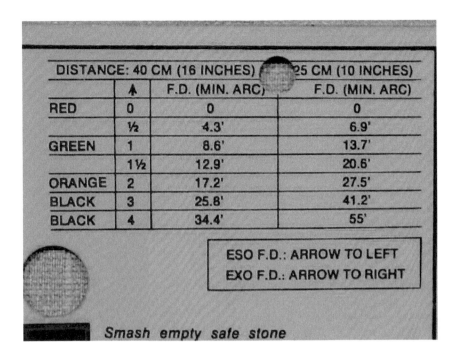

| DISTANCE: 40 CM (16 INCHES) | | | 25 CM (10 INCHES) |
	↟	F.D. (MIN. ARC)	F.D. (MIN. ARC)
RED	0	0	0
	½	4.3'	6.9'
GREEN	1	8.6'	13.7'
	1½	12.9'	20.6'
ORANGE	2	17.2'	27.5'
BLACK	3	25.8'	41.2'
BLACK	4	34.4'	55'

ESO F.D.: ARROW TO LEFT
EXO F.D.: ARROW TO RIGHT

Smash empty safe stone

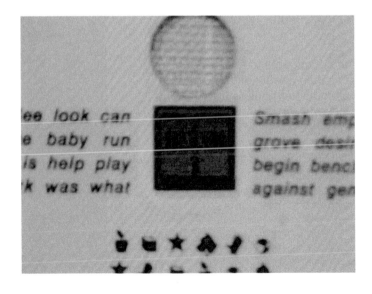

ee look can
e baby run
is help play
k was what

Smash emp
grove desi
begin bench
against gen

VISION AND BALANCE

Evaluates: Visual factors involved in maintaining gross motor balance under various conditions.

Set - up: Standard room illumination is used and test distance is not applicable except for the eye movement sequence and then a 40 cm distance should be used. The athlete should remove his/her shoes and stand on the flat edge of a standard 4 X 4 (3 5/8″ X 3 5/8″ X 10 ft.). The athlete should place feet heel to toe, parallel to the long dimension of the beam.

Critical Factors: The examiner should read and memorize the scaling definitions in order to avoid the need for reference during screening. Use different colored targets to test eyes.

Scaling Definitions:

1. Highly stressed, tremendous body wavering and struggling. Obvious difficulty staying on the beam. Unable to stay on any longer than 2-3 seconds during tasks.

2. Stressed, with considerable struggling and wavering present; falls off the beam two or more times during the task.

3. Significant wavering, but able to recover. Falls off the board no more than one time during a task. Excessive wavering and struggling (to the point where barely recovers) with no falls.

4. Slight noticeable lean with minimal wavering. No falls or near falls. Maintains a high level of stability during the majority of the task.

5. No wavering and no falls. Maintains a high level of stability throughout the task.

Instructional Set:

The vision and balance testing consists of five subtests, each of which should be carefully scored in accordance with the criteria listed above.

A. "Stand heel to toe and maintain balance while looking straight ahead with arms at your side (demonstrate). You may use whichever foot you prefer in the forward position." Score 10 seconds.

B. "Now close your eyes." Score for 10 seconds beginning the moment the athlete closes his/her eyes.

C. "Open your eyes. I want you to follow this target (bead) with your eyes only. Do not use head movement." Use the following four eye movement probes:

1. Two slow NPC's to nose (break and recovery) over 15 seconds total. One slow NPC 6" from the patients right to nose (break and recovery) over 8 seconds and one slow NPC 6" from the patients left to the nose (break and recovery) over 8 seconds.

2. Rapid saccades between opposite cardinal points at a test distance of 40 cm with the beads separated by approximately 75 cm. Two times each point.

3. Rapid near-far saccades, 3 feet away to 6" away.

4. Smooth eye movements at a 40 cm target distance. Lateral pursuits 2 X 2 round trips full range, oblique pursuits 2 X each, vertical pursuits 2 X each, rotation 1 X each.

D. Dynamic: Eyes open - "Walk forward to the end of the beam and back using heel to toe. Try to keep your eyes pointed straight ahead."

E. Dynamics: Eyes closed - "Walk forward to the end of the beam, I will tell you when you are at the end, then reverse and stop.

Recording: Record the performance scale rating on each subtest.

Criterion: The athlete should score a grade 3 on all phases of the screening. The total score is related to computer averages.

Mean = 18
Standard Deviation = 2

Scoring criteria:
(low) 1　2　3　4　5(high)

Example:　　An athlete shows good balance with slight wavering during the first test. When the patient closes his/her eyes, he/she has to use a toe touch to keep balanced, but then shows steady balance for the remainder of the test. The athlete falls once when performing eye movements. The athlete uses two toe touches when walking with eyes open, and wavers and struggles to keep balance when walking with eyes closed. The athlete also falls twice during the last test.

Record:
1. 5
2. 3
3. 3
4. 3
5. 2
TOTAL = 16

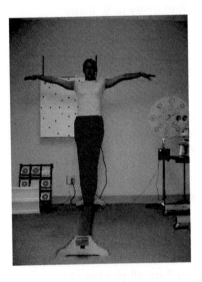

Appendix B

SAMPLE BASEBALL SCREENING

Name: _____   Date: _____   Athlete #:_____

Position:_____   Throwing hand? R   L

Case Hx:
LEE: _____Do you wear CL or glasses: Y   N   do you wear them while you play? Y   N
___Difficulty seeing/blurry vision   ___Double vision

___Difficulty following moving objects   ___Reduced performance as stress builds

___Poor depth perception   ___Reduced peripheral vision

___Dry eyes   ___Watery/Itchy eyes

___Eye/head injury   ___Eye surgery

___Blurred vision after near work   ___Headaches

___Lack of consistency of play (ex: day/night, early/late in competition)

___Any other concerns/problems with eyes?

Concussions? Y   N How many/when did they occur _____

Testing:
VA: sc_____cc

OD: _____   OS: _____   OU: _____

Contrast (Vectorvision) Circle the last one that the athlete stated correctly:

	1	2	3	4	5	6	7	8
Row B:	B	B	T	B	T	T	B	B
Row C:	B	T	B	T	B	B	T	T
Row D:	T	T	B	T	B	T	B	T

MOART and BASSIN: (2 demos, then 5 runs with random delay)

MOART (glove hand)   Basin (speed: 50 mph)

Attempt 1_____/_____   attempt 1: _____/_____
Attempt 2_____/_____   attempt 2: _____/_____
Attempt 3_____/_____   attempt 3: _____/_____
Attempt 4 _____/_____   attempt 4: _____/_____
Attempt 5_____/_____   attempt 5: _____/_____

Binovi: Go No/Go

correct/ late_____/_____

Howard Dolman stereo acuity test OU: (Every athlete begins with the 4 cm separation distance, if ¾ were correct move down to the 2 cm separation distance, if ¾ were NOT correct move up to the 6 cm separation. Put an "X" through each wrong answer. Circle the smallest separation distance and its corresponding stereoacuity.)

Primary gaze

	1	2	3	4					
4 cm	L	R	R	L					
2 cm	R	L	R	R	OR	6 cm R	L	L	L
1 cm	L	R	R	L		9 cm R	R	L	R

Batters stance

	1	2	3	4					
4 cm	R	R	L	L					
2 cm	R	L	L	R	OR	6 cm L	R	R	L
1 cm	L	L	R	L		9 cm R	L	R	L

Results

Sep Dist	Stereoacuity
9 cm	30.94″
6 cm	20.73″
4 cm	13.75″
2 cm	6.88″
1 cm	3.44″

Cover test at distance (if needed): _____

Haynes Distance Rock: 30 sec time- 20/25 lines (small letters) (have the patient warm up with calling out the first lines on the near and far card of the bigger letters (20/80). Next time the pt for 30 seconds while they call out the smaller letters starting with the far card first. Ciircle the last one called out after 30 seconds. Put a line through any letters that they call out incorrectly.)

Total number correct: _____

Start on **far card first**
V N C O Z H R D N K S C V V O R K Z C S N O O K H Z S D Z N C R V H
C O K V S S H V S C K N D R Z N O K H O R H Z S C D

Notes/comments:

Appendix C

**SPORTS VISION
EVALUATION REPORT**

DATE

Patient Name: Parent:
Date of Birth: Address:

NAME was evaluated in our Vision Therapy Service at NAME on DATE following a referral from NAME. The main reason for this visit was a sports vision evaluation for softball. Other problems mentioned were LIST. The medical and developmental histories were unremarkable. The following is a summary of our findings:

VISUAL ACUITIES & REFRACTIVE STATUS:
   NAME's distance visual acuity (clarity of eyesight) without correction was 20/15 right eye, left eye, and with both eyes. His/her near visual acuity without correction was 20/20 right eye, left eye, and with both eyes. NAME was found to be slightly hyperopic (farsighted). NAME's vision was found to be adequate for her current seeing needs.

CONTRAST SENSITIVITY:
   This is a measure of visual sensitivity to subtle differences in black-white contrast. Contrast sensitivity is related to visual acuity and provides a qualitative index of the athlete's visual sensitivity to detail. NAME had excellent contrast sensitivity at lower spatial frequencies, but only average performance on high spatial frequency (18cpd). This is a critical skill in softball for helping to judge the flight and timing of a pitch.

OCULAR MOTILITY (Eye Movement Skills):
   NAME's eye movement performance was evaluated using the Visagraph Computerized Reading Eye Movement Test and the NSUCO Oculomotor Test. Overall results indicated appropriate eye movement ability.

   The NSUCO assesses gross fast (saccadic) and slow tracking (pursuits) eye movements. These data help rule out motor dysfunctions that can hinder information processing. Results indicated that extra ocular motilities were full (without restriction) in both eyes. NSUCO gross pursuits, the ability to track a moving target, were full, smooth, and accurate. NSUCO gross saccades, the ability to make rapid movements of the eyes from one target to another, were accurate and efficient. Visagraph infrared-oculography was used during the NSUCO test to provide an objective measure of eye movements.

ACCOMMODATIVE SKILLS (Focusing):
   NAME's ability to focus clearly on near objects as well as to sustain this focus for an extended period of time, such as required in reading, was adequate. Accommodative facility, the ability to make rapid and accurate changes in focus for different distances, was excellent.

BINOCULAR STATUS (Eye Teaming):

NAME's eye teaming strength and sustaining ability were adequate. Vergence facility, the ability to make rapid and accurate changes of eye posture for different distances, was also better than average. Tests to assess NAME's eye posturing indicated adequate functioning. NAME's stereopsis (two-eyed depth perception) was assessed at far and was found to be good.

SPAN OF RECOGNITION:

This test measures the speed and breadth of visual information processing, where a series of random numbers is presented for a brief moment in the center of the visual field. This test may be interpreted as an indicator of "visual quickness." NAME's ability to quickly process numbers flashed before her and recall what numbers were seen was at a level expected for an elite-level athlete.

REACTION TIME:

These are measures of visual reaction and motor response times, consisting of an accurate hand movement in response to a visual stimulus in the center of the visual field. Reaction time is defined as the time required to mentally determine the presence of visual information and to formulate the motor response. Motor response time is defined as the time required to complete the motor response. Reaction time relates to overall *quickness*, while motor response time relates to overall *speed*. NAME demonstrated performance at a level expected for an elite-level athlete.

PERIPHERAL REACTION/RESPONSE:

This is a measure of speed and accuracy of visually-guided hand movements for all areas of the visual field. The score reflects overall efficiency of the visual motor eye-hand response loop and is related to performance in any sport requiring quick eye-hand responses. In *Self Paced*, athlete responds as quickly as they can at their own pace. In *Instrument Paced*, the athlete responds as quickly as they can at a predetermined pace. The score reflects performance under stress. NAME demonstrated performance at a level expected for an elite-level athlete.

COINCIDENCE-ANTICIPATION:

This is a measure of precision, accuracy, and sensitivity of timing a motor response to a rapidly approaching visual stimulus. NAME's ability to anticipate the arrival of the stimulus lights traveling at speeds relevant for softball was at a level expected for an elite-level athlete.

OCULAR HEALTH STATUS:

The internal and external health examination of the eyes and surrounding structures revealed no evidence of ocular disease or abnormality.

RECOMMENDATIONS:

In summary, our evaluation revealed excellent performance in all of the areas assessed. NAME's performance on the high spatial frequency contrast sensitivity testing indicates an opportunity to elevate her performance. As mentioned previously, this skill is a critical element for judging the spin, speed and trajectory of a pitched softball. One simple method recommended to help improve contrast sensitivity on the field of play was to use sunglasses to challenge contrast judgments. It was suggested that NAME start with lightly tinted sunglasses in a batting cage and with a pitchback for 10 to 15 minutes; she should then remove the sunglasses and continue practicing. Once this becomes easy, she can gradually move to darker tinted sunglasses and live pitches.

A strobe light provides a method for the development of visual information processing speed, increasing visual-motor reaction and response speed, and anticipation skills. A strobe light in a darkened room reduces the availability of visual information to the brief periods when the strobe light illuminates the room. The faster the flash rate of the strobe light, the greater the amount of information available to the athlete. Ultimately NAME is encouraged to maintain performance of an activity with progressively less visual information as the flash rate on the strobe light is reduced. The pitchback activity (eg, throwing a ball into a pitchback net and attempting to catch it on the return flight) is a good starting activity for the strobe light. As the ability to catch improves, the ball is thrown faster into the net. To add a level of unpredictability to the task, the ball can be thrown by another person, thereby requiring the athlete to rapidly judge the speed and trajectory of the ball during flight. The flash rate of the strobe light is gradually reduced so that the athlete must perform with less and less visual information. The pitchback activity can be replaced with other motor tasks such as fielding and batting drills, however care must be taken to protect the athletes from injury when conducting strobe activities.

If you have any questions regarding NAME's vision care, please feel free to contact us any time.

Sincerely,

SPORTS VISION
EVALUATION REPORT

DATE

Patient Name: Address:
Date of Birth:

NAME was evaluated in our Vision Therapy Service at the Forest Grove Family Vision Center on DATES following a referral by NAME. The main concern was inconsistent depth perception resulting in reduced accuracy and consistency of tennis swing. The following is a summary of our findings:

VISUAL ACUITIES & REFRACTIVE STATUS:
    NAME's distance visual acuity (clarity of eyesight) without correction was normal (20/17 right eye, 20/13 left eye, and 20/9 with both eyes). Her near visual acuity was normal at 20/20 with both eyes, indicating clear eyesight.

BINOCULAR STATUS (Eye Teaming):
    NAME manifests normal eye posture; orthophoria at 6 meters, and 4^Δ exophoria at 40cm. NAME's ability to converge the eyes on a near object was found to be adequate. NAME's ability to quickly switch focus was found to be below average on the Senaptec Sensory Station (1st percentile). Accommodative facility testing revealed 10 flips per minute of a ±2.00 flipper, with some difficulty clearing the plus lenses (relaxing focus). Vergence facility testing showed 8 flips per minute of a 4^Δ BI/BO flipper, with some difficulty clearing the BI prism (relaxing convergence). NAME's ability to converge and diverge eyes were found to be reduced with the following results of in-phoroptor prism ranges: at 6 meters, BI x/12/6, BO x/6/2; at 40cm, BI x/4/2, BO x/6/2.

    NAME shows normal stereopsis (depth perception) at near, however her ability to judge stereopsis for distant targets (6 meters) in real space with the Howard-Dolman test showed a minimum detectable offset of 7cm. This level of depth perception is not as strong as the average ability of athletes. NAME did better with depth perception testing on the Senaptec Sensory Station assessment, but this is an area that should be strengthened.

Sports Vision Testing
    NAME completed a visual performance assessment battery with the Senaptec Sensory Station (see attached). Her results were compared to the database of female high school tennis players. Compared to this database, her superior skills were visual clarity (acuity) and perception span. The skills that were close to average were depth perception, reaction time and eye-hand coordination. The skill areas that should be considered for enhancement include contrast sensitivity, near-far quickness, multiple object tracking, target capture (dynamic visual acuity), and Go/No Go.

    On the Bassin Anticipation timer, NAME was consistently late by ~100ms for a target approaching at 20mph, and ~20ms early for a targets approaching at 40mph.

RECOMMENDATIONS

1. To improve contrast sensitivity, it was recommended that NAME use the UltimEyes app, found at https://ultimeyesvision.com. In addition, a nutritional supplement with Lutein & Zeaxanthin is recommended to increase contrast sensitivity; particularly, the NAME products should be considered.

2. It was recommended that a program of vision therapy be considered at NAME Center with the goal of improving near-far quickness. In addition, the vision therapy program may also be able to improve dynamic visual acuity and go/no-go skills. Since NAME is not involved in team sports that demand strong multiple object tracking skills, this is not suggested for her therapy program.

If you have any questions regarding NAME's vision care, please feel free to contact us anytime.

Sincerely,

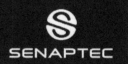

SENSORY PERFORMANCE REPORT
Kiana Pielli

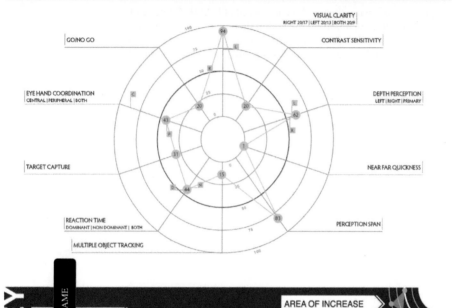

SPORT & POSITION
TENNIS
N/A

CURRENT LEVEL
HIGH SCHOOL

COMPARED TO
TENNIS
HIGH SCHOOL

STRENGTHS
VISUAL CLARITY
PERCEPTION SPAN
DEPTH PERCEPTION

OPPORTUNITIES
NEAR FAR QUICKNESS
MULTI-OBJECT TRACK
GO/NO GO
TARGET CAPTURE

IMPROVEMENT PLAN
NEAR-FAR SHIFT
DYNAMIC VISION
STROBE TRAINING
LIGHTBOARD

SCORE
44

Appendix D

CASE HISTORY

- Last Eye Exam: Unknown
- Athlete wears glasses and contact lenses. Athlete reports history of multiple concussions.

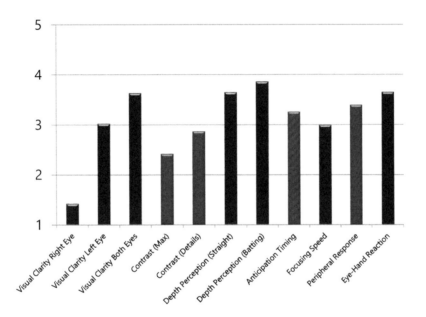

VISUAL STRENGTHS

- Depth perception
- Eye-hand reaction

AREAS OF OPPORTUNITY

- Visual clarity (right eye)

RECOMMENDATIONS

- Consider scheduling a comprehensive eye exam to determine if right eye clarity can be improved.

DEFINITIONS OF VISUAL PERFORMANCE SKILLS
Visual Clarity

- Visual clarity, or visual acuity, is one of the most basic, fundamental measures of a person's vision, telling how clearly a person sees the world and the details he or she is able to see in routine tasks.
  - This is what people are referring to when they talk about 20/20 vision.
- The average collegiate or professional baseball player will have a visual acuity that is better than 20/20.
- This is the first three bars on the athlete graphs (Right Eye, Left Eye, and Both Eyes).

Contrast Sensitivity

- This test is used to evaluate the athlete's ability to distinguish subtle differences in contrast between different objects.
  - It is the ability to detect details in various light settings and/or in moving objects (e.g., judging the spin and trajectory of a baseball).
- Similar to visual acuity, contrast sensitivity is a fundamental attribute of visual performance.
- The athlete graphs display performance at levels of peak human sensitivity (peak) and with detailed resolution demand (detailed), which is the most visually challenging.

Depth Perception

- The test measures the ability of the athlete to accurately judge the distance of a target.
  - Baseball requires the ability to judge the depth and distance of targets (i.e., the baseball, teammates, plates, and boundaries).
- We assessed depth perception in both a straight-ahead posture and a batting stance.

Anticipation Timing

- This measures the accuracy and consistency in judging the timing of an approaching object moving at speeds similar for baseball pitches.

- This is a critical skill for accurate timing in batting as well as catching a baseball.

Focusing Speed

- This measures the ability to shift focus between distant and near objects.
- This is important when looking quickly between the ball, teammates, and opponents who are away at varying distances.

Peripheral Response Time

- This measures how quickly the athlete is able to identify objects in his or her side vision and react to them.
- This is critical for base running, fielding, and picking off base runners.

Eye-Hand Reaction

- This measures how quickly the athlete is able to identify objects in his or her central vision and react to them.
- This is critical for batting and fielding.

Index

Note: Page numbers followed by "f" indicate figures, "t" indicate tables and "b" indicate boxes.

Printed and bound by CPI Group (UK) Ltd, Croydon, CR0 4YY

03/10/2024

01040300-0005